Obesity and Disease in an Interconnected World:

A Systems Approach to Turn Huge Challenges into Amazing Opportunities

Editors

Judith Wylie-Rosett

Atran Foundation Chair in Social Medicine, Professor and Division Head for Health Promotion and Nutrition Research, Department of Epidemiology and Population Health, Albert Einstein College of Medicine, Bronx, NY, USA

Sunil S. Jhangiani

Division of Gastroenterology and Clinical Nutrition, Department of Medicine (Wakefield Campus), Montefiore Medical Center, Clinical Assistant Professor of Medicine and Family and Social Medicine, Albert Einstein College of Medicine, Bronx, NY, USA

Founder & Medical Director, Doctors for a Healthier Bronx, NY, USA & www.NutritionVista.com

Bentham Science Publishers Ltd.
Executive Suite Y - 2
PO Box 7917, Saif Zone
Sharjah, U.A.E.
subscriptions@benthamscience.org

BENTHAM SCIENCE PUBLISHERS LTD.

DEDICATIONS

To all of the people who have shared their personal stories about how obesity has affected their health and lives. I have learned so much from their experiences as too often they have encountered bias and discrimination in so many of the systems that form our global society. My deepest appreciation goes to my daughter, Renee Rosett, from whom I have learned so much. Most importantly, she taught me to listen and know that my view is limited by my perspective.

Judith Wylie-Rosett

To my parents for their unstinting devotion to their kids, my wife, Mrinal and our two kids, Nikhyl and Tasha for their love and support, my sister, Hiroo for always being there for the family, & my teacher, Dr. CS Pitchumoni for sparking my interest in the field of Nutrition.

Sunil S. Jhangiani

CONTENTS

CHAPTERS

Section I: Health Risks Assessment: A Systematic Approach

contd…..

Section II: Prevention & Reduction of Risk Factors: A Targeted Approach

contd…..

Section III: Building Stronger Health Systems Globally: A Shared Responsibility

FOREWORD

I recall a lecture about prevention early in medical school, given by a wise, silver-haired professor, in which he made the provocative remark, "If we could only get people to stop smoking, drink less, be physically active and eat right, half of you could go home and do something else with your lives: we wouldn't need so many doctors." While one could argue with his math, thirty years of providing medical care in the United States-though this would be increasingly applicable to the developing as well as the developed world-have convinced me of the truth which was highlighted by this offhand comment. Despite-or rather in parallel to-a quarter century of progress in medical management and pharmacotherapeutics, a few basic interventions, affecting how people eat, engage in physical activity, and use substances, can have a profound impact on the health of patients and communities. A recent meta-analysis in the British Medical Journal confirmed the equivalence or superiority of exercise *vs* standard medical therapy in improving disease outcomes and even mortality in patients with stroke, cardiovascular disease, and diabetes [1]. This study echoed the landmark findings of the Diabetes Prevention Program (DPP), which demonstrated the superiority of lifestyle interventions *vs* metformin in preventing the progression of pre-diabetes to diabetes [2]. The YMCA now offers the DPP intervention as the Y-DPP which could potentially be available at any YMCA across the globe. Yet if these basic interventions are so effective, why have they not been more widely implemented? Basic, but perhaps not simple, in terms of how behavior is influenced and ultimately determined and changed. The factors that influence health-related behaviors have an impact at the individual patient, family, local community, and larger societal levels. Likewise, any strategies that would hope to change these behaviors must be thoughtfully pursued and engaged at each of these levels as well. Fortunately, this volume, Obesity and Disease in an Interconnected World: A Systems Approach to Turn Huge Challenges into Amazing Opportunities!, edited by Judith Wylie-Rosett, EdD, RD & Sunil S. Jhangiani, MD, MBA, FACP, AGAF, is a welcome and useful tool to help elucidate and frame this multi-level strategy. Specifically, as implied by the title, this is a systematic and systems-oriented examination of how to address the global epidemic of obesity and related chronic disease prevention and mitigation, in a comprehensive and coordinated way.

Recent advances in the basic science of fat metabolism, and adiposity, the related endocrinopathies and disease pathogenesis, and the multi-morbidity that affects even some organ systems not traditionally believed to be affected by obesity, have broadened the basis for understanding both the clinical impact of this epidemic and potential biomedical approaches for intervention. At the individual patient level, advances in behavioral science-for example, recent work in the area of motivational interviewing and behavior change [3]-have helped increase clinicians' skills and sensitivity in the area of health-promotion. Local community interventions, including the promotion of local coalitions of health care providers, public health agencies, local governmental officials, and community-based organizations and advocates, have been found to improve local conditions and increase resources for healthy eating, active living, and smoking cessation and prevention [4]. An important challenge to be overcome is in encouraging and supporting the coordination between clinical (*i.e.*, medical, health care delivery-related) and public health (*i.e.*, population-level) systems, since these two arena have traditionally been disconnected and even potentially discordant. The advent of the Accountable Care Organization (ACO) model in the United States, particularly the beginning of an era in which population-level health outcomes become part of the measurable goals and priorities of large ACOs, provide a structural opportunity to promote this broader approach to health promotion, extending beyond the medical exam room into the local community where patients' behaviors are largely determined and expressed [5, 6]. This approach will start to focus on creative and potentially powerful collaborations across sectors, such as strategies to implement the standardized Y-DPP educational program not only within health care delivery sites but also local community agencies, faith-based organizations, and schools, as outlined in this volume as well.

Beyond the individual and local community level, as suggested by the chapters in this eBook that address larger societal and even global issues, advocacy and coordinated policy development are essential in helping to shape the broad social priorities that have such an important impact on these health-promoting behaviors. Urban planning, local zoning, financing (from micro-finance to venture capital), health insurance incentives, taxation, marketing and the communications industry, all are examples of the kinds of key factors and areas for strategic intervention that can help determine the health of individuals, and societies. With the United Nations and World Health Organization estimating that over 50% of the chronic disease morbidity and mortality in the world is now due to non-communicable diseases [7], it is clear that one of the unintended consequences of development is to import the familiar array of obesity- and lifestyle-related diseases to many countries that had not previously experienced this-Mexico, India, and China are only a few examples of this phenomenon.

While the behaviors that need to change are basic -- again, how we eat, move, and use substances- and while the impact of behavior change on disease outcomes is clear-cut, it is the challenge of this decade and perhaps this century to create the kind of environments and communities in which these changes can and will take place. As scientists, as clinicians, as public health advocates and educators, and as citizens of our communities and the world, there is no more pressing agenda with the potential of impacting the health of billions of people worldwide. This eBook is an important addition to our efforts to accomplish this agenda for our own and future generations.

REFERENCES

[1] Naci H. Comparative effectiveness of exercise and drug interventions on mortality outcomes: metaepidemiological study. BMJ 2013;347:f5577 doi: 10.1136/bmj.f5577 (Published 1 October 2013)

[2] Diabetes Prevention Program Research Group. Reduction in the incidence of type 2 diabetes with lifestyle intervention or metformin. N Engl J Med 2002; 346:393-403.

[3] Lakerveld *et al.* International Journal of Behavioral Nutrition and Physical Activity 2013, 10:47. Available at http://www.ijbnpa.org/content/10/1/47

[4] Cantor J, *et al.* Community-centered health homes: bridging the gap between health services and community prevention. Prevention Institute, 2011. Available at http://www.preventioninstitute.org/component/jlibrary/article/id-298/127.html

[5] Gourevitch *et al.* The challenge of attribution: Responsibility for Population Health in the Context of Accountable Care. Am J Prev Med 2012;42(6S2):S180-S183.

[6] Noble DJ, Casalino LP. Can accountable care organizations improve population health? Should they try? JAMA, 2013; 309(11):1119-20.

[7] Global status report on noncommunicable diseases 2010. World Health Organization, April, 2011.

Peter A. Selwyn, *MD, MPH*

Professor and Chairman

Department of Family and Social Medicine

Director, Office of Community Health

Montefiore Medical Center

Albert Einstein College of Medicine

Bronx, NY, USA

Tel: (718) 920-8434

Emails: peter.selwyn@einstein.yu.edu, pselwyn@montefiore.org

PREFACE

A 20-something woman, on over-the-counter appetite suppressant pills for an overweight condition, stays up all night to complete a paper due the next day. To stay alert she takes a stimulant drug along with a few beers. She then takes an herbal sleep aid and sends an email to her professor at 4 am that she will hand deliver the paper herself later that morning. A few hours later, she begins to feel sick with vomiting, dizziness and calls poison control for help. She arrives at a local hospital by ambulance and is given a sedative that puts her in deep sleep. Later that evening she is found to have brain damage, is put on life support and dies six days later. After five years and a four week trial, the jury finds the hospital and its staff not negligent and in the jury's opinion the 20-something had "an overexerted lifestyle" with lack of sleep and a cocktail of drugs.

While tragic indeed, not a day goes by that we don't hear about an illness, condition or even death brought on all as a result of the way we live, work and go about our everyday lives; what we call "Lifestyle Diseases". In a world which is "hyper-connected", urbanized, technologically advanced, and scientifically enriched; sleep, alcohol abuse, drug and tobacco use are usually an after-thought and where physical activity and healthy eating have become an exception rather than the norm. As per the World Health Organization (WHO), our altered lifestyles that result in chronic non-communicable diseases (NCDs) such as obesity, diabetes, heart disease, metabolic syndrome, chronic lung and many cancers account for 50% of the global burden of disease. Furthermore, of the sixty million global deaths that will occur this year, nearly two-thirds or forty million will be secondary to NCDs.

In large parts of the world, especially middle and low income countries, many of these diseases are detected late requiring more expensive and extensive medical care. With most if not all of this care covered through out-of-pocket payments, millions get pushed into poverty year after year. Clearly then, lifestyle diseases are a consequence of man's inability to adapt to this rapidly and constantly changing environment, where immediate gratification takes precedence over everything else, and where affluence and material possession are a fight to the finish line. Can we then change our behaviors, our environments and the way we deliver health care services that would help us ward off these illnesses? Research clearly indicates that lifestyle illnesses all share common risk factors, with unhealthy diets, physical inactivity, overweight, obesity and tobacco and alcohol abuse leading the way. So, prevention strategies aimed at reducing the incidence of any one chronic malady, will not only help lower the incidence of that particular condition, but also the incidence of many other chronic illnesses.

With this epidemic of NCDs showing no signs of abating, we find ourselves in the midst of the most challenging times ever - with our financial, climate and health systems in total disarray. And, the problem is expected to get even worse, with the WHO projecting 2.4 billion overweight and 700 million obese individuals worldwide by the year 2015. With "total inaction", WHO estimates the total cost to the global economy in the range of $ 50 Trillion through 2030 mainly secondary to productivity losses and medical treatments for lifestyle ailments. We, therefore consider the World Economic Forum's projected annual global price tag to fight these ailments at $15 Billion a real steal. We must begin now!

We are deeply indebted to Dr. Selwyn who in his foreword sets the stage by highlighting obesity and related diseases as the global challenge of this century. He calls on us to create the kinds of environments and communities in which we promote health, prevent disease and create a healthier world for one and all. This eText; "Obesity & Disease in an Inter-connected World: A Systems Approach to Turn Huge Challenges into Amazing Opportunities," sets out to provide a roadmap to help turn the tide, by addressing first in Section One, the global burden of highly prevalent but easily preventable risk factors and related conditions, their epidemiology, and the complex biological processes for some of the different disease states, and then going on to highlight in Section Two, the evidence-based opportunities available to prevent and address risk factors *via* health and nutrition education, individual and group counseling, promotion of physical activity and active living, and the importance of adequate sleep, stress management, yoga, meditation and the proper use of pharmacological medications. It is in Section Three that the eBook delves into the much-needed systems approach required to strengthen health systems globally; provision of universal health insurance, the importance of greater investments in community, workplace and life-course health programs, the leveraging of health information technology for the greater good and the global leadership and accountability that will be required for the proper implementation of NCD interventions to achieve the post-2015 Millennium Development Goals (MDGs). As members of the global health community, the contributing authors toward this eBook hope to make the case that better health is a basic fundamental right of every human being, and that enhanced investments in health will help us move forward toward achieving the thus-far elusive goals of health equity, social justice, and financial protection. While the action plans and the resulting key objectives, as outlined by the various authors, may appear to be similar and at times repetitive, this was indeed our intention such that each and every chapter is complete and fully justified as a "stand-alone" and as part of the entire publication.

ACKNOWLEDGEMENTS

We thank our colleagues for sharing their insights as contributing authors. Their chapters address the challenges posed by the global rise in obesity and related co-morbidities and explore opportunities for innovative solutions using a systems approach.

Our sincere appreciation goes to Guy Laufer, MPS, who designed the eBook cover, to illustrate the interconnections we need to consider in dealing with obesity.

Our deepest gratitude goes to Maryellen P. Brucato, DPM, AACFAS, who made it all possible. She tirelessly read and made valuable editing suggestions. Her contributions also included helping us consider the widely varying systems involved in obesity prevention and control.

We thank Bentham Science with a special appreciation to Ms. Hira Aftab of the eBooks Publications Department for her valuable assistance towards the completion of this eBook.

Judith Wylie-Rosett, *EdD, RD*
Atran Foundation Chair in Social Medicine, Professor and Division Head for Health Promotion and Nutrition Research, Department of Epidemiology and Population Health, Albert Einstein College of Medicine, Bronx, NY, USA

Sunil S. Jhangiani, *MD, MBA, FACP, AGAF*
Division of Gastroenterology and Clinical Nutrition, Department of Medicine (Wakefield Campus), Montefiore Medical Center, Clinical Assistant Professor of Medicine and Family and Social Medicine, Albert Einstein College of Medicine, Bronx, NY, USA

LIST OF CONTRIBUTORS

Jason Baker, *MD* — Weill Cornell Medical Associates. Assistant Professor of Clinical Medicine Weil Cornell Medical College New York, NY, USA

Jeannette Beasley, *PhD, RD* — Assistant Professor of Epidemiology and Population Health, Albert Einstein College of Medicine, Bronx, NY, USA

Richard Bernstein, *MD, FACP* — Associate Clinical Professor of Clinical Preventive Medicine and Geriatrics & Palliative Medicine, Icahn School of Medicine at Mount Sinai, New York, NY, USA

Chloe Cheng, *MPH* — Director of Wellness Frenkel Benefits, LLC, New York, NY, USA

Beth E. Conlon, *MS, RD* — Department of Epidemiology and Population Health, Albert Einstein College of Medicine, Bronx, NY, USA

S. Davuluri, *MD* — Division of Geriatrics, Montefiore Medical Center (Wakefield Campus) University Hospital of Albert Einstein College of Medicine, Bronx, NY, USA

Nichola Davis, *MD, MS* — North Bronx Healthcare Network, Associate Professor OF Clinical Medicine and Clinical Epidemiology and Population Health, Albert Einstein College of Medicine, Bronx, NY USA

L. Dharmarajan, *MD, FACP, FACC, FAHA* — Professor of Clinical Medicine, Weill Medical College of Cornell University, New York, Chief, Division of Cardiology, Lincoln Medical and Mental Health Center, Bronx, New York, USA

T.S. Dharmarajan, *MD, MACP, AGSF* — Vice Chairman, Department of Medicine, Clinical Director, Geriatrics, Montefiore Medical Center (Wakefield Campus), Bronx, New York, Professor of Clinical Medicine, University Hospital of Albert Einstein College of Medicine, Professor of Medicine and Associate Dean, New York Medical College, Valhalla, NY, USA

Lindy Fenlason, *MD, PNS, MPH* — Division of General Pediatrics, Department of Pediatrics, Assistant Professor of General Pediatrics, Vanderbilt Children's Hospital, Nashville, TN, USA

Yvette Fruchter, ***MA*** — Department of Psychology, Ferkauf Graduate School of Psychology of Yeshiva University, USA

Lauren Hagemann, ***MA*** — Ferkauf Graduate School of Psychology of Yeshiva University, USA

Philip Haberstro — Founder and CEO of the Wellness Institute of Greater Buffalo and WNY, Inc and the Director of the Be Active New York State initiative, Buffalo, NY, USA

Meredith Hawkins, ***MD, MS*** — Professor of Medicine (Endocrinology), Director, Global Diabetes Institute, Albert Einstein College of Medicine, Bronx, NY, USA

Douglas Heimburger, ***MD, MS*** — Professor of Medicine, Associate Director for Education and Training, Vanderbilt Institute for Global Health, Nashville, TN, USA

K. Indulekha, ***M.Sc*** — Department of Diabetology & Epidemiology, Madras Diabetes Research Foundation & Dr. Mohan's Diabetes Specialties Centre, Chennai, India

Sunil Jhangiani, ***MD, MBA, FACP, AGAF*** — Division of Gastroenterology and Clinical Nutrition, Department of Medicine, Montefiore Medical Center (Wakefield Campus), Clinical Assistant Professor of Medicine and Family and Social Medicine, Albert Einstein College of Medicine, Bronx, NY, USA

Harmit Kalia, ***DO*** — Assistant Professor, Division of Gastroenterology and Liver Diseases, Marion Bessin Liver Research Center, Albert Einstein College of Medicine and Montefiore Medical Center, Bronx, NY, USA

Kristie Lancaster, ***PhD, RD*** — Associate Professor, Department of Nutrition, Food Studies & Public Health, New York University, New York, NY, USA

Guy Laufer, ***MPS*** — Global Digital Learning Director for McCann Worldgroup, New York, NY, USA

David Lounsbury, ***PhD*** — Assistant Professor of Epidemiology and Population Health, Albert Einstein College of Medicine of Yeshiva University, Belfer Building, Bronx, NY USA

Carlos Marquez, ***MA*** — Ferkauf Graduate School of Psychology of Yeshiva University, Bronx, NY, USA

V. Mohan, *MD, PhD*
President & Chief of Diabetes Research, Department of Diabetology & Epidemiology, Madras Diabetes Research Foundation & Dr. Mohan's Diabetes Specialties Centre, Chennai, India

Yasmin Mossavar-Rahmani, *PhD, RD, CDN*
Associate Professor of Clinical Epidemiology and Population Health, Albert Einstein College of Medicine of Yeshiva University, Bronx, NY, USA

Marcelle Pigananelli
Universidad Iberoamericana, Santo Domingo, Dominican Republic, USA

C.S. Pitchumoni, *MD, MACP, MACG, FRCP(C), AGAF, MPH*
Clinical Professor of Medicine, Rutgers University, New Jersey, Adjunct Professor of Medicine, New York Medical College, NY, Chief, Gastroenterology, Hepatology & Clinical Nutrition, St. Peter's University Hospital, NJ, USA

Pooja Raghavan, *MD, MS*
Clinical Endocrinology Fellow, National Institutes of Health (NIH), Bethesda Maryland, USA

Dhyan Rajan, *MD*
Division of Gastroenterology, Nassau University Medical Center, East Meadow, NY, USA

Kathryn J. Reid, *PhD*
Research Associate Professor, Department of Neurology, Northwestern University, Feinberg School of Medicine, Chicago, IL, USA

Sarah Litman Rendell, *PhD*
Postdoctoral Fellow, Southold Center for Development, Southold, NY, USA

Lynn Rivera, *DPT*
Associate Professor and Chair Department of Physical Therapy, D'Youville College, Buffalo, NY, USA

Anthony Santoro, *MA*
Ferkauf Graduate School of Psychology of Yeshiva, University, Bronx, NY, USA

Mary Stottele, *BS*
AmeriCorps VISTA, Buffalo, NY, USA

Sonia Suchday, *PhD*
Professor, Chair of Department of Psychology, Pace University, New York, NY, USA

Charles Swencionis, *PhD*
Associate Professor of Psychology, Ferkauf Graduate School of Psychology of Yeshiva University; Associate Professor of Epidemiology and Population Health, and Psychiatry, Albert Einstein College of Medicine of Yeshiva University, Bronx, NY, USA

Denise Tahara, ***MBA, MPhil, PhD***

Associate Professor of Public Health Practice and Director of MPH Studies in the Department of Health Policy and Management at the School of Health Sciences and Practice at New York Medical College Valhalla, NY, USA

Sirakarn Tejavanija, ***MD, MS***

Division of Clinical Nutrition, Department of Internal Medicine, Phramongkutklao Army Hospital and Medical College, Bangkok, Thailand

Allan Wolkoff, ***MD***

The Herman Lopata Chair in Liver Disease Research, Professor of Medicine and Anatomy and Structural Biology, Associate Chair of Medicine for Research, Chief, Division of Gastroenterology and Liver Diseases, Director, Marion Bessin Liver Research Center, Albert Einstein College of Medicine and Montefiore Medical Center, Bronx, NY, USA

Judith Wylie-Rosett, ***EdD, RD***

Division of Health Promotion and Nutrition Research, Professor of Epidemiology and Population Health, Albert Einstein College of Medicine, Bronx, NY, USA

BIOGRAPHIES

Judith Wylie-Rosett, EdD, RD, is Professor and Head of the Division of Health Promotion and Nutrition Research in the Department of Epidemiology and Population Health at Albert Einstein College of Medicine where she is the Atran Foundation Chair in Social Medicine. Dr. Wylie-Rosett's research addresses the role of lifestyle in relation to health disparities including diabetes, heart disease and cancer. Much of her work has focused on optimizing resources to provide better nutritional care for underserved populations. Her research collaborations have addressed how community, clinical and personal factors are related to health care delivery, lifestyle and health outcomes. Dr. Wylie-Rosett's research has examined acculturation, health behaviors and disease biomarkers among Chinese immigrants in New York City; her research collaborations have examined global culture and health behavior among students in India. Dr. Wylie-Rosett has focused on strategies for tailoring interventions using a social ecological framework to promote healthier lifestyle choices by individuals considering their life context. Her research has also addressed issues related to implementing guidelines to reduce obesity and concomitant rise in non-communicable disease. Dr. Wylie-Rosett's multi-center research trial collaborations include the Diabetes Control and Complications Trial, the Diabetes Prevention Program and the Women's Health Initiative. She has served on the editorial boards of several journals and is currently Associate Editor of the journal Diabetes Care. Dr. Wylie-Rosett has over 200 peer-reviewed research papers and 75 book chapters in addition to five books on lifestyle and weight. Dr. Wylie-Rosett earned her master's and doctoral degrees from Columbia University Teachers' College in New York City.

Sunil Jhangiani, MD, MBA, FACP, AGAF, is board certified by the American Board of Internal Medicine, Clinical Nutrition and Gastroenterology. He is a fellow of the American College of Physicians (FACP), the American Gastroenterological Association (AGAF), and has memberships in the American College of Gastroenterology (ACG) and the American Society of Parenteral and Enteral Nutrition (ASPEN). To get a better understanding of how the clinical practice of medicine interacts with the broader and global issues of health care policy, delivery and economics, Dr. Jhangiani obtained a Master's in Business Administration degree (MBA) in 1998 followed by board certification in Managed Care/Population Medicine in 2001. He then moved on to practical health-related training under two very eminent experts in the fields of health care operations and business strategy; Dr. Richard Bernstein and Mr. Kenneth Abramowitz. Dr. Jhangiani is the Founder and Medical Director of "Doctors for a Healthier Bronx" a non-profit community-organization focused on improving the health and wellness of the citizens of the Bronx. Founded in 2007 with just 3 physicians, it has since grown to over 350 Bronx doctors with such strategic partners as Montefiore Medical Center, Albert Einstein College of Medicine, the Bronx Chamber of Commerce, numerous New York City public schools, and several local businesses in the New York City area. Dr. Jhangiani has authored several articles and book chapters in the field of clinical nutrition, gastroenterology and health care management. His keen insights into health care trends and strategy have resulted in numerous interviews on TV, radio, and the print media. He has delivered speeches on a wide range of health related issues with publications in "Vital Speeches of the Day" and "Vital Speeches International". Dr. Jhangiani holds faculty appointments in the departments of Medicine and Family and Social Medicine at the Albert Einstein College of Medicine. He is on the medical staff at Montefiore Medical Center, Bronx, NY and currently serves on the institution's Medical Executive Committee.

SHORT SUMMARY WITH SALIENT FEATURES

The eBook examines how the rising epidemics of obesity and other lifestyle diseases are changing health guidelines globally; from directing health care professionals on how to care for individuals to encompass the interconnected systems involved in chronic disease risk management, prevention and treatment. With a focus on systems, the text serves as an excellent resource on how to develop a more comprehensive approach to population health. Starting with a systematic approach to risk assessment, followed by a targeted approach to risk reduction and prevention, the eBook moves along seamlessly into section three calling for a shared responsibility toward strengthening health systems globally that can help determine and improve upon the health of individuals, and societies across the world.

2

CHAPTER 1

Lifestyle Diseases in the Modern Era: A Major Threat to Global Health!

Sirakarn Tejavanija[1] and Sunil S. Jhangiani[*,2]

[1]Division of Clinical Nutrition, Department of Internal Medicine, Phramongkutklao Army Hospital and Medical College, Bangkok, Thailand; and [2]Division of Gastroenterology and Clinical Nutrition, Department of Medicine, Montefiore Medical Center, Clinical Assistant Professor of Medicine and Family and Social Medicine, Albert Einstein College of Medicine, Bronx, NY, USA

Abstract: Lifestyle diseases, a subset of non-communicable diseases (NCDs) are a result of the way we live, work and go about our everyday lives. Over the last several decades, our diets have become unhealthy, our lifestyles sedentary and many of us still use tobacco and abuse alcohol. These four risk factors have resulted in an ever-increasing prevalence of five lifestyle diseases; namely obesity, diabetes, cancer, chronic lung disease and cardiovascular disease (CVD). As per the World Health Organization (WHO), NCDs have become the major contributors to higher morbidity, mortality and at the same time the single biggest obstacle to development globally. Furthermore, NCDs continue to increase in virtually every region of the world with the WHO reporting a higher burden in middle and low-income countries. Health promotion and preventive health approaches are proven effective strategies in reducing disease burden with lower costs compared to the cost of NCD treatment. However, NCD prevention and control cannot be done with diet control and increased physical activity alone. It requires action at multiple levels with health care providers and governments as leaders, along with stronger health care systems and multi-stakeholder involvement. To ensure that the interventions meet set targets; regular reporting, global monitoring and accountability are important.

Keywords: Alcohol, behavior, cardiovascular disease, cervical cancer, crisis, DALY, diabetes, diet, disability, exercise, global health, health care, HIV-AIDs, intervention, IOM, life expectancy, lifestyle diseases, lifestyle, NCD, non-communicable diseases, physical activity, physical inactivity, premature death, smoking, United Nations.

***Corresponding author Sunil S. Jhangiani:** 2425 Eastchester Road, Bronx, NY 10469, USA; Tel: (718) 231-5100; Fax: 1-718-515-8885; E-mail: sjgimd@aol.com

INTRODUCTION

"*A crisis is a terrible thing to waste*". This is something we have heard repeatedly over the last decade by economists, climate change experts, and politicians alike, all looking for a ray of hope amidst the now familiar worldwide threats. Today, the same could be said about the dramatic alteration occurring in the landscape of global health. We are witnessing a profound change so much so that non-communicable diseases are becoming more common than communicable diseases [1]. This alteration, although greater in high-income countries, is also occurring and moving rapidly across low and middle-income countries [2]. If not addressed and tackled, these conditions could very soon overwhelm health systems worldwide, and virtually negate all of the gains made over the last several decades.

And, rightfully indeed, Dr. Margaret Chan, the Director-General at the World Health Organization (WHO), called these non-communicable lifestyle diseases (NCDs) a "Slow Motion Disaster" in her address at a 2011 High Level United Nations (UN) General Assembly Meeting in New York City [3]. She concluded her speech calling for more focused international and country responses to NCDs, declaring that with appropriate interventions, these diseases can be controlled, treated and largely prevented as well.

To put this in context; one begins to wonder as to how we got here despite the amazing advances in medicine, biotechnology and food security of the last several decades that have resulted in transformational health gains globally. Countries such as India and Ethiopia [4] have doubled the life expectancy of its citizens, and in the United States, we have now over 6 million individuals over the age of 85 [5] with that number expected to rise to 20 million by 2050. Furthermore, in the U.S., economists at the University of Chicago have been able to show that health does deliver wealth. The increased life expectancy in the U.S. between 1970 and 2000 contributed to a wind-fall $3.2 Trillion annual increase in national GDP (Gross Domestic Product) [6]. Further advances in medicine, genetics and pharmaceuticals to slow down the ageing process itself has led some experts to boldly predict that the first humans to live to 150 and beyond may have already been born [7, 8].

Are we then at a crossroads when it comes to global health? We could move along the path toward improving health, longevity and prosperity for all or fall prey to the onslaught of obesity, diabetes, and related diseases. Being driven largely by the forces of globalization and urbanization, these lifestyle illnesses are spreading rapidly across the world; a world where geographic boundaries are blurred and economic time zones have lost their meaning. But then what exactly does the term "global health" convey? As adopted by Fineberg and Hunter, in simple terms it would come to mean "public health for the world" [9]. In 2008, the U.S. Institute of Medicine (IOM) put out a detailed description of what one can call a definition of the term "Global Health" [10] which runs as follows:

> "*Global health is the goal of improving health for all people in all nations by promoting wellness and eliminating diseases, disabilities, and deaths. It can be attained by combining clinical care at the level of the individual person with population-based measures to promote health and prevent disease. This ambitious endeavor calls for an understanding of health determinants, practices, and solutions, as well as basic and applied research concerning risk factors, disease, and disability* [10]".

With an emphasis on disease prevention, health promotion, and improving lives for all people globally; the importance of "lifestyle diseases" comes into sharp focus.

DEFINITION

Lifestyle

A simple meaning of "Lifestyle" is "a way of life" (how one lives) on a day-to-day basis by an individual, group (*e.g.*, family, a particular neighborhood), or society (*i.e.*, social class, culture) [11, 12]. It is influenced by both tangible and intangible factors. Tangible factors are mainly demographic-related. For example, populations that live along the sea are more likely to have a surfing lifestyle and consume more seafood. On the contrary, intangible factors are mainly psychological aspects. One's lifestyle reflects not only the social, physical, psychological, and economic environments an individual is exposed to, but also his or her self-image and attitudes. As a result of these complex interactions, lifestyle eventually expresses itself in many different ways including health, work, behavior, leisure patterns, activities, attitudes, interests, opinions, and values. However, lifestyle can also be learned by experience. Therefore, lifestyle is modifiable.

Many recent studies have shown that one's lifestyle can transfer its effect across generations. The data suggests that the health of the parents, especially that of the mother plays a significant role in the overall expression of an offspring's lifestyle [13, 14]. Economic issues such as total family income may also have a great effect on the physical and mental health of the parents. Parents with lower income are more likely to have unhealthier lifestyles (such as smoking, poor living conditions, *etc.*), be stressed and more often be depressed. In all likelihood, how parents and other family members react and deal with these issues can get easily transferred to their children through the learning processes [15].

The concept of lifestyle management/intervention has developed and significantly broadened in many aspects over the past decade. For instance, in terms of business, the analysis of consumer lifestyles aims to create a detailed customer profile (termed "Psychographics") [16], a very important factor in determining how consumers make their purchasing decisions. Similarly, by a careful analysis of an individual's lifestyle factors, one could develop and implement interventions that help prevent, delay or ameliorate a lifestyle-related illness.

Lifestyle Diseases

Lifestyle has a great impact on an individual's heath including physical, mental and social well-being. Lifestyle diseases with a few exceptions are those conditions brought on all as a result of the way we live, work and go about our everyday lives. They have at least one risky life style as a causative factor. Conditions such as obesity, type 2 diabetes, heart disease, and certain forms of cancer are contracted from the way we live. Smoking, excess alcohol, poor diet and, sedentary lifestyles may all either contribute to these illnesses or be their primary cause (Table **1**). Insomnia and a range of sleep disorders by themselves are much more prevalent today and are being blamed on the way we work and live. To summarize, a lifestyle disease has the following characteristics:

1. Non-infectious in nature.

2. Late-onset. It needs a longer life expectancy in order to become the cause of death.

3. Long natural history. The progression of the disease is usually slow.

4. Lifestyle interventions that alter behaviors or exposures can prevent or delay the occurrence of the disease.

Table 1. List of lifestyle diseases [18, 19].

Body Systems	Lifestyle Diseases/Conditions
Endocrine system	Type 2 diabetes, obesity, metabolic syndrome, osteoporosis
Cardiovascular system	Coronary heart disease, stroke
Respiratory system	Asthma, COPD[a]
Gastrointestinal system	NAFLD, [b] liver cirrhosis, gastroesophageal reflux disease (GERD)
Renal system	Chronic kidney disease
Nervous system	Alzheimer's disease
Others	Insomnia, other sleep disorders, certain types of cancers

[a]COPD; chronic obstructive pulmonary disease; [b]NAFLD; Non-alcoholic fatty liver disease.

Studies have very clearly shown that almost 80 percent of heart disease, stroke and type 2 diabetes and over a third of all cancers are preventable [17].

Non-Communicable Diseases (NCDs)

In general, NCDs are defined as chronic diseases which are not infectious. Such diseases result from either genetic or lifestyle factors [18, 19]. Therefore, lifestyle diseases are a subset of NCDs. Genetic factors are non-modifiable, whereas lifestyle factors are modifiable. This means that the majority of NCDs are preventable by eliminating lifestyle-related risk factors. In general, the term “NCDs” is usually used to refer to lifestyle diseases.

And, because, some lifestyle related cancers (stomach, liver, and cervix) can be secondary to infections, WHO generally considers the term “NCDs” to be a misnomer [18].

EXTENT OF THE PROBLEM

The global burden of NCDs continues to rise and spread worldwide. The WHO projects that the absolute number and proportion of global deaths from NCDs will rise to about 70% by 2030 [20]. The total number of years lost due to ill-health, disability or premature death is used as an indicator of the overall disease burden, termed “disability-adjusted life-years” (DALYs). One DALY is thought of as one lost year of healthy life. During the past two decades, total mortality and calculated DALYs from NCDs have increased by 8% [1, 21] and 11% [2], respectively. According to WHO global estimates in 2008, close to 36 million people die each year (63% of the total number of deaths worldwide) as a result of

NCDs [18, 22] (Fig. **1**). Based on data from death certificates, about 80% of all deaths from NCDs (29 Million) were in the following four major groups of diseases, *i.e.* cardiovascular diseases (17.3 million), cancers (7.6 million), chronic pulmonary diseases (4.2 million) and diabetes (1.3 million) [21] (Fig. **2**). In addition, the Global Burden of Diseases, Injuries, and Risk Factors Study 2010 (GBD 2010) estimated that the percentage of DALYs due to NCDs had increased from 43% in 1990 to 54% in 2010 [2]. Unsurprisingly, cardiovascular diseases accounted for the highest numbers of both global deaths and global DALYs. As per WHO data, all of these four major NCDs are more prevalent in low- and middle-income countries and account for approximately 45% of disability-adjusted life years (DALYs) [23]. Hunter and Reddy have suggested that as we see an increase in the size and age of the world's population, we are more likely to see an increase in the overall prevalence of and the proportion of NCD deaths globally [24].

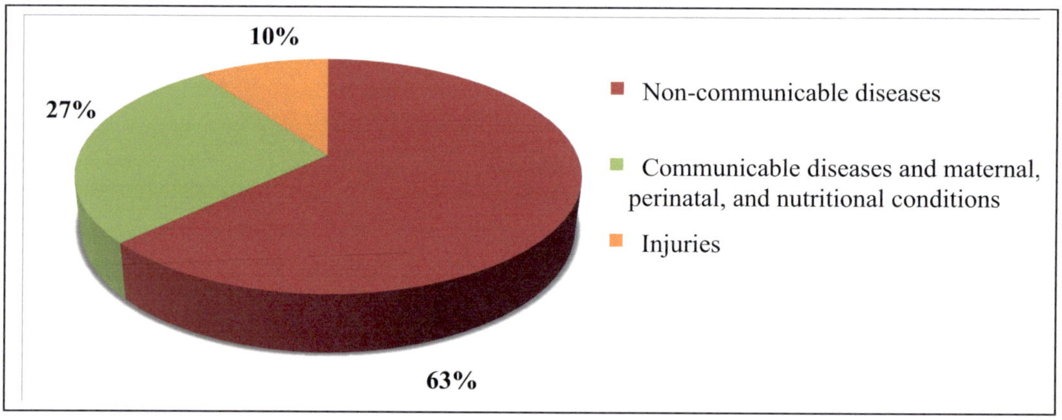

Fig. (1). Causes of global deaths (WHO 2008, adapted from refs. [22, 24]).

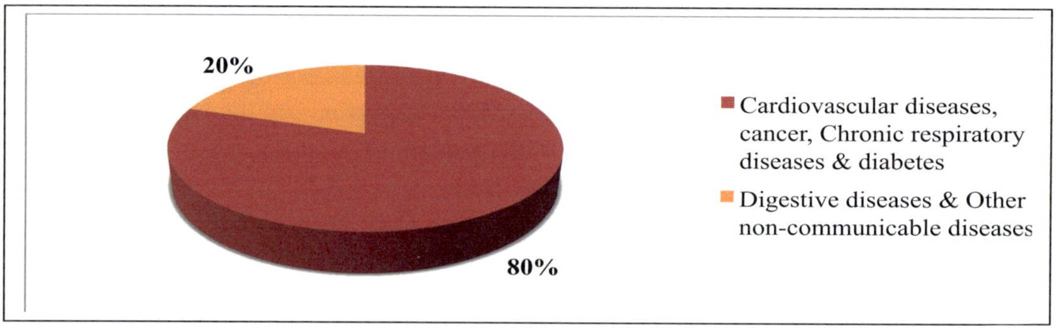

Fig. (2). Major NCD deaths globally by cause & < age 70 years (WHO 2008, adapted from ref. [21]).

This rapidly growing burden is being accelerated by the negative effects of insufficient physical activity and unhealthy diets rich in processed foods, saturated fats, trans fats, sugar and salt resulting in rising prevalence of overweight and obesity. These two major risk factors for NCDs along with tobacco use and alcohol misuse not only contribute to more than two-thirds of all new cases of NCDs, but also result in a higher risk of complications in people with preexisting NCDs [25]. According to 2008-2010 world, regional and, country-specific data available from WHO, the percentage of people age 15 years or older with insufficient physical activity, rates of overweight/ obesity and the number of NCD-related deaths per 100,000 of the population in some select countries are shown in Figs. (**3**, **4** and **5**) respectively. The annual and attributable deaths from each common risk factor are summarized in Table **2**.

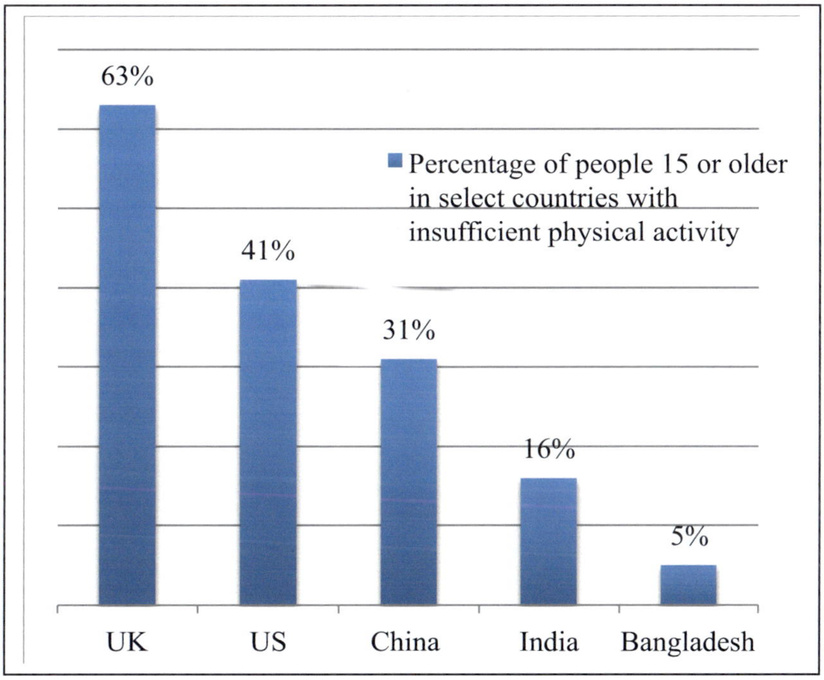

Fig. (3). Percentage of people aged 15 years or older in select countries with inadequate physical activity (sources: WHO, adapted from refs. [10, 23]).

In addition, the current NCD crisis has become a major barrier to developmental goals such as poverty reduction, and the provision of universal healthcare, food and income security, and clean air and water to population groups across the globe as shown in Fig. (**6**).

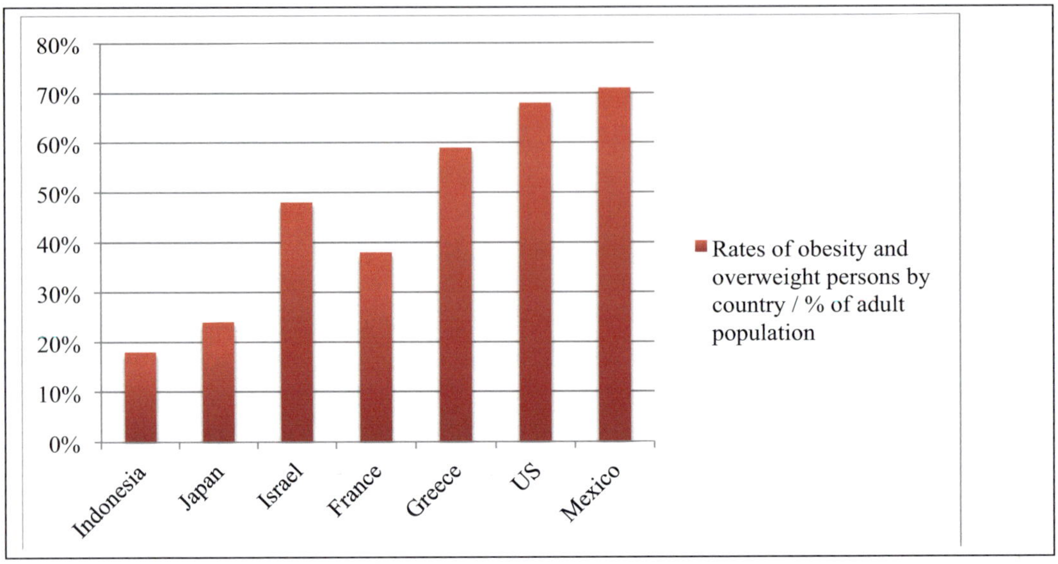

Fig. (4). Rates of obesity/overweight by country (Sources: WHO, adapted from refs. [10, 23]).

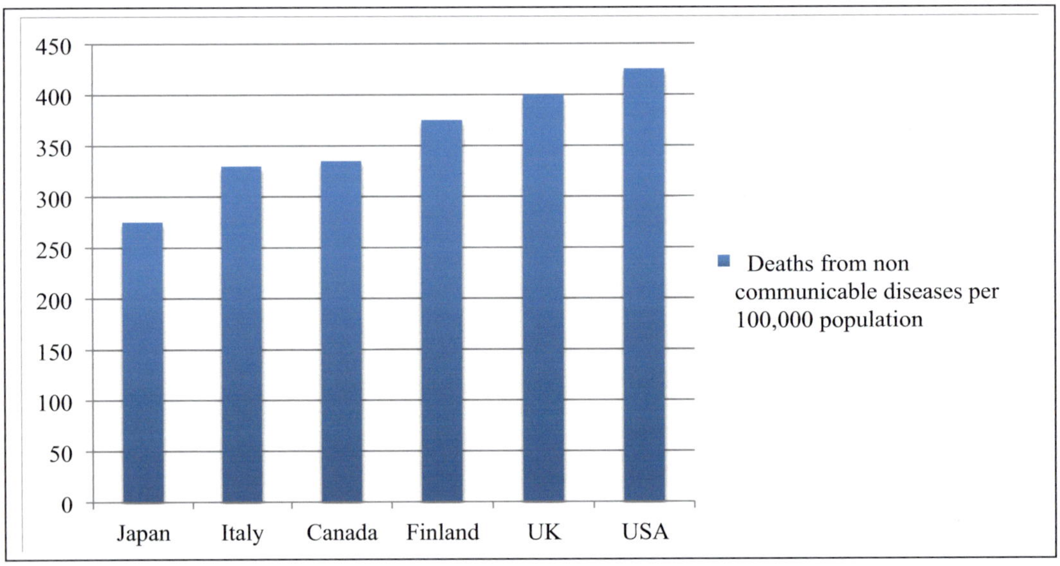

Fig. (5). Deaths from non-communicable diseases per 100,000 population (sources: WHO, adapted from refs. [10, 23]).

Table 2. The annual and attributable deaths from common lifestyle factors (WHO [18]).

Lifestyle Factors	Approximate Annual Deaths from NCDs	Attributable Deaths
Tobacco	6 million[a]	9%
Unhealthy diets	1.7 million	N/A[b]
Physical inactivity	3.2 million	6%
Alcohol abuse	1.15 million	N/A

[a]10% of deaths are from exposure to second-hand smoke; [b]N/A indicates data not available.

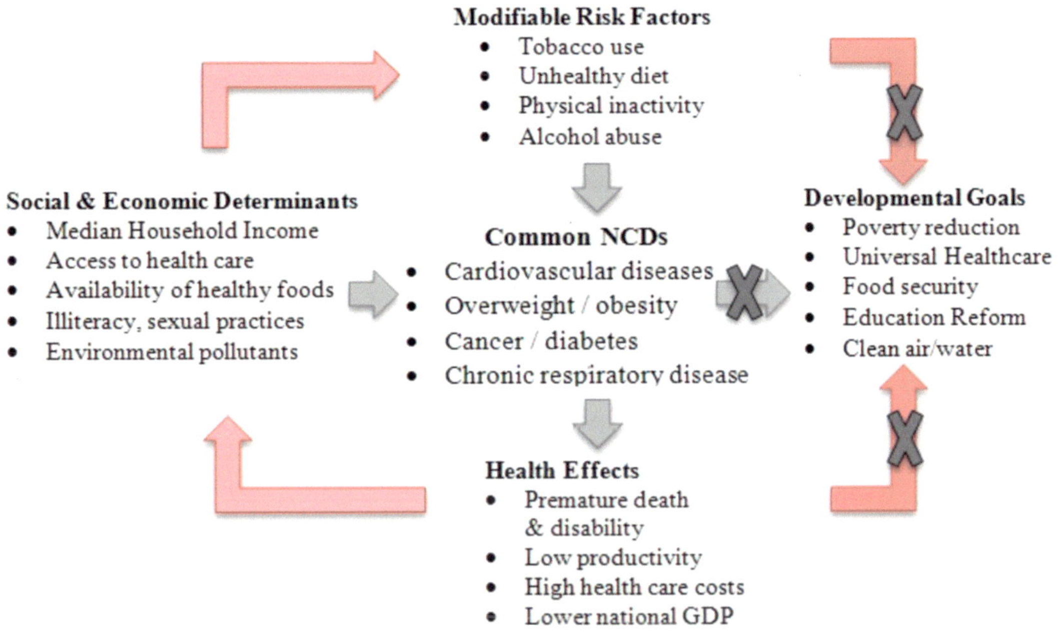

Fig. (6). Association between NCDs and development goals (adapted from refs. [25, 26]). X represents barrier to.

ROOT CAUSES

The root causes of the vast majority of lifestyle diseases are multifactorial in origin. They are a result of the interactions between social factors, environmental issues, and some specific risky behaviors. The four common risk factors that contribute to the development of major NCDs are tobacco use, alcohol abuse, unhealthy diets and, physical inactivity. These factors are believed to be behind the deaths of 100,000 people every day [27].

These harmful behaviors lead to four major metabolic changes which are the components of the metabolic syndrome (Fig. **7**, also see CHAPTER 5 on Moving Beyond Metabolic Syndrome). These are raised blood pressure, overweight/obesity hyperglycemia, and dyslipidemia. The hyperglycemia and overweight/obesity-attributable deaths are estimated to be 6% and 5%, respectively [18]. Furthermore, these lifestyle factors are more likely to cause disease and premature deaths if individuals also lack the basic knowledge with regards to prevention and early detection and have little or no access to standard treatment options [27]. We now know that NCDs with specific and unique risk factors such as cervical and liver cancers require a more targeted approach so as to manage all aspects of these conditions comprehensively [24].

Common modifiable risk factors		Resulting metabolic changes		Main NCDs
Unhealthy Diet	➡	High blood pressure	➡	Heart disease, stroke
Physical inactivity		High blood sugar		Diabetes
Tobacco use		High body weight		Chronic respiratory diseases
Improper alcohol use		Dyslipidemia		Cancer

Fig. (7). Causes of non-communicable diseases (WHO, adapted from refs. [18, 22, 23]).

As globalization spreads, NCDs affect populations across all age groups, every income level, and all regions of the world. According to the characteristics of NCDs, these conditions should be more prevalent in older age groups. What is indeed surprising is that approximately 25% of all NCD deaths are now premature which means that they occur before the age of 60 (Fig. **8**). This may imply exposure to risk factors since a very young age. Recent evidence on epigenetics (see CHAPTER 2 on Overweight & Obesity), a new research area regarding gene science, indicates that there is a link between gene, environment and lifestyle [28]. If someone is healthy, this means that the structures and functions of all genes or programs in cells are working optimally. Gene expression (turning on) /silence (turning off) mechanism is a signal-dependent process. There are two types of signals. Firstly, metaphysical signals which are intangible signals *e.g.*, feelings, beliefs, faith, attitudes, values, perception, *etc.* Secondly, material signals, which are tangible chemical signals *e.g.*, foods, drinks, drugs, medications, enzymes, hormones, neurotransmitters, *etc.* Interestingly, both metaphysical and material signals are largely influenced by our daily lifestyles. This means that if we have a healthy lifestyle and good living conditions, these healthy signals affect our genes in a way that get transmitted to cell programs to positively direct our body functions. On the contrary, if we have a risky lifestyle, the unhealthy signals will negatively affect our bodies.

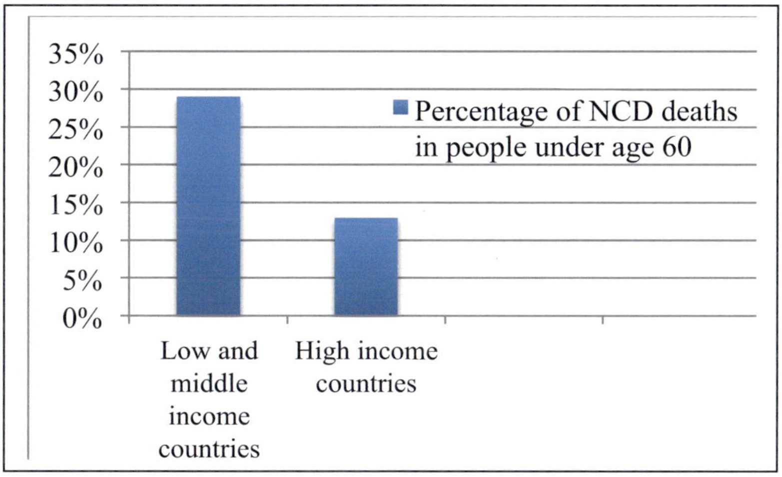

Fig. (8). Percentage of NCD deaths in people under age 60 years (WHO 2010, adapted from refs. [23, 24]).

GLOBAL PATTERNS AND TRENDS

The patterns of the global change in the incidence of NCDs vary between and within regions of the world, whether rich or poor and in accordance to the prevalence of risk factors [29]. People with a lower socioeconomic status [30] are more likely to be exposed to harmful products and environments which cause them to be sicker and even die sooner than people from a higher socioeconomic stratum of society. Moreover, many of them have limited access to necessary medicines and health services. Four out of five people diagnosed with cancer, diabetes, cardiovascular or respiratory diseases live in poor countries [27]. About 80% of all NCD-related deaths occur in low- and middle-income countries with 90% of them being premature [31] (Fig. **9**), and responsible for about 45% of disability-adjusted life years (DALYs) [23]. Although maternal and child mortality are much higher in low- and middle-income countries as compared to high-income countries, cardiovascular deaths still account for the largest proportion of deaths from NCDs in these countries [2].

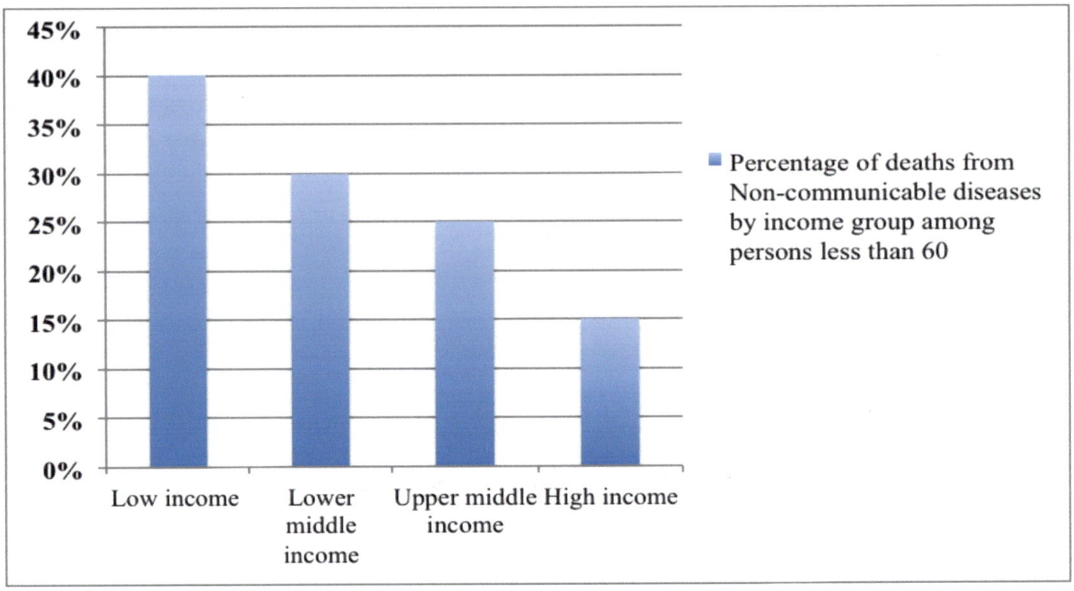

Fig. (9). Percentage of deaths from NCDs by income group among persons aged less than 60 years (adapted from refs. [24, 31]).

In many high-income countries, such as the U.S., NCD-related death rates have been substantially reduced [32]. However, when you take in to consideration the growth and ageing of the population, the annual absolute number of deaths from NCDs has not changed significantly.

ECONOMIC BURDEN

With improvements in health care and modern medical treatment modalities, life expectancy of people globally has been steadily rising. As a result, health care costs across the globe have increased significantly over the last several years. If one were to take a high income country as an example, total health spending in the United States stood at $2.6 trillion in 2010, which was ten folds greater than in 1980 ($256 billion) [33]. Hospital care and physician services accounted for approximately half of the total costs; and in overall terms, health spending accounted for 17.9% of the nation's Gross Domestic Product (GDP) [34]. Current estimates suggest that the costs of treatments for chronic diseases alone account for over 75% of national health expenditures [35] in the U.S.

One of the driving factors of ever-increasing health care spending globally is the increased incidence of NCDs. Across the globe, more of national health care spending is going toward the treatment of cardiovascular disease, diabetes, cancer, and chronic respiratory disease. NCDs can further exacerbate the economic burden from large-scale losses in productivity as a result of higher rates of absenteeism by the work force and their inability to put in a full days' worth of work. This results in a decline in the national Gross Domestic Product (GDP). Across the globe today just diabetes costs can range from 1.5% of GDP in Venezuela to 5.9% of GDP in Barbados [23]. Furthermore, evidence suggests that globally NCDs will cause an estimated cumulative output loss of US $47 trillion over the next two decades, of which about US $30 trillion will be attributable to cardiovascular diseases, diabetes, cancers, and chronic pulmonary diseases [24, 36, 37]. It thus becomes abundantly clear that NCDs cause a huge economic burden not just in low and middle-income countries, but in high-income countries as well. This is directly as a result of high direct health care costs and loss of economic productivity due to premature disability and deaths (also see CHAPTER 16: Using Systems Thinking to Understand the Dynamics of Obesity In Low and Middle Income Countries).

MOUNTING CHALLENGES

Effective strategies to reduce and control overall health care costs in the long term are health promotion and disease prevention. In addition, health promotion is a proven cost-effective method in improving overall health and wellbeing, reducing the burden of NCDs, addressing health inequities, facilitating the better use of resources and enhancing economic productivity [38-41]. The advanced treatment of NCDs is not a major key to success for achieving behavioral change. Therefore, a major component of health system reform is to find a balance between investments in health promotion for preventable NCDs, particularly for vulnerable communities and populations, and investments in medical treatment. This would require a collaborative approach amongst health, education, food and agriculture, finance, and planning sectors of the economy to promote such preventive interventions.

Encouraging a healthier lifestyle can be very challenging. It requires comprehensive, multi-disciplinary and multi-level preventive system to drive a new paradigm shift towards healthy lifestyles at all levels; individual, community, and societal. This strategy is aimed for better long-term health outcomes. Today, we have a wide range of potential lifestyle interventions, ranging from education at the individual level to policy changes at the national level.

At Individual and Community Level

Being healthy is everyone's business. Effective lifestyle changes depend a lot on personal motivation and individual preferences. The International Federation of Red Cross and Red Crescent Societies (IFRC) whose strength lies in its volunteer and community-based network across 190 countries have always advocated the important role that women can have toward promoting healthy lifestyle in their families and then across their communities. The IFRC has furthermore invested in women's participation toward this effort for the simple reason that the majority of caregivers are female [27].

Lifestyles are also influenced by social environments. Communities have the right to receive appropriate information as to the health risks of NCDs and the steps they could take to mitigate those risks. Community-based prevention will require volunteers to work as leaders to create the required healthy environments and to encourage people to choose and maintain healthy living choices [27]. In addition, health education through mass media and health promotion in specific settings, such as schools, workplaces and community centers, are also important and discussed throughout this eBook.

On Government Response

Government has an essential role in disease prevention. A multidisciplinary approach that involves health and other non-health ministries within the government, such as finance, education, sports, and agriculture can all contribute toward reversing the underlying socioeconomic causes of the problem. Governments should promote rapid scale-up of NCD interventions and health services access to raise the priority of NCDs on the national public health agendas globally.

All governments are expected to design appropriate health care systems for their countries. A national action plan that mobilizes many sectors of the economy requires strong political leadership, ensuring accountability and at the same time having the processes in place that monitor progress. Health care systems for industrialized countries which can readily access most if not all essential medicines may have to focus more on the ageing population. In low and middle-income countries, health care systems must address infectious diseases, malnutrition, and maternal and child health along with NCDs. Therefore, human and financial resources for NCDs in such countries will be limited. In addition, about one-third of the world's population still has no regular access to many essential medications [42]. Majority of these neglected communities live in sub-Saharan Africa. Countries with rapidly emerging economies such as the Philippines and Thailand are witnessing huge "societal conflicts" due to the wide gaps between the "haves" and the "have-nots". These countries face huge challenges when it comes to developing early and cost-effective intervention programs to lessen the spread of NCDs.

Multiple Stakeholder and Sector Response

Prevention of NCDs requires a broader community-based engagement and a sustained impact. Only governmental action is not enough. It requires multi-stakeholder partnership, either public, private, civil society or volunteers to build and actively promote a conducive environment in every aspect. Healthy choices must be easy and not expensive. Multi-stakeholder efforts can make major contributions to achieve the WHO global target of a 25% reduction in premature deaths from NCDs by 2025 [43].

Today, many international, national, and regional foundations and societies partner with governments and private stakeholders to combat the burden of NCDs. They set their visions and strategies to facilitate NCD interventions. A good example is the "Charter of Healthy Living" which came down from the World Economic Forum's Healthy Living Initiative [36]. It was developed in 2012 as the outcome of a one-year process engaging leaders of governments, businesses, local communities and international organizations worldwide to invest toward the transformation of the current health landscape where NCDs have become the major cause of morbidity, mortality and lost economic output. In addition, the IFCR has set NCDs prevention as a major component of its Strategy 2020 Initiative; a collective plan of action to tackle major health and development challenges facing mankind today. It encourages partnerships at the community and national levels with the underlying goal being to achieve the development of a framework that provides universal health insurance and a more inclusive public health system. To break the barriers that limit access to medications necessary for the primary and secondary prevention of a disease, *e.g.*, cardiovascular disease in developing countries, "Access to Medicine Index" was set up by an independent initiative in 2004. This serves as a vehicle to encourage pharmaceutical companies to make their products available at affordable prices in low and middle income countries. This index has been used to evaluate and rank the pharmaceutical companies every two years [44]. This reflects the responsibility of the pharmaceutical industry to public health.

Primary Health Care Approach

Primary health care also has a significant role in both primary and secondary prevention of NCDs with early detection and timely treatment targeting low socioeconomic communities. This is another way to diminish the high impact of NCDs by reducing morbidity, disability and premature death. Moreover, such effective primary health care systems reduce the need for more expensive treatments. As seen in Fig. (**10**), high-income countries are about four times more likely to have NCD services covered by national health insurance than low-income countries. Communities with inadequate health insurance coverage are more likely to have a sub-optimal access to essential NCD interventions, resulting in higher out-of-pocket expenses which exacerbate poverty and impair developmental goals.

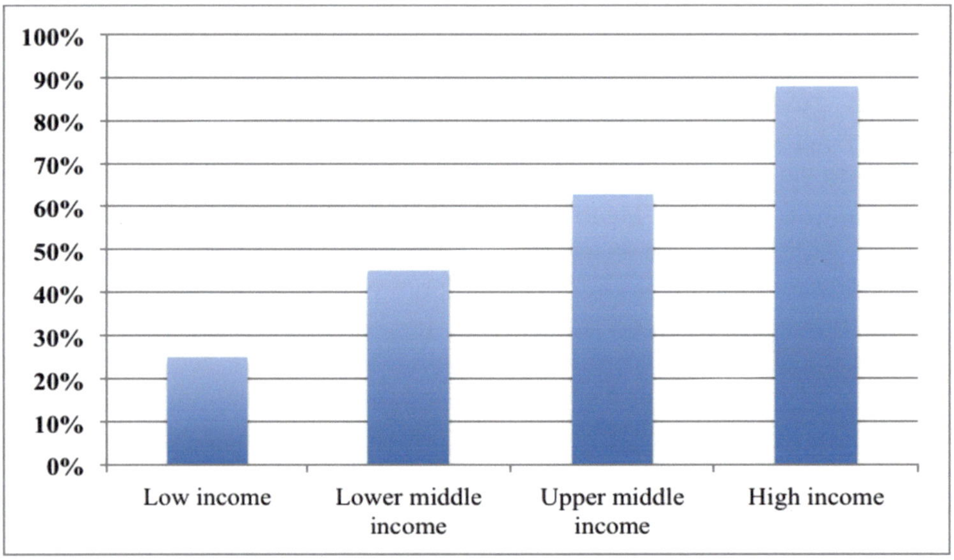

Fig. (10). Proportion of countries where NCD-related service and treatments are formally covered by health insurance by world bank income group (adapted from WHO, 2010, adapted from refs. [36]).

WHO Response

Since the year 2000, WHO has become the lead organization at advocating and implementing policies for the prevention and treatment of NCDs globally, with a special emphasis on developing countries. Approximately five years ago [43], it set a "2008-2013 Action Plan of the global strategy for the prevention and control of NCDs". Recently, an updated 2013-2020 Action Plan has been set to continue to take action against NCDs. This Action Plan provides practical steps on how to address NCDs with 6 multilevel objectives and actions.

1. To strengthen international cooperation and advocacy to raise the priority accorded to prevention and control of NCDs in the development agenda and in internationally-agreed development goals.

2. To strengthen national capacity, leadership, governance, multi-sectoral action and partnerships to accelerate country response for prevention and control of NCDs.

3. To reduce exposure to the four most common modifiable risk factors for NCDs; tobacco use, unhealthy diets, physical inactivity and harmful use of alcohol through creation of health-promoting environments.

4. To strengthen and reorient health systems to address prevention and control of NCDs through people-centered primary health care and provision of universal health coverage.

5. To promote and support national capacity for high quality research and development for prevention and control of NCDs.

6. To monitor trends and determinants of NCDs and evaluate progress in their prevention and control.

The following five key recommendations are intended to reduce NCDs by countries and international agencies, and the approach is illustrated in Fig. (**11**).

1. **Leadership**: develop global and national leadership with high-level and sustained political commitments and supports. The aim is to reduce NCD death rates by 2% per year.

2. **Prevention**: choose the cost-effective interventions with a high impact on health and high feasibility to yield the greatest benefit. The Lancet Series [45-48] address five major risk factors targets including (1) smoking, (2) high dietary salt intake, (3) obesity, unhealthy diets and physical inactivity, (4) harmful alcohol intake, and (5) cardiovascular risk. The Interventions,

implementation costs, feasibility and WHO targets to deal with specific lifestyle risk factors are shown in Tables **3-6**.

3. **Treatment**: deliver cost-effective and affordable essential drugs and technologies for all priority disorders in primary health care across different levels of the health system.

4. **International Cooperation:** cooperate with all relevant multiple sectors and stakeholders to facilitate the actions and increase funding.

5. **Monitoring, reporting, and accountability**: regularly assess progress and report such commitments.

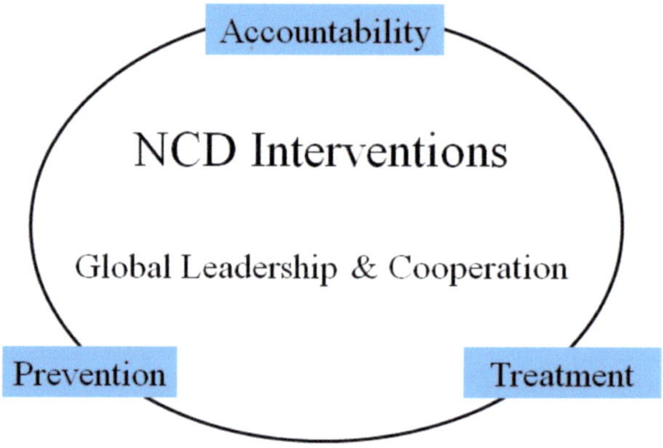

Fig. (11). Approach to non-communicable diseases interventions (WHO, adapted from ref. [5]).

These strategies appear clearly targeted toward the shared risk factors for the major four disease clusters, namely cardiovascular diseases, cancers, chronic pulmonary disease, and diabetes which are considered high priorities. They do not comprehensively cover every topic in global heath, but are a welcome starting point. And, in many ways these strategic interventions mimic the one taken by various agencies across the globe such as the Centers of Disease Control and Prevention (CDC), the National Institutes of Health (NIH) and the Food and Drug Administration (FDA) in the U.S., along with WHO, its many affiliates and several other international organizations to come up with a collective and strategic response to understand not only the biology of the disease, but also the prevention, disease surveillance and treatment of HIV-AIDs [50]. Those invaluable lessons learned from HIV-AIDs could and are being applied for risk

Table 3. Interventions, implementation costs, feasibility: WHO tobacco and alcohol targets [49] a. DALY is disability adjusted years of life.

Risk Factors (DALYs[a] in Millions; % of Global Burden)	Interventions [45, 47]	Implementation Costs	Feasibility	WHO Targets by 2025 [43]
Tobacco use (DALYs > 50 m; 3.7% global burden)	– Protect people from tobacco smoke – Warnings about the dangers of tobacco – Enforcing bans on advertising – Raise taxes on tobacco – Offer counseling to smokers	Very Low Quite Low	High Feasible (primary care)	A 30% relative reduction in prevalence of current tobacco use in persons aged 15+ years
Harmful use of alcohol (DALYs > 50 m; 4.5% global burden)	– Restrict access to retailed alcohol – Enforce advertising bans – Raise taxes on alcohol – Enforce drunk driving laws (breath tests) – Counseling services -	Very low Quite low	High Interventional (primary care)	At least a 10% relative reduction in the harmful use of alcohol, as appropriate, within the national context

Table 4. Interventions, implementation costs, feasibility: WHO physical inactivity targets [49]. Physical inactivity results in more than 30 million DALYs and 2.1% of global burden.

Interventions [46]	Implementation Costs	Feasibility	WHO targets by 2025 [43]
Public Service Announcements (PSAs), Mass media promoting physical activity	Very low cost	Highly feasible	– Halt in the rise in diabetes and obesity – A 10% relative reduction in prevalence of insufficient physical activity
Promote physical activity (Communities)	Not assessed globally	Inter-sectoral action	
Support active transport strategies	Not assessed globally	Inter-sectoral action	
Counseling-Primary care	Higher cost	Feasible-Primary care	
Work site promotions	Higher cost	Very feasible	
Physical activity in schools	Higher cost	Very feasible	

Table 5. Interventions, implementation costs, feasibility: WHO unhealthy diet targets [WHO, 49]. Unhealthy diets result in 15-30 million DALYs and represent 1-2% of global burden. [a]WHO's recommendation is less than 5 grams of salt or 2 grams of sodium per person per day.

Interventions [45, 46]	Implementation Costs	Feasibility	WHO Targets by 2025 [43]
• Replace trans fats with polyunsaturated Fats • Promote public awareness about healthy eating • Reduce salt intake	Very Low	High	– Halt in the rise in diabetes and obesity – A 30% relative reduction in mean population intake of salt/sodium intake[a]
• Replace saturated fat with unsaturated fats • Restrict marketing of unhealthy food and beverages to children • Manage food taxes and subsidies	Very low	High	
• Promote healthy eating in schools • Promote healthy eating at worksites	Very low Quite low	High High	
• Counseling-services - diet	Higher costs	Feasible	

Table 6. Interventions and WHO targets for cardiovascular risk reduction [43, 48].

Risk factor	Interventions [48]	WHO Targets by 2025 [43]
Cardiovascular risk	Combination of drugs for individuals at high risk of NCDs	– A 25% relative reduction in the prevalence of raised blood pressure or contain the prevalence of raised blood pressure according to national circumstances – At least 50% of eligible people receive drug therapy and counseling (including glycemic control) to prevent heart attacks and strokes. Essential Non-communicable disease medicines and basic technologies to treat major NCDs – An 80% availability of the affordable basic technologies and essential medicines, including generics, required to treat major NCDs in both public and private facilities.

factor mitigation, control and treatment of NCDs. Statistical modeling suggests that 44 to 76% reduction in coronary heart disease mortality can be explained by risk factor manipulation and another 23 to 47% from improvements in treatments and access to treatments [51].

21st CENTURY AMAZING OPPORTUNITIES

Over the last decade, policy makers globally were not totally convinced at the growing burden of NCDs. But, this has changed since WHO set the 2008-2013 action plan for NCDs' focused on 4 major NCDs (cardiovascular diseases, diabetes, cancer, and chronic pulmonary disease) and their 4 shared risk factors (tobacco use, physical inactivity, unhealthy diets, and alcohol abuse) on the global health agenda. Similarly, various United Nations agencies and other international organizations have now begun to recognize the importance of addressing NCDs at the global level and have joined the band wagon to set the prevention and control of NCDs as a health goal. The main goals are reductions of NCD-related premature deaths and health care costs.

In the midst of all the limits we see today when it comes to health care infrastructure [24], public financing and health insurance, there are ongoing health care related-interventions which when adopted on a large scale can prove to be cost-effective and realistic. One of the first nationwide diabetes "mHealth" initiatives in a developing country was launched at the 2011 Clinton Global Initiative (CGI) annual meeting in India, *via* an innovative collaboration between Arogya World, a non-profit organization and cellphone maker Nokia [52]. Using text messages in multiple languages, the partnership's principal aim has been to reach out people across rural and urban India to raise awareness about diabetes and its prevention. (See also CHAPTER 20, *From Technology to Innovation*). Similarly, another advanced mHealth system, Project UDAY, utilizes Decision Support Software applications that incorporate evidence-based medicine and management algorithms for physicians and other health care providers to screen, diagnose and formulate a treatment and management plan for the individual patient for both diabetes and hypertension across two states in India [53]. The evidence-based interventions for diabetes are shown in Table 7. Due to the fact that billions across the world now possess a mobile phone, several such mobile phone applications can be developed for frontline health care workers in many developing countries not just for screening, diagnosis and treatment but also for data collection, monitoring, and surveillance [52, 53].

Additionally, WHO has also developed the WHO Cardiovascular Risk management package that has indeed been found to be quite useful in the low and medium-resource settings [55]. Similarly, another excellent innovation that emerged from what was clearly a global collaboration with funding provided by

Table 7. Evidence-based interventions for diabetes [54].

Diabetes: Evidence-Based Interventions
• Lifestyle changes in all cases
• A1C test at least 2 times a year
• Lowering BP to < 140 / 80 mmHg
• Patients with diabetes and hypertension should receive a regimen that includes either an ACE inhibitor[a] or an angiotensin receptor blocker (ARB)
• LDL-cholesterol goal < 100 mg/dL if without overt CVD; < 70 if with overt CVD[b]
• Statin therapy, regardless of baseline lipid levels for all diabetic patients – with overt CVD or – without CVD who are over the age of 40 and have ≥ 1 one of other CVD risk factors
• Aspirin therapy (75-162 mg/day) as: – Primary prevention strategy in those with increased cardiovascular risk (10-year risk >10%) – Secondary prevention strategy in those with history of CVD
• Annual comprehensive eye exams
• Annual comprehensive foot examination

[a]ACE, angiotensin converting enzyme; [b]CVD, cardiovascular diseases.

the Gates Foundation came from India where utilizing visual inspection of the cervix following application of simple vinegar (acetic acid) was seen to be a more cost-effective alternative strategy to the standard cervical cytology screening (Pap smears) for the early detection of cervical cancer. This low-cost and simple method has now been shown to decrease the mortality from cervical cancer by nearly 30% at the population level. Experts predict that over 22,000 deaths in India and 72,600 deaths worldwide would be prevented as a result of this new method of screening [56-58]. Many such low-cost innovations could be easily shared across our inter-connected globe, helping countries cope with rising health care expenditures. With the constraints that many developing countries face when it comes to availability of trained medical specialists the most appropriate response that has worked very well, has been to train non-physicians such as community health worker and nurses to screen and manage common NCDs, such as hypertension and diabetes based on standard country-specific guidelines [59].

GRAND AMBITIONS LOOKING FORWARD

In their 2014 Gates Annual Letter, Bill & Melinda Gates make a bold prediction that by the year 2035, there will be almost no poor country left in the world and that over 70% of the countries globally will have a higher per-person income than China does today [60]. Having put their words and billions of dollars into action over the last several years across many parts of the globe, this prediction for the next twenty years is extremely timely and strategically importance. To put this in perspective, one has to look at the last twenty years where health gains and economic development have gone along hand in hand with the number of people living in low income countries down by over two-thirds between 1990 and 2010 and life expectancy up almost across the board. Engstrom *et al.* correctly argue that an additional US$5 (equivalent to just 2% increase over current levels) per person per year investment in 74 high-burden countries would yield up to 9 times more value in terms of economic and social benefits with gains in GDP growth, productivity, labor participation and higher savings [4]. Murphy and Topel [6] also argue that in a developed country such as the U.S., a 1% reduction in cancer mortality would be worth almost $500 billion to the U.S. economy. One can only imagine the world-wide benefits if this could be accomplished globally.

In a world where we went through a "Nutrition Transition", we are now facing a "Disease Transition" with more deaths and disability from non-communicable diseases, while we still fight off the perils of communicable diseases; especially tuberculosis, malaria and HIV/AIDs. Today, a billion people are either overweight or obese, and millions more suffer and die prematurely from malnutrition [61] a vast majority before the age of five. As we enter 2015, three countries; Nigeria, Afghanistan and Pakistan still prevent us from calling the world "poliomyelitis-free" [62]. And, although now largely regarded as a chronic illness thanks to the universal availability of potent retroviral agents, new cases of HIV/AIDs still occur across most parts of the globe. Furthermore, cardiovascular diseases, despite a marked decrease in morbidity and mortality still remain the number one cause of death and disability worldwide with huge numbers of new cases in low and middle-income countries. The rising incidence of diabetes, a major risk factor for cardiovascular diseases further threatens to negate most of the gains made in this arena. So, what then are we in the health care community to come up with, so as to put a dent in the increasing prevalence of NCDs and at the same time remain vigilant against the known and hitherto unknown communicable diseases that might strike at any time? As we read along the rest of the chapters which follow in sections one, two and three, we clearly see that this will require a huge commitment across many stake-holders with physicians leading the way at taking stewardship of the health care arena and working with public, private and non-profit organizations toward halting the progression of lifestyle diseases and promoting health and wellness globally. This crisis is too big of a threat to be left alone. We must take action now.

ADDITIONAL RESOURCES & LINKS

International Federation of Red Cross and Red Crescent Societies (IFRC). Noncommunicable diseases. http://www.ifrc.org/en/what-we-do/health/diseases/noncommunicable-disease/

Cause-specific mortality, 2008: WHO region by country. Geneva: World Health Organization, 2011. http://apps.who.int/gho/data/node.main.887?lang=en

Noncommunicable diseases. Geneva:World Health Organization, 2013. http://www.who.int/mediacentre/factsheets/fs355/en/

Health, United States, 2011: with special feature on socioeconomic status and health. Hyattsville, MD: National Center for Health Statistics, 2012. http://www.cdc.gov/nchs/data/hus/hus11.pdf

Charter for Healthy Living. A report from the World Economic Forum's Healthy Living Initiative: Prepared in collaboration with Bain & Company http://www3.weforum.org/docs/WEF_HE_HealthyLiving_Charter_2013.pdf

Bloom DE, Cafiero ET, Jané-Llopis E, *et al.* The global economic burden of noncommunicable diseases. Geneva: World Economic Forum 2011

http://www.weforum.org/reports/global-economicburden-non-communicable-diseases

The world medicines situation report. Geneva:World Health Organization,2011. http://www.who.int/medicines/areas/policy/world_medicines_situation/en

WHO. Action plan of the global strategy for the prevention and control of non-communicable diseases 2013-2020: http://www.iogt.org/wp-content/uploads/2013/03/IOGTInt-Response-draftGAP-Feb2013.pdf

ACKNOWLEDGEMENTS

Declared none.

CONFLICT OF INTEREST

The authors confirm that this chapter contents have no conflict of interest.

REFERENCES

[1] Murray CJL, Lopez AD. Measuring the global burden of disease. N Engl J Med 2013; 369(5): 448-57.

[2] Murray CJL, Vos T, Lozano R, *et al.* Disability-adjusted life years (DALYs) for 291 diseases and injuries in 21 regions,1990-2010:a systematic analysis for the Global Burden of Disease Study 2010. Lancet 2012; 380: 2197-223.

[3] Rosenbaum L, Lamas D. Facing a "slow motion disaster"-The UN meeting on non-communicable diseases. N Engl J Med 2011; 365(25): 2345-8.

[4] Engstrom H, Khin PT, Coll-Seck A *et al.* Reinvesting in health post-2015. Lancet 2013; 382:1861-4.

[5] U.S. Census Bureau, Population Division, 2011. [Cited February 17, 2014]. Available from http://www.census.gov/population/socdemo/statbriefs/agebrief.html

[6] Murphy KM, Topel RH. The value of health and longevity. J of Political Economy. 2006; 114(5): 871-904

[7] Dawn of a New Era: The first person to reach 150 is already alive...and soon we'll live to be a thousand, claims scientist. Mail online [newspaper online]. 2011 July 6 [cited 2014 Feb 15]. Available from: http://www.dailymail.co.uk/sciencetech/article-2011425/The-person-reach-150-alive--soon-live-THOUSAND-claims-scientist.html

[8] Greens B. Would you want to live to 150? CNN Global News View [newspaper online]. 2013 Jun 23 [cited 2014 Feb 22]. Available from: http://edition.cnn.com/2013/06/23/opinion/greene-living-to-150/

[9] Fineberg H, Hunter D. A global view of health-an unfolding series. N Engl J Med 2013; 368(1):78-79

[10] Institute of Medicine, Committee on the U.S. Commitment to Global Health. The U.S. commitment to global health: recommendations for the public and private sectors. Washington DC: National Academics Press, May 2009.

[11] BusinessDictionary.com [homepage on the Internet]. No date [cited 2013 July 30]. Available from: http://www.businessdictionary.com/definition/lifestyle.html

[12] Merriam-Webster [homepage on the Internet]. c2013 [cited 2013 July 13]. Available from http://www.merriamwebster.com/dictionary/lifestyle

[13] Case A, Lubotsky D, Paxson C. Economic status and health in childhood: the origins of the gradient. The American Economic Review. 2002;92(5):1308-34.

[14] Khanam R, Nghiem HS, Connelly LB. Child health and the income gradient: evidence from Australia. J Health Econ 2009; 28(4): 805-17.

[15] Ponthiere G. Mortality, family and lifestyles. Journal of Family and Economic. 2011;32(2):175-90.

[16] BusinessDictionary.com [homepage on the Internet]. No date [cited 2013 July 30]. Available from: http://www.businessdictionary.com/definition/psychographics.html

[17] WHO. 2008-2013 Action plan of the global strategy for the prevention and control of noncommunicable diseases. [homepage on the Internet]. No date [cited 2013 July 27]. Available from: http://whqlibdoc.who.int/publications/2009/9789241597418_eng.pdf

[18] WHO fact sheet. Noncommunicable diseases. [homepage on the Internet]. c2013 [updated 2013 March; cited 2013 July 26]. Available from: http://www.who.int/mediacentre/factsheets/fs355/en/

[19] International Federation of Red Cross and Red Crescent Societies (IFRC). Noncommunicable diseases. [homepage on the Internet]. No date [cited 2013 July 27]. Available from: http://www.ifrc.org/en/what-we-do/health/diseases/noncommunicable-disease/

[20] Mathers CD, Loncar D. Projections of global mortality and burden of disease from 2002 to 2030. PLoS Med. 2006;3(11):e442.

[21] Lozano R, Naghavi M, Foreman K, *et al.* Global and regional mortality from 235 causes of death for 20 age groups in 1990 and 2010: a systematic analysis for the Global Burden of Disease Study 2010. Lancet 2012; 380: 2095-128.

[22] Cause-specific mortality, 2008: WHO region by country. Geneva: World Health Organization, 2011. [Cited February 20, 2014]. Available from: http://apps.who.int/gho/data/node.main.887?lang=en

[23] WHO. Data and statistics [homepage on the Internet]. c2013. [cited 2013 July 27]. Available from: http://www.who.int/research/en/

[24] Hunter DJ, Reddy KS, Noncommunicable diseases, N Engl J Med 2013;369(14):1336-43.

[25] Geneau R, Stuckler D, Stachenko S, *et al.* Raising the priority of preventing chronic diseases: a political process. Lancet 2010;376: 1689-98.

[26] Beaglehole R, Bonita R, Horton R, *et al.* Priority actions for the non-communicable disease crisis. Lancet 2011; 377: 1438-47.

[27] International Federation of Red Cross and Red Crescent Societies (IFRC). Community-based prevention of noncommunicable diseases: Key messages. [homepage on the Internet]. No date [cited 2013 July 27]. Available from: http://www.ifrc.org/en/what-we-do/health/diseases/noncommunicable-disease/community-based-prevention-of-non-communicable-diseases---key-messages/

[28] Latham KE, Sapienza C, Engel N. The epigenetic lorax: gene–environment interactions in human health http://www.ncbi.nlm.nih.gov/pmc/articles/PMC3471221/pdf/nihms-406065.pdf

[29] Ezzati M, Riboli E. Behavioral and dietary risk factors for noncommunicable diseases. N Engl J Med, 2013;369(10):954-64.

[30] Health initiatives in poor countries: what can we learn from them? BMJ 2004;328:894.

[31] Noncommunicable diseases. Geneva:World Health Organization, 2013. [Cited February 17, 2014]. Available from: http://www.who.int/mediacentre/factsheets/fs355/en/

[32] Health, United States, 2011: with special feature on socioeconomic status and health. Hyattsville, MD: National Center for Health Statistics, 2012. [Cited February 18, 2014]. Available from: http://www.cdc.gov/nchs/data/hus/hus11.pdf

[33] Centers for Medicare and Medicaid Services, Office of the Actuary, National Health Statistics Group, National Health Care Expenditures Data, January 2012.

[34] Martin AB, Lassman D, Washington B, Catlin A and the National Health Expenditure Accounts Team. Growth In US Health Spending Remained Slow In 2010: Health Share Of Gross Domestic Product Was Unchanged From 2009. Health Aff 2012;31(1): 208-19.

[35] Centers for Disease Control and Prevention. Rising health care costs are unsustainable. April 2011.

[36] Charter for Healthy Living. A report from the World Economic Forum's Healthy Living Initiative: Prepared in collaboration with Bain & Company [homepage on the Internet]. c2013 [cited 2013 July 28]. Available from: http://www3.weforum.org/docs/WEF_HE_HealthyLiving_Charter_2013.pdf

[37] Bloom DE, Cafiero ET, Jané-Llopis E, *et al.* The global economic burden of noncommunicable diseases. Geneva: World Economic Forum, 2011. [Cited July 28, 2013]. Available from: http://www.weforum.org/reports/global-economicburden-non-communicable-diseases

[38] The evidence of health promotion effectiveness. Shaping public health in a new Europe. A report for the European Commission by the International Union for Health Promotion and Education 2002.

[39] World Health Report 2008. Primary health care-now more than ever. World Health Organisation, Geneva.

[40] Harper T, Oldenburg B. Call for a national charter for health. Issue paper, February 2009.

[41] McQueen DV, Jones CM, editors. Global perspective on health promotion effectiveness. International union for health promotion and education. Springer, New York; 2007.

[42] The world medicines situation report. Geneva:World Health Organization,2011. [Cited June 30, 2013]. Available form: http://www.who.int/medicines/areas/policy/world_medicines_situation/en

[43] WHO. Action plan of the global strategy for the prevention and control of noncommunicable diseases 2013-2020: revised draft [homepage on the Internet]. Updated 2013 February 11; cited 2013 August 1. Available from: http://www.iogt.org/wp-content/uploads/2013/03/IOGTInt-Response-draftGAP-Feb2013.pdf

[44] Hogerzeil HV. Big pharma and social responsibility-the access to Medicine Index. N Engl J Med 2013; 369(10):896-9.

[45] Asaria P, Chisholm D, Mathers C, Ezzati M, Beaglehole R. Chronic disease prevention: health effects and financial costs of strategies to reduce salt intake and control tobacco use. Lancet 2007; 70: 2044-53.

[46] Cecchini M, Sassi F, Lauer JA, *et al.* Tackling of unhealthy diets, physical inactivity, and obesity: health effects and cost-effectiveness. Lancet 2010; 376:1775-84.

[47] Anderson P, Chisholm D, Fuhr D. Effectiveness and cost-effectiveness of policies and programmes to reduce the harm caused by alcohol. Lancet 2009; 373:2234-46.

[48] Lim SS, Gaziano TA, Gakidou E, *et al*. Prevention of cardiovascular disease in high-risk individuals in low-income and middle-income countries: health effects and costs. Lancet 2007; 370: 2054-62.

[49] World Health Organization. CHOosing Interventions that are Cost Effective (WHO-CHOICE) [homepage on the internet]. c2014 [cited 2014 Feb 28]. Available from: www.who.int/choice

[50] Narayan KMV, Ali, MK, Del Rio C, Koplan JP. Global Noncommunicable Diseases-Lessons from the HIV-AIDS Experience. N Engl J Med 2011; 365(10): 876-78.

[51] Habib SH, Saha S. Burden of non-communicable disease: global overview. Diabetes & Metabolic Syndrome: Clinical Research & Reviews 2010;4:41-7.

[52] Arogya World. Arogya world launches new diabetes prevention mHealth program in India with Nokia Life Tools [homepage on the internet]. c2011 [updated 2011 Sep 20; cited 2014 Feb 24]. Available from: http://www.arogyaworld.org/arogya-world-launches-new-diabetes-prevention-mhealth-program-in-india-with-nokia-life-tools/

[53] Improving prevention, treatment and management of diabetes in India. Impact global health news and commentary [serial online] 2013 Nov 14 [cited 2014 Feb 24]. Available from: http://blog.psiimpact.com/2013/11/improving-prevention-treatment-management-diabetes-india/

[54] American Diabetic Association. Standards of medical care in diabetes-2014. Diabetes care. Diabetes Care 2014;37(1):s14-80.

[55] Cardiovascular risk programme. WHO Cardiovascular Risk management package for low- and medium-resource settings. World Health Organization, Geneva, 2002. Printed in France. Available from: http://whqlibdoc.who.int/publications/2002/9241545852.pdf

[56] Jeronimo J, Bansil P, Lim J, *et al*. A multicountry evaluation of care HPV testing, visual inspection with acetic acid, and Papanicolaou testing for the detection of cervical cancer. Int J Gynecol Cancer 2014; 24(3):576-85.

[57] Qiao YL, Sellors JW, Eder PS, *et al*. A new HPV-DNA test for cervical-cancer screening in developing regions: a cross-sectional study of clinical accuracy in rural China. Lancet Oncol 2008; 9(10):929-36.

[58] Narayan KMV, Ali MK, Koplan JP. Global Noncommunicable Diseases-Where Worlds Meet. N Engl J Med 2010; 363(13): 1196-98.

[59] Mills A. Health Care Systems in Low- and Middle-Income Countries. N Engl J Med 2014; 370(6): 552-57.

[60] Bill & Melinda Gates foundation. 3 Myths that block progress for the poor. Annual letter 2014 [document on the internet]. No date [cited 2014 February 18]. Available from: http://annualletter.gatesfoundation.org/~/media/Annual%20Letter%202014/PDFs/2014_GatesAnnualLetter_ENGLISH_1.pdf

[61] Tejavanija S, Jhangiani S. Nutritional evaluation: a paradigm shift in the twenty-first century. In Segal I, Pitchumoni CS, Sung J (Eds.), Gastroenterology and Hepatology Manual: a clinician's guide to global phenomenon. McGraw Hill Australia Pty Ltd; 2011; p. 242-56.

[62] Mundel T, Orenstein W. No country is safe without global eradication of poliomyelitis. N Engl J Med. 2013; 369(21): 2045-6.

CHAPTER 2

Overweight and Obesity: It All Starts Here

Lindy Fenlason[*,1] **and Doug Heimburger**[2]

[1]*Division of General Pediatrics, Vanderbilt Children's Hospital, Nashville, TN, USA; and* [2]*Vanderbilt Institute for Global Health, Nashville, TN, USA*

Abstract: The prevalence of obesity has markedly increased worldwide. We confront it daily: in our social interactions, in our work, everywhere we turn. It is an issue that has significant effects on our health as reinforced by the ruling of the American Medical Association in June of 2013 to classify obesity as a disease. Although it is essential to address this condition, it is extremely intimidating and difficult to manage due to its multifactorial causation, potential for comorbidities, associated stigma, and the need for lifestyle change- never easy to recommend or to do. This chapter will provide an overview: the What, Who, Why, and How of obesity etiology and management. Our goal is to provide the reader with a basic understanding and tools to enable him/her to participate in addressing this critical public health issue.

Keywords: Activity, behavior, BMI, body mass index, comorbidities, diet, global health, health status, lifestyle modification, metabolism, motivational interviewing, noncommunicable disease, nutrition transition, nutrition, obesity, overweight, risk.

INTRODUCTION

Obesity has multifactorial causation and is associated with health and social co-morbidities. Yet an increasing proportion of the population worldwide is overweight and at high risk for becoming obese. Approaching obesity from a public health perspective poses a challenge, but the clinical capacity for addressing the associated co-morbidities is limited. This chapter will provide an overview: the What, Who, Why, and How of obesity etiology and management. Having a basic understanding of obesity helps health professionals and the broader community address the assessment and treatment issues while minimizing the stigma associated with obesity.

***Corresponding author Lindy Fenlason:** Monroe Carell Jr. Children's Hospital at Vanderbilt, 2200 Children's Way, DOT 8241, Nashville, TN 37232, USA; Tel: (615) 936-2425; Fax: (615) 343-7650; E-mail: lindy.fenlason@vanderbilt.edu

Judith Wylie-Rosett & Sunil S. Jhangiani (Eds)

WHAT IS IT?

What is the significance of "overweight" or "obesity"? Are these just subjective classifications or are these terms having significant meaning? Overweight and obesity are most often defined by a calculated Body Mass Index (or weight-for-length percentile in those under two years of age), which incorporates both height and weight. It is not a perfect measure of body fat, but is highly correlated and feasible in clinical settings. Tables **1** and **2** present the BMI chart from the Centers for Disease Control and Prevention (CDC) [1, 2] and the World Health Organization (WHO) [3] respectively. Of note, WHO has proposed additional cutoff points of for public health action and has subsequently recommended lower clinical BMI cutoff points of particular Asian populations due to higher risk of certain comorbidities at lower BMI levels in these demographics. Similar changes have been proposed for other ethnicities as well [4].

Table 1. Centers for disease control and prevention Body Mass Index (kg/m^2) classifications.

Weight Status	Children	Adults
Underweight	<5th percentile	<18.5
Healthy weight	5th -84th percentile	18.5-24.9
Overweight	85th-94th percentile	25-29.9
Obese	> 95th percentile	>30.0
Severely Obese	>99th percentile	>40.0

WHO IS AFFECTED?

The Scope

In the last three decades, the world has seen a dramatic rise in rates of overweight and obesity across all age ranges. The United Stated has led to the rise. According to data from the National Health and Nutrition Examination Survey (NHANES) over one-third (37.5%) of U.S. adults are obese, and an additional one-third are overweight. One third of children and adolescents are overweight or obese, with a majority of these (total 17%) classifying as obese. In fact, one-third of U.S. children are overweight before they reach 5 years of age [5, 6].

Table 2. World Health Organization Body Mass Index (kg/m^2) classifications.

Weight Status	Principal Cut-Off Points	Additional Cut-Off Points
Underweight	*<18.50*	*<18.5*
Severe thinness	<16.00	<16.00
Moderate Thinness	16.00-16.99	16.00-16.99
Mild Thinness	17.00-18.49	17.00-18.49
Normal Range	*18.50-24.99*	*18.5-22.99*
		23.00-24.99
Overweight	*>25.00*	*>25.00*
Pre-obese	25.99-29.99	25.00-27.49
		27.50-29.99
Obese	*> 30.00*	*>30.00*
Obese Class 1	30.00-34.99	30.00-32.49
		32.50-34.99
Obese Class II	35.00-39.99	35.00-37.49
		37.50-39.99
Obese Class III	>40.00	>40.00

Yet, this situation is not unique to the United States. Prevalence of overweight and obesity has also been rising in low and middle-income countries. These settings, which were previously marked only by undernutrition, are experiencing a "Nutrition Transition" as rates of undernutrition are decreasing and rates of obesity are increasing [7, 8]. Indeed, there is a global spectrum of poor nutrition involving both under- and over-nutrition, at times even within the same household [9]. There are an estimated 868 million undernourished people in the world, and globally there are over 1.4 billion adults who are overweight or obese, and over 40 million children [10]. Among these children, more than 35 million reside in developing countries (Fig. **1**) [7].

Disparities

In an attempt to evaluate for disparities in this epidemic, researchers have examined variables such as age, gender, ethnicity, socioeconomic status, educational level, and urban *versus* rural, but it is difficult to find consistent

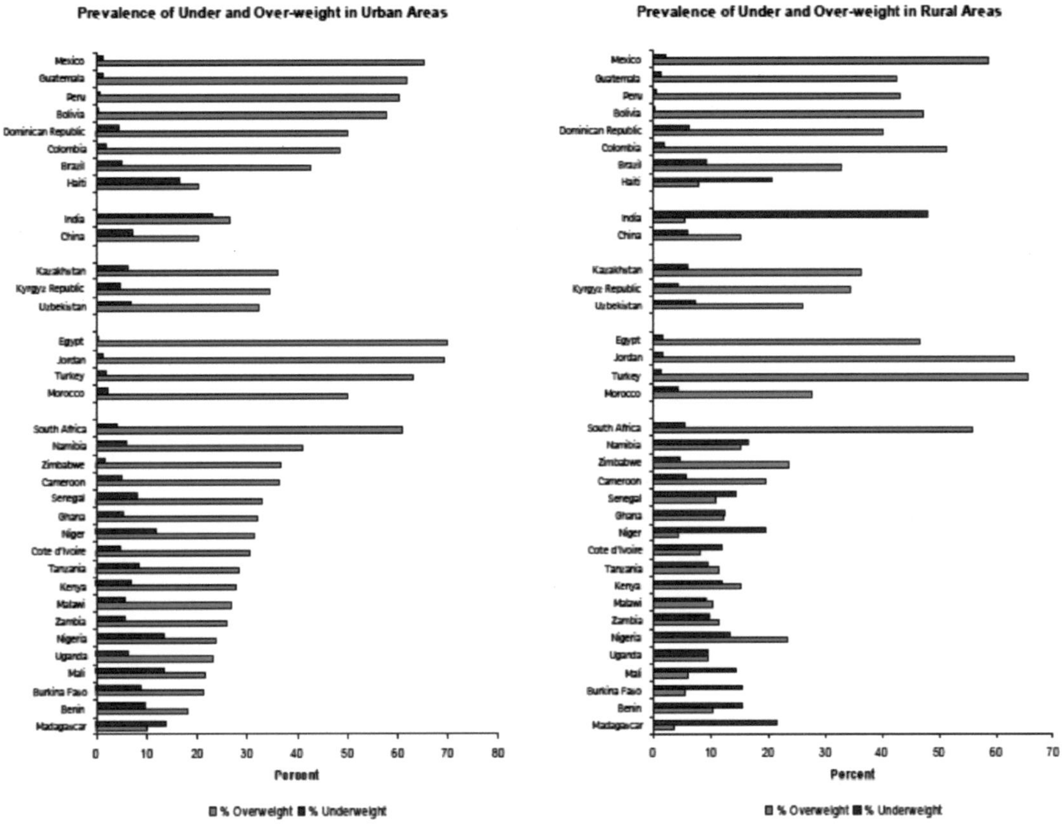

Fig. (1). Prevalence of overweight and underweight [7].

correlations. For example, data from the United States National Center for Health Statistics http://www.cdc.gov/nchs/data/databriefs/db131.htm show that obesity is increasing across all income levels; the increase appears to be greater in lower socioeconomic groups, but not across all ethnicities. Higher educational levels also seem to have some protective effects. Obesity rates are inversely correlated with the educational levels of the heads of households, but again, not across all ethnicities [11, 12]. Studies have also been done to evaluate overall global trends and trends in high-income *versus* low- and middle-income countries. Again, some trends can be seen but data are imperfect and results are inconsistent. It is clear that while there may be subtle variations, obesity appears to be rising in all populations [8]. Moreover, it is also clear that complex systems of individual and societal factors influence risk for developing obesity.

WHY: WHY IS OBESITY AN IMPORTANT ISSUE?

Comorbidities

Individuals with obesity are at high risk for physical and social repercussions. This excess weight affects every body system, increasing morbidity and mortality, and placing one at risk for severe and chronic diseases and diminished quality of life. Obesity is a major risk factor for noncommunicable diseases (NCDs); while it is not seen as an NCD in its own right, obesity contributes to the NCD burden. Globally, 44% of diabetes, 23% of cardiovascular diseases (23%), and 7-41% of particular cancers can be attributed to obesity [13]. Abdominal or central obesity in particular is associated with increased morbidity and mortality. The 2012 World Health Organization (WHO) Global Status Report on NCDs found that annually 2.8 million lives are lost as a consequence of overweight and obesity. This risk for NCDs can even be seen in childhood. In one study, 70% of obese children had at least one cardiovascular disease risk factor, and 39% had two or more. Data also indicate that not only the prevalence of obesity is increasing, but the degree of obesity is increasing as well. More people are becoming obese, and they are becoming more obese [5, 6, 11]. Ludwig noted that this may be the first generation of children who have shorter lifespans than their parents as a result of the consequences of overweight and type 2 diabetes [14].

Additional Costs

Beyond the immediate physical effects, obesity carries additional costs, which play out at individual and societal level. These costs may be direct (medical) or indirect (non-medical). Direct costs refer to obesity-related evaluations and treatments, and health insurance coverage. These costs are rising due to the frequency and severity of illness and higher insurance premiums for persons with obesity. Forecasting models have predicted that by 2030, over 50% of the US population will be obese, leading to additional medical costs of nearly $550 billion [15]. Indirect costs include absenteeism (loss of work time), presenteeism (loss of work productivity), worker's compensation, disability, and premature mortality [16]. These costs are also rising, placing added pressure on the global economy.

WHY: WHY IS IT HAPPENING?

Etiology

At its core, the cause of obesity is quite simple: positive energy balance in an individual over time. However, the interplay of contributing factors is complex.

Many frameworks have been designed in attempts to explain these factors; Figs. (**2** and **3**) depict two of them. Each model provides a slightly different way of looking at the issue, but in its most basic form it involves three levels of influence: 1) biological, 2) environmental/societal, and 3) behavioral. Our environment acts on us through our circumstances, and we act on our environment based on our genetics and choices.

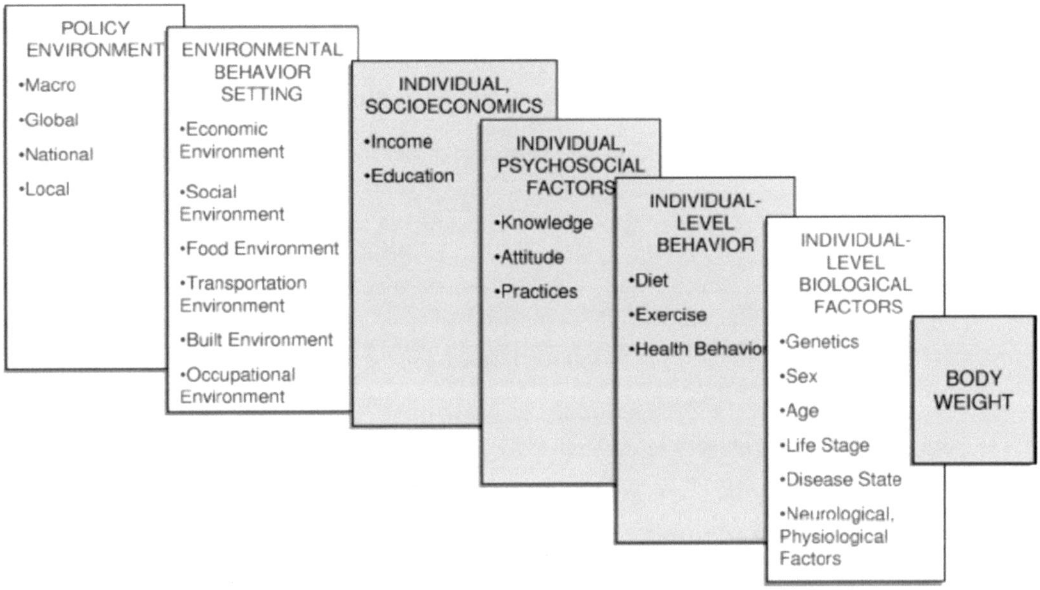

Fig. (2). Systems and environments underlying obesity [17].

Biological (Endogenous) Factors

The human body has systems of absorption, metabolism, and signaling pathways in place to maintain energy balance (energy intake and energy expenditure). These can be altered by genetics, epigenetics, medical conditions, medication usage, *etc.* or overridden by our behaviors (in the case of obesity: excess energy intake and decreased energy expenditure).

Metabolism

The body's metabolism comprises of three major components (see Fig. **4**): basal metabolic rate (energy need for normal body functions at rest), thermic effect of food (energy needed to process food), and activity-related thermogenesis (energy

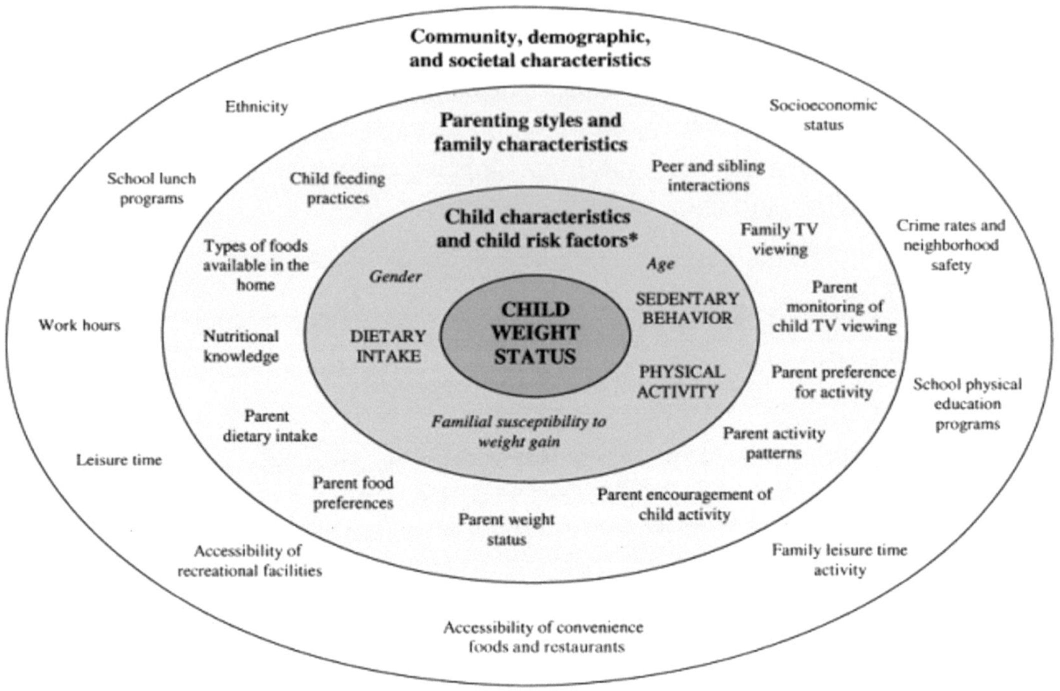

Fig. (3). Factors influencing obesity in children [18].

expended through specific exercise and non-exercise daily activities). These components determine how much daily energy an individual needs for ideal body functioning. Calorie intake above what is required results in positive energy balance and a tendency to store body fat. The question is often raised: Does the metabolism of obese individuals differ from that of healthy-weight individuals? Basal metabolic rate differs by amount of lean body mass, gender, ethnicity and age, but it is unclear if there is a genetic anomaly in obese individuals. In fact, energy expenditure increases in obese individuals, who have greater lean body mass as well as fat mass, and therefore require more energy for the same activities than do lower-weight individuals [19].

Neuroendocrine Signaling Pathways

A complex network of signaling pathways exists in the body and acts on the brain (primarily hypothalamus) to help direct the body to meet its energy balance. These signals act in three main ways: adipose tissue feedback, satiety, and reward. Examples include the following: Leptin is produced by body fat in proportion to the adipose tissue mass. It acts on receptors in the hypothalamus to discourage

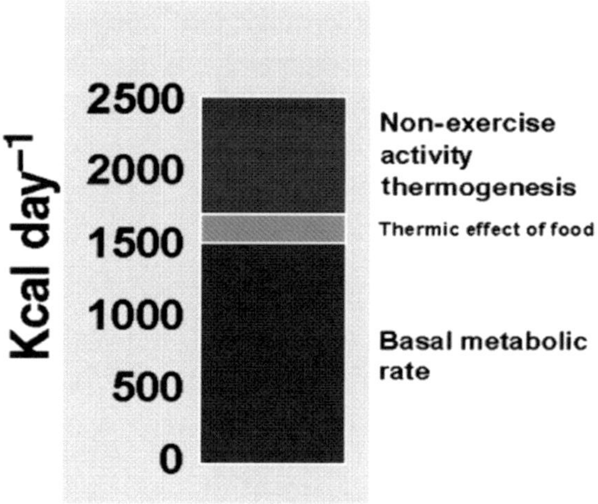

Fig. (4). Components of total daily energy expenditure in a free-living sedentary adult [19].

further food intake and encourage breakdown of stores for energy use. Ghrelin, on the other hand, promotes food intake. It is produced by the stomach and is increased during fasting and decreased with meals. The dopaminergic pathways in the brain also influence food intake, encouraging food intake by acting on centers that influence the emotions, memories and reward of food intake [20].

Genetics

While the obesity epidemic cannot be entirely explained by a genetic shift in the population, research has clearly demonstrated that genetics plays a role through effects on signaling, metabolism, and behavior [21-24]. This is a growing area of research, and as newer techniques are being used, more information is being generated. The role of genetics in obesity, particularly severe obesity, is apparent. Family, adoption, and twin studies have demonstrated that up to 45-75% of inter-individual differences in BMI can be explained by heredity [22].

Single Gene Mutations

It is accepted that only 5% of obesity can be attributed to single-gene mutations. Investigations into the signaling pathways have identified mutations that affect the mediators, which influence hunger and satiety. Leptin was one of the first mediators whose gene was identified, and mutations involving the leptin gene have since been explored in depth [21]. One of these, the MC4R mutation [22] is thought to be the most common obesity-related single gene mutation. MC4R influences leptin's regulation of food intake and body weight, and disruption of the MC4R gene in mice leads to increased energy intake and severe obesity. Multiple mutations in the human MC4R gene are associated with obesity and related traits [21].

Genetic Syndromes

There are multiple syndromes that involve obesity as a manifestation (see Table **3**). Prader-Willi syndrome, one of the most well known, is characterized by poor feeding and failure to thrive in the first 1-2 years of life followed by hyperphagia with consequent obesity by early childhood.

Genome-Wide Association Studies (GWAS)

A more recent advance in research technology, GWAS allows for large-scale exploratory studies of single nucleotide polymorphisms (SNPs) and traits associated with obesity. GWAS has identified many potential genetic loci, among which the strongest is the fat mass and obesity-associated (FTO) gene [21]. Most studies have been done in populations of European origin, so further research will determine clinical applicability and relevance to non-white populations [22].

Epigenetics

While genetics is the study of changes in the DNA sequence, epigenetics is the study of factors that do not alter the underlying DNA, but modulate the expression of the genes. A key example pertaining to obesity epidemic is the theory of "thrifty genes" or "fetal programming". There is an evidence that the nutritional environment during fetal growth can affect the expression of genes, resulting in structural and physiological changes in metabolism. Thus, a fetus that develops in an undernourished mother during a time of famine may develop the ability to store energy more efficiently. While enabling survival in times of food scarcity, this becomes problematic when these individuals food is abundant. This ability to hoard energy puts them at higher risk for obesity [23, 24].

MEDICAL CONDITIONS AND TREATMENTS

Other medical conditions and treatments affect our metabolic balance and risk for adiposity (Table **3**).

Table 3. Genetic and medical contributors to obesity [21-26].

Medical Conditions	
Syndromes: Single Gene Mutations	*Other*
• Prader-Willi • Alstrom • Bardet-Biedl • Borjeson-Forssman-Lehmann • Carpenter • Cohen • Prohormone Convertase • Beckwith-Wiedemann • Nesidioblastosis • Pseudohypoparathyroidism (Type 1A) • Leptin deficiency	• Hypothyroidism • Hypopituitarism • Polycystic Ovarian Syndrome • Castration or Ovarian Failure • Insulinoma • Hypothalamic lesion- trauma, cancer • Depression • Anxiety
Medications	
Anti-depressants Anti-psychotics Anti-seizure medications Diabetes medications Steroids Beta-blockers	

Societal/Environmental (Exogenous) Factors

Our environments have the potential to predispose us to obesity. Policies, trends, and the people around us affect our food and physical activity environments, influencing our options and perceptions of what is normal and desirable. There is a controversy regarding which of these aspects is the most responsible for the obesity epidemic but there is an agreement that changes in environmental factors have occurred and the majority of the world's population now finds itself living in an "obesogenic" environment [8]. Policy changes range from government subsidies for certain crops like corn and soy and foreign direct investments to city planning to budget allocation for physical and nutritional education in schools (Table **4**) [27].

The Physical Activity Environment

Multiple changes have taken place worldwide which make a less physically active life readily available and commonplace. The community and "built environment"

Table 4. Environmental influencers of obesity.

Large-Scale Societal Policies and Trends		
Policy examples	▪ Crop subsidies ▪ City planning ▪ Physical and nutrition education ▪ Food availability	▪ Incentives to grow corn and soy ▪ "suburban sprawl", trends towards "unwalkable" cities that require motorized transport ▪ Budget cuts that limit time and teaching for physical activity, nutrition and health ▪ Contracts with food companies for unhealthy vending machines in schools
Trends	Technology Globalization Urbanization	▪ Food processing, resulting in less nutritious food options ▪ Mechanization that decreases manual labor needs ▪ Media: global advertising of food products; availability of "screens" (tv, computers, video games, *etc.*) ▪ Global export of food products, food chains and media. Rise in foreign direct investment and transnational food companies ▪ Move to rural to urban settings
Community and Family Influences		
People	Cultural Social Networks/Family	▪ Traditions around food and activity; perceptions of healthy weight ▪ Support, weight of those in social circle
Additional	Socioeconomic status Time Stress	▪ Financial access to food and activity. Food Insecurity. ▪ Time to prioritize food and activity ▪ Effect on eating behaviors and body response

of one's city and neighborhood has changed. Rural, walkable communities with ready access to safe recreational space have been replaced by trends of "urbanization" and "suburban sprawl". More of the world's population is moving to urban and peri-urban areas, which are characterized by reliance on motorized transport and less access to safe recreation. Changes in physical activity levels are also seen in our work and schools, where much of the population spends a majority of its time. Due to advances in technology and mechanization, jobs involving strenuous manual labor have become a rarity, being replaced by employment that requires very little physical effort. In schools, funding and time for physical education courses have been drastically reduced. Due to these and other changes, little physical activity is demanded in homes, work and school. Instead, sedentary behaviors are promoted through the means mentioned above as well as the ready access to screens: television, video games, cellular telephones, computers, *etc*. The influence of family, friends and culture also directs physical activity levels. Factors such as time, financial access, social support, *etc*. can promote or deter physical activity levels [7].

The Food Environment

The above environmental changes have promoted an obesogenic food environment. With the help of advancing technology and subsidies, the world is producing more food per capita, much of which is highly processed and less nutritious (energy-dense but nutrient-poor), but has a longer shelf-life and is less expensive. Shifts towards urbanization have decreased reliance on home/locally-grown fresh foods. Instead, trends such as globalizations, foreign direct investments, transnational food companies, rise in food retailers and chains have increased access to processed foods worldwide. Food industry marketing promotes its benefits and availability, should one forget. Just as with physical activity, family, friends and culture also influence dietary habits and feeding practice through parental modeling, accepted traditional foods, cultural beliefs on breastfeeding, *etc*. [7].

Behavioral Issues

As seen above, there are many biological and environmental factors that can influence one's predisposition towards obesity. All of these factors are influential: body signaling, genetics, culture, social circles, finances, access, time, sleep routines, disordered eating habits, supervision, boredom, knowledge, understanding, support, *etc*. Yet the elements of individual behavior, motivation, and choice cannot be ignored. We must be cognizant of these factors when we consider how to approach obesity.

HOW DO WE APPROACH IT?

In The Clinic: Assessment

Anthropometrics

Clinical assessment of the obese patients begins with identifying the presence and degree of the condition, and its associated risk factors. Patient assessments should include body mass index (BMI), which calculated as body weight (kg)/height (m^2). It is an imperfect measure, but it serves as a valuable test for screening and follow-up because it is predictive of health risk and it is easily performed in the clinical setting. BMI classifications are based on a score or percentile (Tables **1** and **2**). In children greater than two years of age, it is based on a BMI percentile. Waist circumference is another measure of adiposity, particularly central adiposity. A waist circumference of > 40 inches in males or > 35 inches in females is associated with a greater risk of diabetes and cardiovascular disease. As with BMI, lower cutoffs have been recommended in Asian populations [4]. In children, waist circumference has not been shown to be a reliable predictor and is not recommended as a screening measure. Bioimpedance analysis (BIA), which estimates body fat *vs* lean mass, can also be easily performed in the clinic with modestly priced tools. There are more precise measures of adiposity such as dual energy x-ray absorptiometry (DEXA), computed tomography (CT), magnetic resonance imaging (MRI), and deuterium labeled water, but these measures require more elaborate technology and training and are not feasible in the typical clinical setting, particularly in under-resourced settings [28, 29].

History: Heritage, Birth, Medical, Family, and Social

A thorough history is also necessary to evaluate for potential causes of the excess weight, to identify factors that might put an individual at risk for co-morbid conditions (discussed in the following section), and to assess readiness for change. The questions asked in this portion of the evaluation should address the patient's ethnicity, birth and early feeding history (in children), past medical conditions and treatments, weight trends, social, environmental and behavioral dynamics (sleep, emotional eating, *etc.*) and presence of obesity and other medical conditions in family members [25-33]. A family history of obesity and related traits may provide clues to the relevance of genetic factors in particular cases of obesity. Ethnic heritage is important as hinted earlier due to the higher prevalence of comorbidities in certain people groups such as those of Asian or Hispanic heritage [4, 30, 31]. Maternal history can provide useful information as well and should include the following: gestational weight gain, gestational diabetes, smoking, stress, depression, *etc.* [32].

Physical Examination

The physical examination also provides important information about potential causation and risk for comorbidities. Certain physical features can indicate conditions such as genetic syndromes, endocrine dysfunction, dyslipidemias, cardiovascular abnormalities, *etc.* (Table **5**).

Table 5. Obesity-specific physical exam.

Anthropometrics	Weight and Height, waist circumference
Vital Signs	Routine: Blood pressure, heart rate, respiratory rate
General	Syndromic features, abnormal facies
Head, Eyes, Ears, Nose, and Throat (HEENT)	Cranial nerves, tonsillar hypertrophy, goiter, nodules
Cardiovascular	Bruits, murmurs, edema, right ventricular heave
Respiratory	Wheezing, effusions, increased work of breathing
Abdominal	Hepatomegaly, tenderness to palpation
Reproductive	Tanner stage
Musculoskeletal	Pain, structure and function; range of motion, gait, flat feet
Skin	Acanthosis nigricans, striae, hirsuitism, acne, xanthomas
Fat distribution	Central, moon facies, dorsocervical fat pad
Psychiatric	Affect

Laboratory Assessment

History and physical examination are crucial in the assessment of obese patients, but cannot detect all abnormalities. Laboratory testing and other assessments add further information that clarifies a patient's degree of risk and best treatment strategies. Serum tests such as fasting glucose, HgbA1C, insulin, lipid panel, and liver enzymes (AST, ALT) can serve as screening tests. Vitamin D levels, thyroid studies, and the patient's age, BMI, history, physical exam, and results of screening tests should guide additional evaluations [28, 29].

Attitudes and Readiness

Lifestyle modification begins with the assessment of attitude, readiness, barriers and support. Individuals who are ready to make change and have the support of family and friends are more likely to achieve initial and sustained success. Directed questions and specific techniques such as motivational interviewing can help in this assessment. Motivational interviewing differs from a traditional prescriptive approach, and has been used to encourage behavior modification in other conditions including alcohol and drug addiction and smoking cessation. It is a patient-centered approach that uses reflective questioning to assess an individual's readiness to change and promote motivation [34].

COMPLICATIONS, COMORBIDITIES AND CONSEQUENCES

Obesity is associated with a number of comorbidities. As such, a thorough assessment is necessary to identify risk factors for the development, and necessary treatment if they are present. Fig. (**5**) lists the most common comorbidities of obesity by body system. In addition to those discussed previously, micronutrient deficiencies such as iron and vitamin D can are often present in obese individuals.

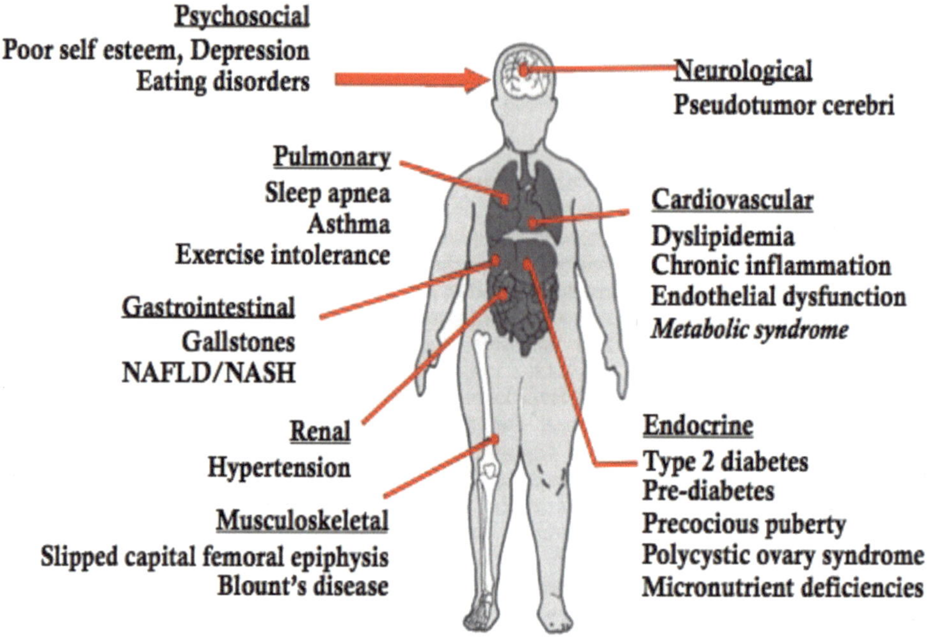

Fig. (5). Body systems affected by obesity [35].

Prevention and Treatment

The treatment of obesity in children and adults differs in some aspects, but the core concepts are the same across the lifespan: Prevention is the ideal, lifestyle and behavior modification is the first course of treatment, and pharmacotherapy and/or surgery follow only when necessary.

Prevention Approaches

The first step in addressing obesity is to prevent it. This section will focus on prevention strategies in the clinical setting and a later section will focus on population-level prevention options.

While prevention of obesity can occur at any age, the fact that obesity is occurring at younger and younger ages makes it imperative to intervene as early as possible. In fact, given the evidence of epigenetics and the effects of maternal nutrition on a child's risk for obesity, one can see the utility of a push for prevention efforts in young, pre-pregnant females. Routine well-child visits make the clinician's office an excellent place for the frequent assessment and education of children and their families. The Expert Committee on childhood obesity produced recommendations regarding the prevention, assessment and treatment of obesity. It is recommended that on a minimum annual basis, all children receive a screen that includes anthropometrics (measurement of weight, height, BMI calculation, and plotting on a growth curve), physical exam, family history, detailed history of dietary and physical activity/sedentary behaviors, and attitudes. It is also recommended that dietary and physical activity education should be given to families as a part of customary anticipatory guidance. In adults, routine screening by the assessment of BMI and risk factors, is recommended, but time intervals are not defined.

Treatment Approaches

Approaches to treatment-lifestyle modification, pharmacotherapy, and surgery are used to terat obesity and its co-morbidities with variability in approach between pediatric and adult populations [29, 35-43]. In the past, pediatric treatment focused primarily on lifestyle modification. However, with increasing prevalence and severity of obesity and its comorbidities in children, pharmacotherapy and surgery are being utilized with more frequency. For both adults and children, the treatment of obesity involves a staged approach, and progression to more intensive levels depends on the patient's age, readiness, degree of obesity, co-existing conditions, and response to interventions.

The goals of treatment also vary slightly between adults and children. In general, they include a sustained reduction in BMI, improvement in comorbidities, and adoption of healthier dietary and activity behaviors. In children, weight loss recommendations are dependent on age and degree of obesity due to the fact that they are still in a stage of active growth and require adequate weight to sustain their development. Thus, weight maintenance rather than weight loss may be appropriate for younger children, but the effect is still a reduction in BMI as height increases. For older children and adults, a safe rate of weight loss is a decrease in 1-2 lb per week, which can be accomplished by a reduction of 500-1000 kcal per day through reduced intake or increased physical activity. More rapid weight loss can result in complications such as gallstone formation.

Lifestyle Modification

Treatment of obesity begins with lifestyle modification, because dietary and activity tendencies and habits of daily life must permanently be altered in order to maintain a more healthful weight and attain an energy balance.

The dietary approach begins with an assessment of the patient's current eating habits (portions, timing, setting, content, *etc.*), risk factors and comorbid conditions. Personalized nutrition goals should be set by taking into account the individual's needs (*e.g.* a diabetic diet) and preferences (to increase acceptability). Barriers such as food insecurity and cultural preferences should be addressed so that recommendations are reasonable and attainable.

Dietary recommendations must also include teaching and planning around age-appropriate portion sizes and calorie goals. In adults, dietary plans of 1,000-1,200 kcal/day for women and 1,200-1,600 kcal/day for men are suitable starting points. Very-low-calorie diets that include less than 800 kcal/day invite complications and are not recommended.

Another approach, which is typically used in children and in adults with less severe obesity and risk factors, is to use focus areas, which address several common dietary habits that are associated with obesity. The major focus areas include eating breakfast, choosing appropriate portion sizes, increasing fruit and vegetable intake, encouraging family meals, and limiting sugar-sweetened beverages and eating out. Helping an individual to make changes in these areas can have profound impact. This approach is particularly useful because it addresses harmful habits directly and avoids the "diet" trap that can lead to patient resistance or weight cycling.

Other dietary interventions exist, but they should be chosen with care. Many fad diets and weight loss programs are on the market and easily accessible, but not all of them are appropriate or safe. Meal replacements (pre-packaged, calorie-restricted meals) can be useful for people who find it difficult to control their portion sizes without assistance. In most cases, specialized and restricted diets should be limited to those with severe or refractory obesity.

Physical activity is an important part of lifestyle modification, as it addresses the energy expenditure portion of energy balance. Yet the benefits of exercise go beyond weight loss, because it can improve cardiovascular and bone health, psychosocial well-being, and glucose control. In 2002, Knowler *et al.*

demonstrated that lifestyle modification involving physical activity as well as reduction in energy intake was more efficacious than pharmacotherapy with metformin [36].

When assessing physical activity levels and making recommendations, it is important to consider the aspects of frequency, intensity, time, and type. Global physical activity recommendations have been issued, by age category (Table **6**) [37]. The type of physical activity can vary from routine child's play, transportation, and activities of daily life to more structured exercise efforts. The frequency, intensity, and time recommendations are listed below.

Table 6. World Health Organization recommendations for physical activity across the lifespan [37].

Age Range	Recommendations
5-17 years of age	• Daily: at least 60 minutes of moderate to vigorous exercise daily • Most activities should be aerobic with strengthening exercises 3 times per week
18-64 years of age	• Weekly: at least 150 minutes of moderate-intensity aerobic physical activity, OR at least 75 minutes of vigorous-intensity aerobic physical activity, OR an equivalent combination of moderate and vigorous intensity activity. • For additional health benefits: Weekly: at least 300 minutes of moderate-intensity aerobic physical activity, OR at least 150 minutes of vigorous-intensity aerobic physical activity, OR an equivalent combination of moderate and vigorous intensity activity. • Activity time may be in smaller bouts (10 minutes minimum) that add up to the above duration • Most activities should be aerobic with strengthening exercises at least 2 times per week
>65 years of age	• Same as above, with the addition of: • Those with poor mobility should incorporate activities that improve balance at least 3 times per week • When health conditions prohibit the ability to meet the above recommendations, individuals should be as active as their abilities and conditions allow

These recommendations should be seen as the goal, not the starting point; otherwise they may be overwhelming, and lead to a sense of failure. In lifestyle modification, safety is of primary importance. An individual's age, risk factors, and overall physical condition must be considered. In some cases, additional medical evaluations will be required before increases in exercise are approved. Personal and cultural preferences and available resources should also be discussed in order to promote the patient's success [38]. Once activities are chosen, a plan for gradual increase can be developed and close follow-up arranged.

Behavior Modification and Psychosocial Support

Beyond making basic changes in diet and physical activity, behavior modification involves counseling in specific strategies that address the underlying issues that affect an individual's attitudes and actions around eating and activity. Helpful techniques include 1) identifying behaviors (eating out of boredom, anxiety, sadness, *etc.*); 2) providing tools for change (self-monitoring, cognitive restructuring, goal-setting, positive reinforcement, problem-solving, barrier identification, contingency management); and 3) encouraging social support (parental modeling, family goals, peer accountability, *etc.*).

Pharmacotherapy

Medications used in treating obesity primarily address the intake side of the energy balance equation through appetite suppression or inhibiting digestion of fats. Additional medications may be necessary for obese individuals when comorbid conditions are present such as medications for high cholesterol or high blood pressure. Most individuals will need to remain on these medications for a lifetime unless improvements in weight loss and lifestyle modification lead significant changes in their laboratory profiles and physical status. Due to side effects of these medications as seen in Table **7**, this can prove quite difficult but necessary for many individuals [39, 40].

Weight Loss Surgery

Bariatric surgery is an alternative treatment for those who have failed lifestyle modification and pharmacotherapy. The most common current surgeries are sleeve gastrectomy, Roux-en-y gastric bypass, and gastric banding. Each of them has advantages and disadvantages, and all effect weight loss through restriction of intake, malabsorption, or a combined effect. Weight loss surgery is increasingly performed in adult and pediatric populations [41, 42], typically in adolescents who weigh 100 kg (BMI of 35 to 40) [41]. It has the potential to be an effective treatment option, but is not without risk. Thus criteria and protocols have been developed to increase probability of patient's success (Table **8**).

Global Approaches

In addition to our individual choices our families' wellbeing, there are opportunities to act at community, regional, national and global levels to affect the obesity epidemic [44-46]. The frameworks discussed previously are relevant

Table 7. Pharmacotherapy in obesity: general guidelines.

Indications	Duration
• BMI>30 • BMI>27 + comorbidities • Lifestyle change x 6 months without improvement • >12-18 years of age	• If less than 2 kg weight loss in 4 weeks, discontinue • If side effects are severe, may need to discontinue • If effective, my need to be lifelong
Options	
Historical	
• Sibutramine: serotonin/norepinephrine reuptake inhibitor -Effect: satiety, appetite suppressant -Risk: myocardial infarction • Fenfluramine/phentermine: serotonin reuptake inhibitor -Effect: satiety, appetite suppressant -Risk: aortic and mitral regurgitation (thickening of leaflets, 20% of women, 12% of men)	
Current	
• Orlistat: inhibitor of fat digestion -Side effects: diarrhea, flatulence, abdominal pain, liver injury • When comorbidities are present: statins, metformin, anti-hypertensives, as indicated	
New	
• Serotonin receptor agonist: Lorcaserin -Effect: satiety, appetite suppressant -Risk: dizziness, headache, constipation, insomnia, drug interactions, teratogenicity • Drug Combinations with phentermine: phentermine (norepinephrine release) + topirimate -Effect: satiety, appetite suppressant, taste, energy expenditure -Risk: dizziness, headache, constipation, insomnia, drug interactions, teratogenicity	

to the causation of obesity in any country. Fig. (**6**) illustrates a framework that also incorporates solutions, and Table **9** breaks down these key policy areas in more detail.

Table 8. Criteria and considerations for bariatric surgery [41, 42].

<table>
<tr><th>Criteria for Bariatric Surgery</th><th>Absolute Contraindications</th></tr>
<tr><td>• BMI ≥ 35 (99th percentile) with severe comorbdities
• BMI > 40 with milder comorbidities
• BMI >50 without comorbidities
• 95% done with linear growth
• Tanner stage of 4 or 5 unless with severe comorbidities (adolescents)
• Attempted comprehensive weight management for at least 6 month
• Maturity to understand risks
• Willingness to maintain physical activity
• Willingness to maintain a healthy diet and behavior monitoring</td><td>• Medically correctable cause of obesity
• Active substance abuse problem
• Medical, psychiatric, or cognitive disability that impairs ability to adhere to postoperative requirements
• Current pregnancy or breastfeeding, or plans for pregnancy within 12 months after surgery
• Inability or unwillingness of patient or parents to undertake lifelong vitamin and mineral supplementation</td></tr>
<tr><th colspan="2">Important Considerations</th></tr>
<tr><td>Favorable
• Numerous Failed Attempts
• Realistic expectations
• Family commitment
• Motivated, no coercion
• Compliance with regimens
• Long-term follow-up
• Decisional capacity
• Understand lifelong change</td><td>Unfavorable
• Unconvincing attempts at weight loss
• Lack of family support
• Major psychoses
• Suicidal ideation
• Lack of insight</td></tr>
<tr><th colspan="2">Disadvantages</th></tr>
<tr><td colspan="2">• Surgical complications: bleeding, leaking, infection, ulcer
• Dumping syndrome
• Hypoglycemia
• Malabsorption and micronutrient deficiencies (iron, calcium, copper, zinc, vitamins D and B_{12}, and potentially others
• Weight regain</td></tr>
</table>

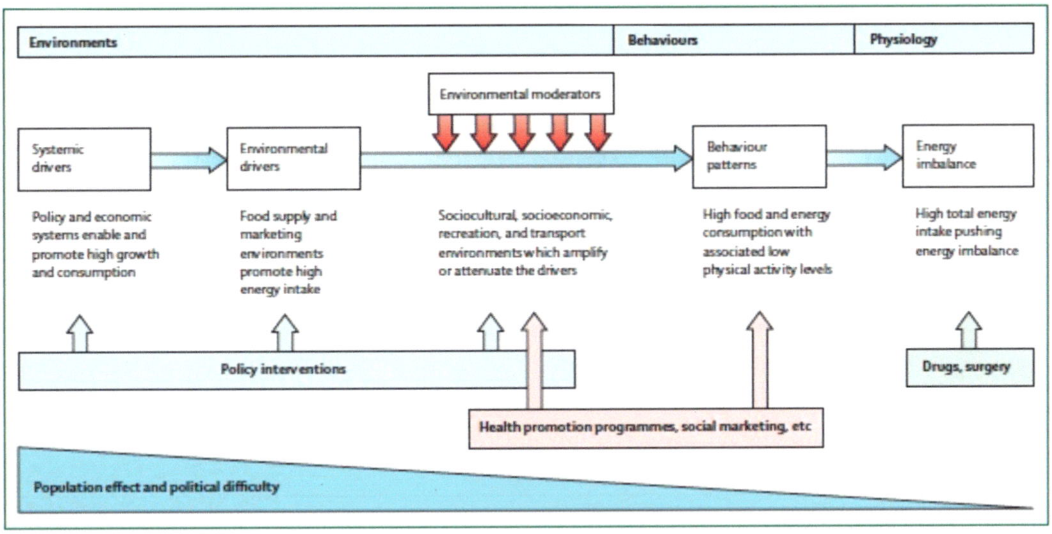

Fig. (6). Obesity determinants and solutions [27].

Table 9. Policies to address the obesogenic environment [44, 46].

Food Environment	Physical Activity Environment
• Food production/subsidies • Food processing • Distribution • Marketing/Media • Retail/access • Catering/Food service • Access and labeling • Financial disincentives	• Infrastructure and planning • Education • Employment • Transport • Sports and Recreation • Safety

CONCLUSION

Obesity is a health condition associated with high morbidity and mortality that is found around the globe in increasing numbers. Ludwig emphasized the importance and urgency of addressing this epidemic by outlining four phases of its trajectory: Phase 1: Increased childhood obesity; Phase 2: Emergence of serious obesity-related comorbidities; Phase 3: Rise in obesity-related life-threatening diseases and Phase 4: Transgenerational transmission, leading to acceleration of obesity [47]. Through raising global awareness, advocacy, research, prevention, and treatment, each of us can play a role in arresting and reversing this cycle.

ADDITIONAL RESOURCES & LINKS

USDA: www.ChooseMyPlate.gov

WHO: "The Three Fives": http://www.who.int/foodsafety/consumer/3x5_SA_en.pdf

CDC: http://www.cdc.gov/obesity/

WHO: http://www.who.int/topics/obesity/en/

American Medical Association: http://www.ama-assn.org/ama/pub/physician-resources/public-health/general-resources-health-care-professionals/roadmaps-clinical-practice-series/assessment-management-adult-obesity.page

Let's move: http://www.letsmove.gov

ACKNOWLEDGEMENTS

Declared none.

CONFLICT OF INTEREST

The authors confirm that this chapter contents have no conflict of interest.

REFERENCES

[1] Centers for Disease Control and Prevention. About BMI for Adults [homepage on the Internet]. c2014. [updated 2011 Sep 13; cited 2014 Feb 17]. Available from http://www.cdc.gov/healthyweight /assessing/bmi/adult_bmi/index.html.

[2] Centers for Disease Control and Prevention (2009a). About BMI for Children and Teens [homepage on the Internet]. c2014. [updated 2011 Sep 13; cited 2014 Feb 17]. Available from http://www.cdc. gov/healthyweight/assessing/bmi/childrens_bmi/about_childrens_bmi.html

[3] World Health Organization. Obesity: preventing and managing the global epidemic. Report of a WHO Consultation. WHO Technical Report Series 894. Geneva: World Health Organization, 2000. [cited 2014 Feb 17]. Available from: http://www.who.int/nutrition/publications/obesity/WHO_TRS_894/en/

[4] World Health Organization expert consultation. Appropriate body-mass index for Asian populations and its implications for policy and intervention strategies. The Lancet, 2004; 157-163.

[5] Ogden CL, Carroll MD, Kit BK, Flegal KM. Prevalence of obesity in the United States. NCHS Date Brief. January 2012, No. 82. (NHANES database).

[6] Ogden, CL, Carroll, MD, Kit, BK, and Flegal, KM. Prevalence of obesity and trends in body mass index among U.S. children and adolescents, 1999-2010. Journal of the American Medical Association 2012; 307(5), 483-490.

[7] WHO Commission on Social Determinants of Health: Globalization, food and nutrition transitions. August, 2007. [cited 2014 Feb 17] Available from: http://www.who.int/social_determinants/resourc es/gkn_hawkes.pdf

[8] Popkin, BM, Adair LS, and Wen Ng S. Global nutrition transition and the pandemic of obesity in developing countries. Nutrition Reviews 2012; 70 (1): 3-21.
[9] Finucane MM, Stevens GA, Cowan MJ, *et al.* National, regional, and global trends in body-mass index since 1980: systematic analysis of health examination surveys and epidemiological studies with 960 country-years and 9.1 million participants. Lancet. 2011; 377:557-67.
[10] Food and Agricultural Association of the United Nations. The State of Food and Agriculture. Rome, 2013. [cited 2014 Feb 17] Available from: http://www.fao.org/docrep/018/i3300e/i3300e.pdf
[11] Flegal, KM, Carroll, MD, Kit, BK, Ogden, CL. Prevalence of obesity and trends in the distribution of body mass index among U.S. adults, 1999-2010. J Am Med Assoc 2012; 307(5), 491-497.
[12] Wang Y. Disparities in pediatric obesity in the United States. Adv Nut 2011; 2:23-31.
[13] WHO Global Status Report on noncommunicable diseases. 2010. [cited 2014 Feb 17] Available from: http://www.who.int/nmh/publications/ncd_report_full_en.pdf
[14] Olshansky SJ, Passaro DJ, Hershow RC, *et al.* A potential decline in life expectancy in the United States in the 21st century. N Engl J Med. 352(11): 1143, 2005.
[15] Finkelstein EA, Khavjou OA, Thompson H, *et al.* Obesity and severe obesity forecasts through 2030. Am J Prev Med 2012; 42(6): 563-570.
[16] Trogdon JG, Finkelstein EA, Hylands T, Dellea PS, and Kamal-Bahl SJ. Indirect costs of obesity: a review of the current literature. Obes Rev 2008; 9:489-500.
[17] Gorden-Larsen P and Popkin BM. Understanding socioeconomic and racial/ethnic status disparities in diet, exercise and weight: underlying contextual factors and pathways. J Am Diet Assoc 2011; 111(12): 1816-1819.
[18] Davison KK and Birch LL. Childhood overweight: a contextual model and recommendations for future research. Obes Rev 2001; 2(3): 159-71.
[19] Levine JA, Vander Weg MW, Hill JO, and Klesges RC. Non-exercise activity thermogenesis- the crouching tiger hidden dragon of societal weight gain. Arteriosclerosis, Thrombosis, and Vascular Biology 2006; 26:729-736.
[20] Hagan S and Niswender KD. Neuroendocrine regulation of food intake. Pediatric Blood Cancer 2012; 58:149-153.
[21] Xia Q and Grant SFA. The genetics of human obesity. Ann NY Acad Sci 2013; 1281: 178-190.
[22] Waalen J. The genetics of human obesity. Transl Res. 2014 May 23. pii: S1931-5244(14)00197-2. doi: 10.1016/j.trsl.2014.05.010. [Epub ahead of print]
[23] Manco M and Dallapiccola B. Genetics of Pediatric Obesity. Pediatrics 2012; 130:123-133.
[24] Bouchard C. The biological predisposition to obesity: beyond the thrifty genotype scenario. Int J Obes 2007; 31: 1337-1339.
[25] Kleinman RE. Pediatric Nutrition Handbook. Elk Grove Village, IL. American Academy of Pediatrics. 2009.
[26] Heimburger DC, Ard JD. *Handbook of Clinical Nutrition.* 4th ed. Philadelphia, PA. Mosby Inc. 2006: 230-261, 371-421.
[27] Swinburn BA, Sacks G, Hall KD, *et al.* The global obesity pandemic: shaped by global drivers and local environments. Lancet 2011; 378: 804-14.
[28] The Practical Guide: Identification, evaluation, and treatment of overweight and obesity in adults. National Heart, Lung, and Blood Institute Obesity Education Initiative. 2000. [cited 2014 Feb 17]. Available from: http://www.nhlbi.nih.gov/files/docs/guidelines/prctgd_c.pdf
[29] Barlow S. Expert committee recommendations regarding the prevention, assessment, and treatment of child and adolescent overweight and obesity: summary report. Pediatrics. 2007; 120: S164.
[30] Caballero AE. Type 2 diabetes in the Hispanic or Latino population: challenges and opportunities. Current Opinion in Endocrinology, Diabetes, and Obesity. 2007; 14(2):151-157.
[31] Torres M, Azen S, Varma R. Prevalence of obesity and associated co-morbid conditions in a population-based sample of primarily urban Mexican Americans. Ethnic Disparities. 2006; 16(2):362-369.
[32] Dixon B, Peña MM, Taveras EM. Life course approach to racial/ethnic disparities in childhood obesity. Adv Nut 2012; 3:73-82.
[33] Spear BA, Barlow SE, Ervin C, *et al.* Recommendations for treatment of child and adolescent overweight and obesity. Pediatrics 2007;120;S254.

[34] Miller WR, Rollnick S. Motivational interviewing: preparing people for change. 2nd ed. New York: Guilford Press; 2002.
[35] Ebbeling CB, Pawlak DB, Ludwig DS. Childhood obesity: public health crisis, common sense cure. Lancet 2002; 360:473-82.
[36] Knowler WC, Barrett-Connor E, Fowler SE, *et al*. Diabetes Prevention Program Research Group. Reduction in the incidence of type 2 diabetes with lifestyle intervention or metformin. N Engl J Med 2002; 346: 393-403.
[37] Global recommendation on physical activity for health [Internet]. Geneva: World Health Organization; 2010 [cited 2014 Feb 17]. Available from http://www.who.int/dietphysicalactivity/factsheet_recommendations/en/
[38] Corsino L, Rocha-Goldberg MP, Batch BC, Ortiz-Melo DI, Bosworth HB, Svetkey LP. The Latino health project: pilot testing a culturally adapted behavioral weight loss intervention in obese and overweight Latino adults. Ethnicity and Disease. 2012; 22(1):51-57.
[39] Sherafat-Kazmzadeh R, Yanovski SZ, and Yanovski JA. Pharmacotherapy for childhood obesity: present and future prospects. Int J Obes 2012; 1-15.
[40] Bray GA and Ryan DH. Medical therapy for the patient with obesity. Circulation. 2012;125:1695-1703.
[41] Pratt J, Lenders CM, Dionne DA *et al*. Best practices updates for pediatric/adolescent weight loss surgery. Obesity. 2009; 17(5): 901-910.
[42] Blackburn GL, Hutter MM, Harvey AM, *et al*. Expert panel on weight loss surgery: a report update. Obesity. 2009; 17(5): 842-862.
[43] Berkowitz RI, Wadden TA, Tershakovec AM, Cronquist JL. Behavior therapy and sibutramine for the treatment of adolescent obesity: A randomized controlled trial. JAMA. 2003;289:1805-1812.
[44] Sacks G, Swinburn BA, and Lawrence MA. A systematic policy approach to changing the food and physical activity environments to prevent obesity. Australia and New Zealand Health Policy 2008; 5:13.
[45] Foltz JL, May AL, Belay B, Nihiser AJ, Dooyema CA, and Blank HM. Population level intervention strategies and examples for obesity prevention in children. Ann Rev Nut 2012; 32:391-415.
[46] Mozaffarian D. Population approaches to improve diet, physical activity and smoking habits: A scientific statement from the American Heart Association. Circulation 2012; 125:1695-1703.
[47] Ludwig DS. Childhood obesity—the shape of things to come. N Engl J Med 2007; 357(23):2325-7.

CHAPTER 3

Physical Inactivity: A Lazy World

Sarah Litman Rendell[1] and Charles Swencionis*[2]

[1]*Ferkauf Graduate School, Yeshiva University, USA;* [2]*Ferkauf Graduate School, Albert Einstein College of Medicine, Yeshiva University, USA*

Abstract: Modern lifestyles in the developed world have led to decreased levels of physical activity. In addition to the contribution, physical inactivity has increased rates of overweight and obesity, physical inactivity has independently been cited as the fourth leading risk factor for non-communicable diseases. In this chapter, we review current guidelines recommended by the Centers for Disease Control, and contrasts them with actual energy expenditures reported in research around the world. We highlight the relationship between physical inactivity, overweight, obesity, and non-communicable diseases. We also identify major contributors to the decline in rates of physical activity in recent years, including availability of public and private modes of transportation, occupational limitations on leisure time, increased time spent in sedentary activities, such as television watching and computer use, and barriers to purposeful exercise. Finally, we review some popular initiatives and recommendations for improving the frequency and quality of physical activity among Americans.

Keywords: Barriers, behavior, CDC, exercise, fitness, global health, health status, lifestyle, nutrition, obesity, overweight, Physical inactivity, public health, risk, weight, wellness.

INTRODUCTION

In 1996, William Dietz [1] reported, "Inactivity represents an understudied behavior that is associated with adverse health consequences. Successful reductions in inactivity may provide the most cost-effective approach to the treatment of obesity and the prevention of cardiovascular disease". Today, many obesity interventions focus on reduction of food intake and an increase in purposeful physical activity. However, physical inactivity does not simply refer to the lack of physical activity, but rather it concerns both a decrease in purposeful energy expenditure and an increase in sedentary behaviors.

***Corresponding author Charles Swencionis:** Ferkauf Graduate School, 1300 Morris Park Ave., Bronx, NY 10461, USA; Tel: (718) 430-3990; Fax: (718) 430-3960; E-mail: charles.swencionis@einstein.yu.edu

Judith Wylie-Rosett & Sunil S. Jhangiani (Eds)

This chapter provides an overview of the guidelines recommended by the Centers for Disease Control and Prevention (CDC), and contrasts them with actual energy expenditures reported in research around the world. After reviewing the relationship between physical inactivity, overweight, obesity, and non-communicable diseases, the chapter describes contributors to the decline in physical activity, focusing on availability of public and private modes of transportation, occupational limitations on leisure time, increased time spent in sedentary activities, such as television watching and computer use, and barriers to purposeful exercise. Initiatives and recommendations for improving the frequency and quality of physical activity among Americans are also discussed.

HISTORY

Today, changes in the ways in which individuals in society conduct personal and professional business have led to alterations in lifestyle and aerobic exercise. Greater access to vehicular transportation, the increase in use of personal devices requiring or promoting sedentary behaviors, such as computers and televisions, and the preponderance of items available to make chores and errands less physically taxing (*i.e.,* robotic vacuum cleaners) has led to decreased physical activity in developed countries. Although the original purpose of such devices was to decrease hardships and increase productivity, it seems that a secondary effect has been a decline in levels of activity [2]. In fact, physical inactivity has been targeted as the fourth leading risk factor for non-communicable diseases [3].

CURRENT PHYSICAL ACTIVITY GUIDELINES: A GLOBAL PICTURE

The World Health Organization (WHO) and the Centers for Disease Control and Prevention (CDC) have published guidelines for physical activity, with the WHO publishing "Global Recommendations on Physical Activity for Health" in 2010 (available at: http://whqlibdoc.who.int/publications/2010/9789241599979_eng.pdf) and the CDC publishing "2008 Physical Activity Guidelines for Americans" (available at: http://www.health.gov/paguidelines/pdf/paguide.pdf) [4, 5]. To accommodate different populations, these organizations break down the guidelines to meet the needs of children, adolescents, adults, older adults, pregnant women and women in the postpartum period, as well as adults with disabilities. They also identify important information for individuals with chronic medical conditions to consider when developing an exercise regimen. Recommendations for children include 60 minutes of daily physical activity.

The WHO and CDC suggest that most of this activity is moderate to vigorous in intensity, and that vigorous-intensity exercise, muscle strengthening, and bone strengthening should be completed at least 3 days per week as part of the 60 minute activity. Adults are recommended to do moderate-intensity activity for at least 150 minutes per week, vigorous-intensity aerobic exercise for 75 minutes per week, or some combination of the two. Muscle strengthening is suggested at least two days of each week. Increasing the amount of exercise is recommended to enhance the health benefits of performing physical activity. Guidelines for older adults are the same as those for adults, but include considerations for adjusting activity to meet the needs and limitations of aging populations. Table **1** provides a condensed summary of the minimum recommended physical activity expenditures suggested by the WHO and CDC.

Table 1. Physical activity guidelines from the CDC [4, 5].

Age Group	Activity Type	Minimum Recommended Activity Level
Children & Adolescents	Overall	60 minutes per day, 7 days per week
	Aerobic	60 minutes per day, at least 3 days per week
	Muscle-Strengthening	60 minutes per day, at least 3 days per week
	Bone-Strengthening	60 minutes per day, at least 3 days per week
Adults	Overall	150 minutes per week of moderate intensity OR 75 minutes per week of vigorous intensity exercise
	Muscle-Strengthening	2 or more days per week

Current Physical Activity Expenditures

In 2012, Hallal, Andersen, Bull, Guthold, Haskell, and Ekelund [2] reported findings of global physical activity levels in 122 countries, representing 88.9% of the world's population, from the WHO global health observatory data repository [6]. They assessed levels of activity and inactivity in adults aged 15 and older and adolescents between 13 and 15 years old. They defined physical activity as meeting either of the three following criteria: 30 minutes of moderate-intensity physical activity for 5 or more days per week, 20 minutes of vigorous-intensity physical activity for 3 or more days per week, or some combination achieving 600 metabolic equivalent minutes per week. In general, this type of physical activity is often described as deliberate exercise. Overall, they reported that 31.1% of adults were physically inactive, and noted that inactivity levels varied between countries and regions. In the Americas, the rate of physical inactivity was 43.3%. The group also found that inactivity increases with age, women are more inactive than men, and inactivity is more common in high income countries than in low income countries.

In terms of lifestyle physical activity, the researchers demonstrated that 64.1% of adults worldwide report walking for a minimum of 10 consecutive minutes for 5 or more days each week. The statistic in the Americas, 65.6%, mirrors the worldwide rate. Fewer than one third of adults worldwide (31.4%) reported engaging in vigorous physical activity for 3 or more days each week. This proportion was smaller in the Americas (24.6%), and vigorous activity rates were lower among women and declined with age.

According to the American Time Use Survey (available at: http://www.bls.gov/news.release/atus.nr0.htm), in 2011, men over the age of 15 reported participating in sports, exercise, or active recreation for an average of 0.35 hours per day on weekdays and 0.49 hours per day on weekends [7]. Women reported participating in such activity for 0.21 hours on weekdays and 0.25 hours on weekends. Those who were employed either full-time or part-time reported engaging in physical activity for less time on both weekdays and weekends than those who were not employed.

Health Risks of Physical Inactivity

Not only does physical inactivity contribute to overweight and obesity among the world's population, but it also significantly contributes to major non-communicable diseases. Lee, Shiroma, Lobelo, Puska, Blair, and Katzmarzyk reported that physical inactivity causes 9% of premature mortality worldwide, and is responsible for 6% of coronary heart disease, 7% of type 2 diabetes, 10% of breast cancer, and 10% of colon cancer [8]. They suggested that the worldwide life expectancy would increase by 0.68 years if physical inactivity was eliminated, and that the life expectancy for individuals who transition from no physical activity to some physical activity may see even greater increases.

Physical Inactivity and Weight

It is common knowledge that physical activity is associated with body weight and that physical activity is a popular way to lose weight or to maintain a healthy weight, but not as well-known is how the body uses energy to balance energy intake. Whereas energy intake consists of what individuals put into their bodies, energy expenditure fits into three categories. Bray described the various means by which the body uses energy [9]. An individual's basal metabolic rate accounts for approximately 70% of energy expenditure, and may be affected by age, sex, fat free mass, drugs, thyroid hormones, and protein turnover. Thermogenesis accounts for another 15% of energy expenditure, and is affected by food intake, cold, stress, and thermogenic drugs. Finally, activity accounts for 15% or more of expenditure, based on the duration and intensity of the physical activity.

THE OBESOGENIC ENVIRONMENT

The Built Environment

Obesity is linked with areas where people reside, their resources, television use, ease of walking, land use, urban sprawl, and level of deprivation [10]. The built environment includes urban design, land use, public transportation, and activity options [11]. These factors can improve or obstruct physical activity and healthful eating [12, 13]. Safer neighborhoods, with a mix of residences, commercial, retail, and recreation, have been associated with more physical and social activity and less obesity [14, 15]. Lower social economic status (SES) neighborhoods have fewer physical activity resources than higher SES neighborhoods and unsafe conditions, but higher levels of walking activity and more use of public transportation [16].

Travel

After World War II, personal automobiles became much more abundant and accessible, as populations began using them not as a luxury, but as a necessity, particularly for commuting, shopping, and socializing [17]. Muller coined the term "Freeway Era" to describe this time from 1945 to present, in which automobile use increased dramatically [17]. Also during this time, the 1956 Interstate Highway Act made commuting in and out of cities easier, encouraging individuals to live in the suburbs. In suburban communities, driving was more efficient than in cities because public transportation was unavailable; therefore walking decreased and driving to and from locations increased.

In 2011, the United States Department of Transportation published the 2009 National Household Travel Survey, which summarized travel information across four decades [18]. From 1969 to 2009, America saw an increase in vehicles and drivers per household. In 2009, the average number of persons per household was 2.50. There were an average of 1.86 vehicles and 1.88 drivers per household. Additionally, there were 0.99 vehicles per driver, indicating that almost all drivers own a vehicle, and 1.39 vehicles per worker, indicating that many workers have more than one vehicle. The increase in use of personal vehicles was associated not only with more time spent in the car and sedentary, but also with less time spent walking or using other active methods to travel from place to place.

The report showed that from 1969 to 2009, the daily number of trips per person increased from 2.02 to 3.79, and the daily mileage per person increased from 19.51 to 36.13 [18]. In 2009, 83.4% of daily trips per person were made by private vehicle, 1.9% were made by public transit, 10.4% by walking, and 4.2% by another mode of transportation, such as bicycle. These statistics included trips to and from work, work-related business, family/personal errands, school, church, social and recreational activities, and other activities. In terms of commuting to and from work in 2009, 89.4% reported using an auto, truck, van, or SUV, 5.1% used public transit, 2.8% walked, and another 2.7% reported using another method, including other passive modes of transportation such as motorcycle, train, and airplane.

In addition to the number of trips made per person each day, the report measured the number of minutes drivers spent in the car each day [18]. The number of minutes per driver increased from 49.35 minutes in 1990 to 55.87 minutes in 2009. Additionally, when the statistics included only persons who drove on their travel day (as opposed to using other forms of transportation), the minutes per day in 2009 increased to 76.37 minutes.

The mileage per year driven by each driver increased from 8,685 miles in 1969 to 13,827 miles in 2001, and then decreased to 12,888 miles in 2009 [18]. Note that this mileage was self-estimated by drivers and included only miles that they drove, not miles for which they were the passenger.

Occupation

Brownson, Boehmer, and Luke described occupational data from the 2000 United States Census and coded occupations as low- or high-activity [19]. They explained that, of the 216.9 million eligible individuals over the age of 16, 63% reported being in the labor force. Out of these individuals, 42.6% described being employed in low-activity occupations, whereas 22.6% were in high-activity occupations. The authors noted significant changes in the percentage of individuals engaged in high- *versus* low-activity occupations over time, such that the rate in high-activity jobs decreased from approximately 30% in the 1950s and the rate in low-activity jobs increased from approximately 23% in the 1950s.

Full-time, employed men worked an average of 8.3 hours and full-time, employed women worked an average of 7.8 hours per workday in 2011 [7]. This was a change even from just eight years earlier, in 2003. At that time, full-time, employed men reported working an average of 8.0 hours and women 7.0 hours [20]. Time Use Surveys from years prior to 2003 were unavailable and we were therefore unable to compare present time use to time use from further back in history.

MEDIA

Television, computer, and internet usage has continued to increase in the United States, with the average American spending about 20% of his or her day watching television [21]. A report released in 2011 showed that all individuals in the United States over the age of two, regardless of whether or not they own the specific technology, watched an average of 35 hours, 37 minutes of traditional live television per week [21]. Additionally, they watched time-shifted television (*i.e.*: DVR or OnDemand television) for another 2 hours, 25 minutes per week, and spent another total of 4 hours, 39 minutes watching television or other video content using the internet on a computer or phone. In total, that sums to 42 hrs, 41 minutes per week spent watching some type of video content or television. The figures differ among varying racial/ethnic groups, with African Americans reporting the greatest television and video viewing of all, at 53 hours, 29 minutes per week. The report suggested that, overall, television viewing increased 22 minutes per month in 2011 over the same period in 2012.

According to the Nielsen report, including television-watching only, females watched more hours than males and television consumption increased with age [21]. For example, while males aged 2 to 17 watched television for an average of 113 hours, 13 minutes and females watched 114 hours, 29 minutes per month, males aged 18 to 49 watched 139 hours, 50 minutes and females watched 151 hours, 18 minutes per month. Finally, males over the age of 50 watched 195 hours, 15 minutes and females in the same age group watched 217 hours, 44 minutes each month. Males reported watching videos on the internet for more time than did females.

The Kaiser Family Foundation published a report in 2010 about the use of media among young people in the previous year [22]. In 2009, 8 to 18 year olds in the United States were reported to spend 4 hours, 29 minutes watching TV, 1 hour, 29 minutes on the computer, 1 hour, 13 minutes playing video games, 25 minutes watching movies, 2 hours, 31 minutes listening to music or other audio, and 38 minutes reading print materials each day. The total media use for these children was 7 hours, 38 minutes per day, but they were reported to have used more than one medium 29% of the time, so their total media exposure was rated at 10 hours, 45 minutes per day. This demonstrates an increase in all forms of media exposure from a decade ago, with the exception of print media. Additionally, the report suggested that 8 to 18 year olds spent 33 minutes per day talking on cell phones and that 7th through 12th graders spent 1 hour, 30 minutes text messaging each day. Furthermore, although computer use was reported as 1 hour, 29 minutes per day in this age group, only 64% of 8 to 18 year olds reported using a computer. Among those who reported using a computer, they spent 2 hours, 17 minutes on the computer each day. Sixty percent in this age group reported playing video games; among those, they spent an average of 1 hour, 59 minutes each day playing video games on either a game console, handheld device, or cell phone.

The most recent available data regarding computer accessibility and use published by the US Census Bureau at the time of print was from the year 2010 [23]. In 2010, 81.4% of individuals over the age of 3 in the United States lived in a household with a computer, including desktops, laptops, handheld devices, and smart mobile phones, among others. 68.0% of those over the age of 15 who reported using a computer stated that they used a computer at home. More than 45% of those between the ages of 25 and 64 reported using a computer at work, and 88.3% of 18 to 24 year olds enrolled in school reported using a computer at school. Individuals between the ages of 15 and 24 reported the greatest amount of computer usage at home, with 77.3% of those with computer access reporting using a computer at home.

Barriers to Exercise

In a study examining barriers to exercise in 1,332 Australians, researchers found that personal barriers to exercise, such as lack of time, other priorities, work, and family commitments were predictive of less time spent engaging in walking or other physical activities, and that environmental barriers, aside from weather, were not strongly related to exercise behaviors [24]. Worries about financial costs of physical activity were associated with increased walking and moderate-intensity physical activity, but with lower levels of vigorous activity, perhaps because vigorous activities, such as most costly sports and gym memberships, may be expensive.

Among 2,912 women aged 40 or older in the United States, factors most strongly associated with inactivity included caregiver duties and lack of energy [25]. Additional factors related to inactivity included older age, less education, and infrequent observation of other exercisers in the community.

Physical activity in childhood and adolescence is particularly important because it paves the way for those individuals to maintain a healthy lifestyle in adulthood. In addition, activity among children, particularly associated with team sports, provides additional benefits such as improved social relationships and self-confidence, among others. Although participation in sports, particularly among children, has a vast number of benefits beyond those of maintaining physical health, lower-income families continue to have children who are less engaged in sports than their higher-income counterparts [26]. This is due in large part to the costs associated with participation on a school or team sport, such as membership or team fees, as well as the cost of equipment. Both Canadian children and their parents reported that involvement in sports is associated with social and personal development [27]. However, despite this understanding, low-income parents reported that financial constraints and scheduling difficulties made it difficult to engage their children in sports activities.

A Canadian study demonstrated differences between the factors associated with participation in physical activity among high socioeconomic status and low socioeconomic status youths [28]. The authors noted that, while both groups cited limited time as a barrier to sports participation, those in the high socioeconomic status group reported work, homework, and other scheduled activities as the most prominent factors, while those in the low socioeconomic status group reported family obligations and homework. Both groups endorsed fun as a major factor influencing their participation, and both also reported perceived competence and skill in a sport as a factor. Low socioeconomic status youths cited a number of environmental barriers not noted by those in the high socioeconomic status group, such as proximity, cost, facilities, and safety. Specifically, their concerns centered on the availability, quality, and safety of areas in which to participate in sports activities. As mentioned previously, if patterns of non-activity become common in youth, those individuals will be less likely to engage in sports or other means of physical activity in adulthood.

INITIATIVES AND RECOMMENDATIONS FOR IMPROVING PHYSICAL ACTIVITY

The Centers for Disease Control and Prevention (CDC) developed the Common Community Measures for Obesity Prevention Project in an effort to identify strategies that can be used at various community and governmental levels to prevent obesity [29]. Among the 24 recommended measures, 12 were comprised of strategies focused on improving rates of physical activity. Four measures were listed under "Strategies to encourage physical activity or limit sedentary activity among children and youth" and eight under "Strategies to create safe communities that support physical activity". With regards to the former set of strategies, the CDC recommended that communities require physical education in schools and provided concrete time requirements for engagement in weekly physical education classes that schools should aim to achieve. Furthermore, they suggested that students should be physically active for at least 50% of time spent in physical education classes. Additionally, the CDC report recommended that communities increase opportunities for extracurricular physical activity, such as through non-competitive games and dance classes in after-school programs, which can be held on school grounds. Finally, they suggested that public community venues reduce the opportunity for children in child care facilities to watch television or movies to less than two hours per day.

The other set of strategies listed by the CDC report focused on creating safe communities to support physical activity among all community members, including youths and adults, by altering the built environment. Firstly, they recommended that communities improve access to outdoor recreational facilities, such as parks, green space, outdoor sports fields, walking and biking trails, public pools, and community playgrounds. They suggested that this strategy be quantified by communities citing the percentage of residences within a half-mile of at least one outdoor public recreational facility. Next, the report suggested that communities enhance infrastructure supporting bicycling, for example by creating bike lanes and shared-use paths on roads and by providing public bike racks. Similarly, they suggested that communities enhance infrastructure supporting walking, such as by creating sidewalks, footpaths, walking trails, and pedestrian crosswalks. Another strategy suggested that communities attempt to locate schools within easy walking distance of residential areas in an effort to increase the number of students who walk or bike to and from school. The CDC report recommended that communities improve access to public transportation so that commuters might engage in physical activity while walking to and from public transportation centers. Another interesting strategy was for communities to zone areas for mixed-use development, such that patrons of shops and businesses would make more trips to stores and other community centers by foot than by automobile because residences would be located in closer proximity to stores. Finally, two more measures recommended that communities enhance personal and traffic safety in areas where individuals might be physically active. Some suggested ideas to implement this include increasing police presence, eliminating abandoned buildings, improving street lighting, lowering the speed limit on surface streets, and improving safety of street crossings.

In addition to governmental policy aimed at increasing energy expenditure among Americans, increasing awareness about the relationship between physical activity and health is imperative in helping individuals increase their own activity levels; two distinct initiatives are discussed here. First Lady Michelle Obama's Let's Move initiative has earned nationwide attention for its goal of improving health and decreasing obesity among America's youth [30]. Specifically, the program aims to focus on five key healthful criteria: creating a healthy start for children, empowering parents and caregivers, providing healthy food in schools, improving access to healthy, affordable foods, and increasing physical activity. A different approach was taken by Activate Omaha, a community-wide health initiative focused on increasing awareness of active living in Omaha, Nebraska [31]. This organization utilized media, such as billboards, television, radio, spokespersons, and grassroots efforts to draw attention to the benefits and availability of physical activity for Omaha residents. The campaign was successful in increasing the percentage of respondents who believed Omaha to be an active community from 63% prior to the study to 78% at the end of the 3-year study period.

For those interested in reading more about or becoming involved in current initiatives to promote healthful physical activity, we direct them to:

ADDITIONAL RESOURCES & LINKS:

- **Let's Move**: http://www.letsmove.gov/
- **Center for Disease Control's National Physical Activity Initiative:** http://www.cdc.gov/nccdphp/sgr/npai.htm
- **National Physical Activity Plan:** http://www.physicalactivityplan.org/

- **President's Council on Fitness, Sports, and Nutrition:** http://www.fitness.gov/participate-in-programs/physical-activity-initiative/

ACKNOWLEDGEMENTS

Declared none.

CONFLICT OF INTEREST

The authors confirm that this chapter contents have no conflict of interest.

REFERENCES

[1] Dietz WH. The role of lifestyle in health: The epidemiology and consequences of inactivity. Proc Nutr Soc. 1996; 55:829-840.
[2] Hallal PC, Andersen LB, Bull FC, *et al*. Global physical activity levels: surveillance progress, pitfalls, and prospects. Lancet. 2012; 380:247-257.
[3] WHO. Global health risks: mortality and burden of disease attributable to selected major risks. [homepage on the Internet]. 2009 [cited 2014 March 23]. Available from: http://www.who.int/healthinfo/global_burden_disease/GlobalHealthRisks_report_full.pdf
[4] World Health Organization. Global recommendations on physical activity for health. Geneva: World Health Organization; 2010.
Available from: http://whqlibdoc.who.int/publications/2010/9789241599979_eng.pdf
[5] United States Department of Health and Human Services. 2008 Physical Activity Guidelines for Americans. Washington, DC; 2008 [cited 2014 March 23].
Available from: http://www.health.gov/paguidelines/pdf/paguide.pdf
[6] World Health Organization. Global health observatory data repository. World Health Organization; 2011. Available from: http://apps.who.int/ghodata/.
[7] American time use survey-2011 results. United States Department of Labor. Bureau of Labor Statistics. Washington, DC; 2012. Available from: http://www.bls.gov/news.release/atus.nr0.htm.
[8] Lee IM, Shiroma EJ, Lobelo F, *et al*. Effect of physical inactivity on major non-communicable diseases worldwide: an analysis of burden of disease and life expectancy. Lancet. 2012; 380:219-229.
[9] Bray, G. Role of physical activity and exercise in obesity. Rose B (Ed). UpToDate. [cited November 13, 2013].
[10] Booth J, Pinkston MM, Walker S *et al*. Obesity and the built environment. J Am Diet Assoc. 2005; 105:S110-117.
[11] Handy SL, Boarnet MG, Ewing R, *et al*. How the built environment affects physical activity: Views from urban planning. Am J Prev Med. 2002; 23:64-73.
[12] Jackson RJ, Kochtitzky C. Creating a Healthy Environment: The Impact of the Built Environment on Public Health. Washington, DC: Sprawl Watch Clearinghouse Monograph Series; 2001.
[13] Giles-Corti B, Macintyre S, Clarkson JP, *et al*. Environmental and lifestyle factors associated with overweight and obesity in Perth, Australia. Am J Health Promot. 2003; 18:93-102.
[14] Saelens BE, Sallis JF, Frank LD. Environmental correlates of walking and cycling: Findings from the transportation, urban design, and planning literatures. Ann Beh Med. 2003; 25:80-91.
[15] Saelens BE, Sallis JF, Black JD, *et al*. Neighborhood based differences in physical activity: An environmental scale evaluation. Am J Public Health. 2003; 93:1552-1558.
[16] Yen IH, Kaplan GA. Poverty area residence and changes in physical activity level: Evidence from the Alameda County study. Am J Public Health. 1998; 88:1709-1712.

[17] Muller, PO. Transportation and urban form: stages in the spatial evolution of the American metropolis. In: Hanson S, Giuliano G, editors. The Geography of Urban Transportation. 3rd ed. New York: The Guilford Press, 2004; p. 59-85.

[18] Santos A, McGuckin N, Nakamoto HY, Gray D, Liss S. Summary of travel trends: 2009 national household travel survey. United States Department of Transportation. Federal Highway Administration; 2011. Available from: http://nhts.ornl.gov/2009/pub/stt.pdf.

[19] Brownson RC, Boehmer TK, Luke DA. Declining rates of physical activity in the United States: What are the contributors? Annu Rev Publ Health. 2005; 26:421-443.

[20] Time use survey-2003 results. United States Department of Labor. Bureau of Labor Statistics. Washington, DC; 2004. Available from: http://www.bls.gov/news.release/archives/atus_09142004.pdf.

[21] State of the media: The cross-platform report. The Neilsen Company; 2011. Available from: http://www.nielsen.com/content/dam/corporate/us/en/reports-downloads/2011-Reports/Nielsen-cross-platform-report-Q1-2011-reissued.pdf.

[22] Rideout VJ, Foehr UG, Robers DF. Generation M^2: Media in the lives of 8- to 18-year-olds: A Kaiser Family Foundation study. [homepage on the Internet]. 2010 [cited 2013 November 23]. Available from: http://kff.org/other/event/generation-m2-media-in-the-lives-of/

[23] Computer and internet use in the United States: 2010. United States Census Bureau. 2010. Available from: http://www.census.gov/hhes/computer/publications/2010.html.

[24] Salmon J, Owen N, Crawford D, *et al.* Physical activity and sedentary behavior: A population-based study of barriers, enjoyment, and preference. Health Psychol. 2003; 22(2):178-188.

[25] King AC, Castro C, Wilcox S, *et al.* Personal and environmental factors associated with physical inactivity among different racial-ethnic groups of U.S. middle-aged and older-aged women. Health Psychol. 2000; 19(4):354-364.

[26] Clark W. Kids' sports. Canadian Social Trends. Component of Statistics Canada catalogue no. 11-088-X. [homepage on the Internet]. 2008 [cited 2013 November 23]. Available from: http://www.statcan.gc.ca/pub/11-008-x/2008001/article/10573-eng.htm

[27] Holt NL, Kingsley BC, Tink LN, *et al.* Benefits and challenges associated with sport participation by children and parents from low-income families. Psychol Sport Exerc. 2011; 12(5):490-499.

[28] Humbert ML, Chad KE, Spint KS, Muhajarine N, Anderson KD, Bruner MW, *et al.* Factors that influence physical activity participation among high- and low-SES youth. Qual Health Res 2006;16:467-483.

[29] Khan LK, Sobush S, Keener D, *et al.* Recommended community strategies and measurements to prevent obesity in the United States. MMWR. 2009; 58(RR07):1-26.

[30] Let's move: America's move to raise a healthier generation of kids [homepage on the Internet]. [updated 2013; cited 2013 Mar 18]. Available from: http://www.letsmove.gov/.

[31] Huberty J, Dodge T, Peterson KR, *et al.* Creating a movement for active living *via* a media campaign. Am J Prev Med 2012; 43(5S4):S390-S391.

CHAPTER 4

From Starvation to Obesity: How Insulin Resistance Affects Global Health

Pooja Raghavan[1], Dhyan Rajan[2] and Meredith Hawkins[*,3]

[1]Albert Einstein College of Medicine, Bronx, New York, USA; [2]Nassau University Medical Center, East Meadow, New York; and [3]Harold and Muriel Block Chair in Medicine, Global Diabetes Institute, Albert Einstein College of Medicine, Bronx, New York, USA

Abstract: Normal quantities of adipose tissue are required in humans, as adipose tissue stores energy and contributes to endocrine and immune functions. Hormones and cytokines secreted by the adipose tissue, collectively known as 'adipokines', include adiponectin, leptin, tumor necrosis factor-α, interleukin 6, and plasminogen activator inhibitor-1. These secretory products play important roles in the maintenance of glucose and energy homeostasis. Both excess and deficiency of adipose tissue can have a negative impact metabolically. In the lipodystrophy syndromes, there is partial or complete loss of adipose tissue, which can lead to insulin resistance, diabetes and hepatic steatosis. Malnutrition due to starvation and anorexia nervosa has also been associated with manifestation of diabetes. In contrast, excess of adipose tissue in obesity has also been associated with insulin resistance, diabetes, fatty liver and cancer. With obesity on the rise globally, non-communicable diseases including cardiovascular disease, cerebrovascular disease, diabetes mellitus, dementia, cancer, and fatty liver disease have increased dramatically in prevalence and are rapidly becoming leading causes of death around the world. Thus, a normal amount and distribution of adipose tissue is required to achieve optimal regulation of metabolism and general good health.

Keywords: Adipose tissue, diabetes, insulin resistance, lipodystrophy, malnutrition, metabolism, obesity, starvation.

INTRODUCTION

Obesity is associated with increased non-communicable disease risk with cardiovascular disease, diabetes mellitus, non-alcoholic fatty liver disease, dementia and many forms of cancer as potential co-morbidities. Insulin resistance contributes to pathogenesis of all of these diseases and associated risk factors such as hypertension, dyslipidemia, abnormal glucose tolerance and systemic

***Corresponding author Meredith Hawkins:** Albert Einstein College of Medicine, Diabetes Research Center, 1300 Morris Park Avenue, Belfer 709, Bronx, NY 10461, USA; Tel: (718) 430-3186; Fax: (718)-430-8557; E-mail: meredith.hawkins@einstein.yu.edu

Judith Wylie-Rosett & Sunil S. Jhangiani (Eds)

inflammation. Ironically, both excess and deficiency of body fat and adipose tissue are associated insulin resistance and diabetes risk. Lipodystrophy syndromes are characterized by partial or complete loss of adipose tissue, which can lead to insulin resistance, diabetes and hepatic steatosis. Alternately, excess of adipose tissue in obesity has also been associated with insulin resistance, diabetes, fatty liver and cancer. This chapter will examine the nature of this paradox.

OBESITY

Obesity was previously a disease of the privileged, occurring in developed countries where food and resources were abundant. With the recent shift in cultural trends and increasing sedentary lifestyles, caloric intake has exceeded energy expenditure, resulting in weight gain. The rise in the rate of obesity is also due to the availability of cheap calories, widespread use of sugar containing drinks and an increased consumption of processed energy-dense foods worldwide [1]. Interestingly, Goran *et al.* showed that countries with higher use of high fructose corn syrup in their beverages and food had a higher prevalence of obesity and type 2 diabetes mellitus (T2DM) than countries that did not use high fructose corn syrup [2]. Thus, in spite of obesity being a complex interplay between environment and genes, an increase in mean caloric intake has significantly contributed to the global epidemic of obesity.

Obesity has been closely linked to several non-communicable diseases, which include cardiovascular disease, diabetes mellitus, non-alcoholic fatty liver disease, dementia and many forms of cancer [3-9]. Insulin resistance has been proposed to be involved in the underlying pathogenesis of all of these diseases and also contributes to the development of cardiovascular risk factors such as hypertension, dyslipidemia, abnormal glucose tolerance and systemic inflammation [10, 11]. Insulin resistance may contribute to the development of hypertension by causing sodium retention by the kidneys and activating the sympathetic nervous system [12, 13]. It has been proposed that insulin resistance is associated with the release of pro-inflammatory cytokines from adipose tissue [14, 15]. Insulin resistance can also result in altered levels of adipokines, which are involved in glucose and energy homeostasis, and ultimately lead to deposition of fat in non-adipose tissues such as muscle and liver.

Increased fat mass in obese individuals could result in decreased sensitivity to the effects of insulin. Normally, insulin has a suppressive effect on adipose tissue lipolysis. When insulin resistance occurs, it leads to an increase in the release of free fatty acids (FFA) into the plasma. These circulating FFA are then free to be deposited in non-adipose tissues such as the liver and skeletal muscle, leading to the development of both hepatic and peripheral insulin resistance [16, 17].

Tissue Fat Deposition

In addition to the impact of BMI and total quantity of body fat, triglyceride deposition in certain tissues seems to confer an increased risk of developing insulin resistance. An excess of subcutaneous fat in areas such as the buttocks, thighs and extremities infers no additional risk. Conversely, an excess of visceral fat, which surrounds intra-abdominal organs such as the liver, is associated with an increased risk of developing insulin resistance and T2DM [18]. Forouhi *et al.* found that levels of the inflammatory marker, C-reactive protein, were strongly correlated with the amount of visceral adipose tissue in South Asians, suggesting that visceral adipose tissue promotes chronic inflammation resulting in insulin resistance [19].

Since an increase in visceral adipose tissue seemed to be associated with insulin resistance, it was of great interest to researchers to see whether removal of visceral fat would lead to an improvement in insulin sensitivity. Barzilai *et al.* observed the effect of removing visceral fat in Sprague-Dawley rats *via* surgery and found that insulin sensitivity increased in these rats compared to the rats who retained visceral fat, though the entire body fat mass was not different between the two groups. In addition, in the rats that had visceral fat removed surgically, there was a decrease in gene expression of both leptin and TNF-α in depots of subcutaneous fat, suggesting that visceral fat negatively impacts the secretory profile of adipose tissue [20]. In obese people with T2DM, evidence shows that insulin sensitivity can be improved by weight loss is a means of improving insulin sensitivity. Though a reduction in overall body weight occurs with weight loss, it can be surmised that a loss of visceral fat and intrahepatic fat content plays a role in the improvement of insulin sensitivity. Petersen *et al.* found that moderate weight loss in obese subjects with type 2 diabetes mellitus results in an improved hepatic insulin sensitivity. This may be attributed to a large decrease in hepatic triglyceride content as shown *via* magnetic resonance spectroscopy [21].

The prevalence of Non Alcoholic Fatty Liver Disease (NAFLD) has increased concomitantly with the rise in prevalence of obesity. NAFLD is defined by excess fat in the liver in the absence of any other liver disease, including alcoholic liver disease [22]. NAFLD and nonalcoholic steatohepatitis (NASH) are projected to be the predominant causes of cirrhosis in the next several years [23, 24]. Hepatic macrovesicular steatosis, defined by an excess of lipid accumulation in hepatocytes, can lead to distortion of the nucleus and this can lead to hepatic insulin resistance [24]. In a study by Kotronen *et al.* subjects with T2DM showed 80% more fat in the liver as well as more intra-abdominal fat when compared to the age and weight matched non-diabetic controls [25]. Eguchi *et al.* found a positive correlation between visceral fat accumulation and the severity of fatty liver disease regardless of the BMI [26]. The severity of liver disease in these subjects was also positively correlated to the degree of insulin resistance [26].

NAFLD in its initial stages is reversible by weight loss. NASH, characterized by damage to hepatocytes and mitochondrial dysfunction, is reversible as well [27-30]. As mentioned previously, this excessive deposition of fat in the liver occurs due to increased insulin resistance in adipose tissue, leading to inefficient suppression of lipolysis and accumulation of triglycerides in the plasma, which are then taken up by hepatocytes. However, nonalcoholic steatohepatitis can eventually lead to liver cirrhosis and hepatocellular carcinoma, thus illustrating the importance of preventing progression of NASH.

Skeletal muscle is another site of fat accumulation that can lead to insulin resistance, as it is largely responsible for whole body glucose disposal. More specifically, mitochondrial dysfunction in skeletal muscle plays a role in the development of insulin resistance and T2DM. There has been much debate in the scientific community about whether mitochondrial dysfunction causes insulin resistance or *vice versa*. Dumas *et al.* suggest that when skeletal muscle becomes inundated with fatty acids in excess of its capability to oxidize them, excessive lipid deposition occurs in the muscles [31]. Reactive oxygen species then accumulate in the skeletal muscle mitochondria, resulting in a decrease in insulin stimulated glucose uptake. On the other hand, one role of insulin in the body is to activate mitochondrial enzymes [32]. In states of insulin resistance, mitochondrial dysfunction occurs. Activity levels also play a role in skeletal muscle mitochondrial function. Lack of exercise leads to a decrease in the number of mitochondria, making it more difficult to sustain normal function [33]. Obesity is also associated with higher plasma triglyceride levels by way of inefficient suppression of lipolysis in states of adipose tissue insulin resistance. This leads to an increased intramyocellular lipid deposition, which overwhelms skeletal muscle mitochondria and their ability to oxidize the fat that is taken up. This eventually results in skeletal muscle insulin resistance. Whichever happens first, continues to be debatable, but skeletal muscle insulin resistance and mitochondrial dysfunction seem to coexist in many people suffering from obesity and T2DM [34].

Intriguingly, recent studies have shown a dissociation of mitochondrial dysfunction and insulin resistance in certain populations. Nair *et al.* studied Asian Indians, a group known to have a high prevalence of diabetes [35]. They found that Asian Indians were more insulin resistant in spite of a higher capacity for oxidative phosphorylation than Northern European American controls, suggesting that mitochondrial dysfunction was not the cause of greater insulin resistance in this group of people [35]. Chandalia *et al.* reported higher subcutaneous fat mass, larger adipocyte size, higher plasma levels of free fatty acids, and lower levels of adiponectin in South Asians as compared to Caucasians, with no differences in the BMI [36]. This is important because evidence shows that large adipocytes are essentially dysfunctional, and can therefore contribute to insulin resistance, regardless of fat mass or BMI [37, 38]. Thus, dysfunctional mitochondria might account for insulin resistance in Caucasians and other populations, but in South Asians, larger adipocytes may be one of the factors causing a higher prevalence of diabetes, regardless of the BMI. Thus, ethnicity seems to play a role in the mechanisms of acquiring insulin resistance.

Adipose Tissue Inflammation and the Immune System

Evidence shows a link between systemic inflammation and the development of insulin resistance [39]. Obesity is associated with increased infiltration of macrophages into the adipose tissue, leading to the formation of inflammatory cytokines [40]. A study performed by DiGregorio *et al.* in normal subjects shows that the quantity of adipose tissue macrophages and pro-inflammatory cytokines is inversely related to insulin action, suggesting that increased inflammation caused by adipose tissue pro-inflammatory cytokines is associated with the worsening of insulin resistance [41].

Stress leads to systemic inflammation by releasing pro-inflammatory cytokines from adipose tissue, which include interleukin-1-β (IL-1β), interleukin-6 (IL-6), tumor necrosis factor-α (TNF-α) and plasminogen activator inhibitor-1 (PAI-1) [14, 42, 43]. Elevated plasma levels of TNF-α have been observed in patients with stressors such as malignancy, infection, trauma and burn injuries [44-47]. It is known that diabetics have higher glucose levels during an infected state. This may be related to the release of proinflammatory cytokines long with other factors, illustrating the effects of inflammation on insulin sensitivity. Lang *et al.*

studied the effects of TNF-α on glucose homeostasis in rats, and observed that both hepatic and peripheral insulin resistance occurred with prolonged infusion of TNF-α [48]. Hotamisligil *et al.* observed a significant decrease in insulin sensitivity in adipocytes treated with TNF-α, thought to be caused by a reduction in the phosphorylation of insulin-receptor-substrate-1, a key step in the insulin signal transduction pathway [49].

Recent studies have attempted to elucidate whether certain infectious diseases can lead to obesity and insulin resistance by the production of pro-inflammatory cytokines. Mehta *et al.* studied infection with *Chlamydia pneumoniae*, a common cause of atypical pneumonia, and showed that it is associated with obesity in humans and also induces production of TNF-α [50, 51]. This in turn leads to diminished action of lipoprotein lipase, resulting in hypertriglyceridemia [50, 52]. Deposition of these excess triglycerides in non-adipose tissues can result in diminished insulin sensitivity. Recently, studies in mice have shown that *Trypanosoma cruzi*, a well-known cause of Chagas disease, can attack and remain in adipocytes for a long-term, allowing the infection to recur [53]. It has been observed that the incidence of diabetes is higher in patients infected with *Trypanosoma cruzi* [54]. The parasite causes an increase in the production of inflammatory cytokines, including TNF-α. TNF-α, in turn, inhibits the production of adiponectin, an adipocytokine produced by and specific to adipose tissue that has anti-inflammatory properties [55]. Desruisseaux *et al.* found significantly decreased levels of adiponectin in mice infected with *Trypanosoma cruzi* [53]. Low levels of adiponectin are associated with obesity and worsening of insulin resistance [56, 57].

Leptin, another adipocytokine predominantly produced by adipose tissue but also produced by immune cells, is also involved in the immune response to infection. Plasma leptin levels are increased significantly during active infection and sepsis, and are also increased in obesity. While adiponectin levels are inversely correlated with the degree of adiposity, leptin has a positive correlation. In the postprandial state, leptin is secreted by adipose tissue and induces satiety by acting on the hypothalamus [58]. During periods of starvation, leptin decreases in the body in order to conserve energy [59]. In both humans and rodents, leptin deficiency resulted in hyperphagia that led to obesity [60]. Ozata *et al.* found that patients with leptin deficiency due to a genetic cause suffered immune system dysfunction and morbid obesity [61]. Without leptin, the brain is unable to sense peripheral energy stores, which can lead to dysfunction of energy homeostasis and immune function. The results of these studies suggest that certain infectious diseases in conjunction with adipocytokine function and other factors may be linked to the development of obesity and insulin resistance.

In obese humans and rodents with a genetic cause for leptin deficiency, leptin administration resulted in satiety and weight loss [62-64]. In obese humans and rodents without a congenital leptin deficiency, serum leptin levels are elevated, as leptin levels typically correlate with the degree of adiposity. In such obese humans and rodents, administration of leptin alone without any other intervention did not induce satiety or result in significant weight loss [65, 66]. Since, leptin levels are elevated but have little effect on satiety or weight loss, such people are thought to be leptin resistant, similar to insulin resistance in obese subjects who have high levels of plasma insulin but whose tissues are resistant to its effects [67]. Current research indicates problems in leptin signaling in these obese subjects with hyperleptinemia. Though leptin administration alone in obese individuals with leptin resistance has shown little promise in achieving weight loss, a recent study by Roth *et al.* showed that administration of leptin along with an amylin analogue in obese humans and rodents resulted in an improvement in leptin sensitivity and signaling that resulted in greater weight loss than that observed by administration of leptin or amylin alone [68]. More research to divulge the reason behind this improvement in leptin resistance may prove useful in finding a successful solution to the global diabetes epidemic. By serving as a signal of the body's nutritional status and adipose tissue reserve, leptin's role is integral in maintaining energy homeostasis and normal metabolic function.

STATES OF NUTRITIONAL DEPRIVATION AND ADIPOSE DEPLETION

Malnutrition

Though obesity has become a global epidemic, nutrient deprivation still exists in many parts of the world. Many developing countries have inhabitants that still suffer from malnutrition due to poverty and inability to acquire food with adequate nutrients. Current estimates suggest that approximately 925 million people suffer from malnutrition globally [69]. Several studies have considered the implications of malnutrition and starvation at critical points throughout life, including during early development. One study assessed the individuals who suffered from malnutrition and starvation due to the Dutch famine in 1944. These individuals were all below the age of 21 during that time period. The results showed that starvation during childhood was associated with an increased risk of developing T2DM in adulthood [70].

Similar to the Dutch famine, another form of diabetes that is not yet well described or understood is malnutrition-modulated diabetes mellitus. Since its first description by Hugh Jones in 1955 in a small group of Jamaican patients, it has been reported in parts of Africa and Asia, including India [71]. This form of diabetes is different from type 1 diabetes mellitus, as patients do have some pancreatic reserve and are able to produce insulin, as indicated by persistent response of c-peptide to nutrient stimuli. These patients are insulin resistant rather than insulin deficient and do not develop ketosis in the absence of insulin therapy. Malnutrition-modulated diabetes mellitus is also different from type 2 diabetes in that patients are lean, typically with a BMI less than 18 kg/m^2 [72]. Common to most patients suffering from this disease is a history of severe malnutrition in utero or during early development, though many may be malnourished throughout most of their lives. A small percentage of patients with malnutrition-modulated diabetes mellitus may have positive serum autoimmune markers such as glutamic acid decarboxylase 65 (GAD 65) and insulinoma antigen 2 (IA-2) autoantibodies.

Onset of disease in patients afflicted with malnutrition-modulated diabetes mellitus is typically between ten to thirty years of age. Blood glucose levels are high at presentation, typically over 250 mg/dl, and fasting insulin levels are elevated. Patients tend to be highly insulin resistant, prompting treatment with high doses of insulin. No evidence of pancreatic pathology was found in imaging studies, differentiating this form of diabetes from fibrocalculous pancreatic diabetes [72]. Fibrocalculous pancreatic diabetes is a type of diabetes also commonly encountered in tropical areas, but differs from malnutrition-modulated diabetes mellitus in which patients have radiologic evidence of pancreatic calculi and/or chronic pancreatitis with no history of alcohol abuse [73]. It is important for the physician to differentiate between these diseases, as the management of each differs. Patients with fibrocalculous pancreatic diabetes should receive replacement of pancreatic enzymes and regular screenings to monitor for the development of pancreatic adenocarcinoma, one of the known complications of chronic pancreatitis [73]. Patients with malnutrition-modulated diabetes mellitus do not present with chronic pancreatitis, and therefore do not require the same follow-up or treatment. However, the metabolic features and body composition associated with this disease have not yet been widely studied or completely understood, limiting the ability to devise an appropriate treatment regimen. Without knowledge of the existence of this disease in tropical areas, patients are often inaccurately labeled as having type 1 diabetes mellitus and treated with insulin. If regular access to nutrition is unavailable and insulin therapy is continued, these patients may suffer from fatal hypoglycemia. Research aiming to understand the metabolic defects of this disease may lead to safer and more effective therapeutic approaches in this patient population. In order to better understand how malnutrition-modulated diabetes mellitus could result in metabolic complications including severe insulin resistance, two well-known models of nutrient deprivation and/or adipose tissue deficiency are discussed below.

Lipodystrophy

Like obesity and malnutrition-modulated diabetes mellitus, lipodystrophy is a condition that also results in metabolic complications. However, unlike those suffering from obesity, people with lipodystrophy have deficient amounts of white adipose tissue and are thus unable to adequately store triglycerides. To compensate for this inability to store excess energy accumulated *via* a meal, lipodystrophic patients will attempt to increase energy expenditure by increasing oxidation of fatty acids [74]. Once they exceed the capacity to increase energy expenditure, excess energy in the form of FFA accumulates in the plasma, resulting in triglyceride deposition in non-adipose tissues similar to their obese cohorts (Fig. **1**). Due to fat deposition in non-adipose tissues, patients with lipodystrophy tend to have associated metabolic complications similar to those seen in obese patients, including hepatic fat accumulation and steatosis, hypertriglyceridemia, insulin resistance and T2DM.

Both a paucity and an excess of adipose tissue causes increased flux of free fatty acids (FFA) to tissues such as skeletal muscle and liver, resulting in insulin resistance. Levels of the adipokines, adiponectin and leptin, which are secreted by adipose tissue, tend to be low in patients with lipodystrophy. Lipodystrophic patients also exhibit hyperphagia, which is thought to be due to low levels of leptin. Shimomura *et al.* found that giving recombinant leptin to mice with congenital lipodystrophy improved insulin sensitivity, while chronically calorie restricting lipodystrophic mice did not show the same effect, suggesting that the insulin resistance in lipodystrophic syndromes is due to a deficiency of leptin [75].

The lipodystrophy syndromes are characterized by the absence of subcutaneous adipose tissue. They are divided into four types, based on the pattern of adipose tissue loss and whether they are inherited or acquired [76]. Generalized lipodystrophy can be acquired or inherited. Patients with the congenital form have

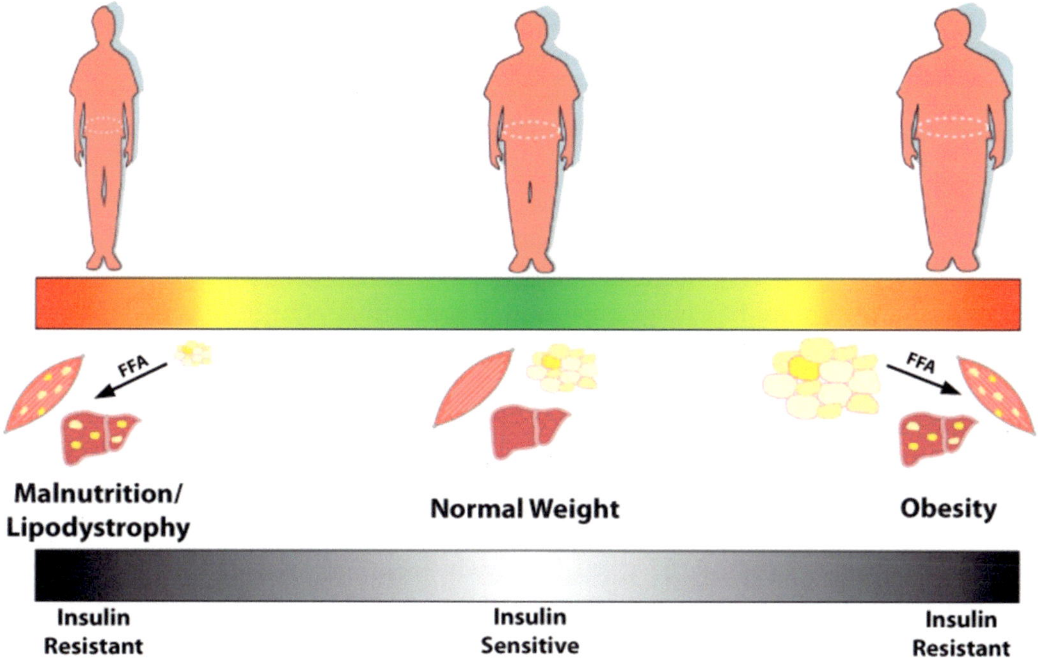

Fig. (1). Relationship between adipose tissue mass and insulin sensitivity.

absence of adipose tissue that manifests in infancy, with the lack of fat involving nearly the whole body, including the upper and lower extremities, face, neck, trunk and abdomen [76, 77]. The acquired form is associated with the loss of adipocytes in similar sites, but does not always involve loss of fat in the abdominal region. Both forms are associated with metabolic complications including insulin resistance, acanthosis nigricans, hypertriglyceridemia and hepatic steatosis [76].

Partial lipodystrophy can also be inherited or acquired, with the inherited form typically beginning with the loss of adipose tissue at or after puberty. The inherited form is associated with the loss of adipose tissue in the upper and lower extremities, while the acquired form is associated with the loss of adipocytes mainly in the upper body, targeting the face, neck, trunk and arms [76, 77]. Both forms of partial lipodystrophy can be associated with increased fat deposition in the abdominal region. HIV infection is associated with the acquired form of partial lipodystrophy [77].

Lipodystrophic patients tend to have severe insulin resistance, often requiring more than 2 units of insulin per kilogram per day. Their serum triglyceride levels tend to be over 500 mg/dl. Complications of inability to lower triglycerides may result, including recurrent pancreatitis and xanthomas [78]. Even with aggressive treatment to combat diabetes and hypertriglyceridemia, these patients have difficulty maintaining good glycemic and lipid control [78]. These patients also suffer from hyperphagia, likely related to low levels of leptin. Thus, Chan *et al.* treated fifty-five lipodystrophic patients with metreleptin, an analog of human leptin, and showed that leptin replacement improved glycemic control and lowered triglyceride levels in these subjects [79]. What science has taught us thus far about lipodystrophy has helped us gain a better understanding of conditions of adipose depletion and nutrient deprivation.

Anorexia Nervosa

Though nutrient deprivation due to poverty is less likely to exist in the United States today, nutrient deprivation due to self-inflicted starvation is of definite concern. Anorexia nervosa is a well-known psychiatric disorder involving a distorted body image, refusal to maintain a normal BMI and a pathologic fear of gaining weight, prompting self-imposed starvation. In light of the metabolic complications that arise from deficient amounts of white adipose tissue, as previously discussed in the lipodystrophic disorders, many studies have assessed the metabolic complications of starvation associated with anorexia nervosa. Mayer *et al.* assessed body fat distribution in anorexic women before and after refeeding and weight normalization and found that visceral fat depots and intramyocellular lipid deposition were greater in women with anorexia nervosa after refeeding compared with controls [80]. One proposed theory for this occurrence is that atrophy of subcutaneous fat depots in anorexic patients may occur during starvation. Subsequently, when the body is reintroduced to food, fat is redistributed to other available tissues, including the truncal region and skeletal muscle [81]. Prioletta *et al.* showed a strong correlation between increased abdominal fat and decreased insulin sensitivity in anorexic patients after weight normalization, but no correlation to BMI [81]. These results are similar to findings from studies involving obese patients and lipodystrophic patients, suggesting that fat distribution is a more accurate gauge of insulin sensitivity than overall BMI in diverse groups of patients at both extremes of the weight spectrum. In addition, the results from the study conducted by Prioletta *et al.* suggest that after weight normalization, anorexic patients develop a body composition and metabolic complications similar to that of lipodystrophic patients, where the absence of adequate subcutaneous fat causes lipids to accumulate in nonadipose tissues, resulting in insulin resistance [81].

Other studies involving subjects with anorexia nervosa have shown no difference or higher insulin sensitivity and higher adiponectin levels in anorexic subjects compared with controls [82, 83]. A possible explanation to these conflicting results is that these studies focused on anorexic patients of lower than normal BMI who had not undergone weight normalization or weight gain. Evidence has shown that fat mass itself may exert negative feedback on the production of adiponectin from fat tissue [83, 84]. In patients with anorexia nervosa who starve themselves to lose weight, lack of negative feedback could result from a significant loss of adipose tissue depots, leading to unrestrained production of adiponectin [83]. Adiponectin has a positive correlation with insulin sensitivity, so perhaps the unrestrained production of adiponectin in anorexic patients serves as a protective mechanism to preserve insulin sensitivity early on in the course of the disease. This could explain the higher insulin sensitivity and adiponectin levels seen in anorexic patients in the studies that assessed anorexic patients prior to weight normalization [82, 83]. However, if extreme fat loss resulted from severe starvation and malnutrition, defects in adipocyte function may develop over time and interfere with the regulation and production of adiponectin. This may result in lower than normal levels of adiponectin, similar to what occurs in the lipodystrophic syndromes. Moreover, with decreased levels of adiponectin, the protective effect on insulin sensitivity may disappear.

Without weight normalization, morbidity and mortality in patients with anorexia nervosa are high due to complications of starvation, including hypoglycemia, dehydration, electrolyte imbalance and dysrhythmias; but with weight normalization comes the possibility of fat redistribution and the burden of associated insulin resistance. Thus, the management of anorexia nervosa becomes a delicate balance of adequate but not over-nutrition and maintenance of energy homeostasis. Again, this model of nutritional deprivation and its metabolic sequelae could be helpful in informing our understanding of the etiology of malnutrition-modulated diabetes mellitus.

CONCLUSION

Access to cheap calories in the form of processed energy-dense foods and over-indulgence in beverages containing large amounts of high fructose corn syrup and empty calories devoid of any nutritional benefit have significantly contributed to the global epidemic of obesity. However, even in this era of epicurism, states of nutrient deficiency also exist in the form of nutrient deprivation due to poverty or self-inflicted starvation due to psychiatric illness. Additionally, states of adipose tissue depletion, such as lipodystrophy have been widely studied in order to understand the metabolic complications of a lack of adipose tissue in comparison to an excess of adipose tissue.

Over the last several years, evidence has shown that adipose tissue serves many roles. It is not only crucial in energy storage, but also has an endocrine function, secreting adipokines, cytokines and hormones that are essential for the maintenance of energy homeostasis. Although obesity and states involving paucity of adipose tissue are at two opposite ends of the weight spectrum, both of them paradoxically result in similar metabolic complications, including insulin resistance. This challenges the over-simplified notion that "weight loss cures diabetes". Weight loss is indeed beneficial in states of overabundance of adipose tissue, but it is not advisable in the lipodystrophy syndromes and other adipose deficient states. Factors determining the development of insulin resistance in both obesity and adipose tissue-deficient states include fat accumulation in non-adipose tissues especially the liver and skeletal muscle due to faulty oxidation of fatty acids, alterations in the levels of adipokines, adiponectin and leptin, and activation of inflammatory cascade in the adipose tissue.

Though the development of insulin resistance and diabetes ultimately represents a complex interplay of environment and genes, knowledge of the various mechanisms resulting in metabolic complications in states of obesity, deficient adipose tissue, and nutrient deprivation during early development, youth, and adulthood can be helpful in investigating various new treatments to improve morbidity and mortality associated with these conditions. Furthermore, it can be relevant in enhancing our understanding of states of malnutrition, such as malnutrition-modulated diabetes mellitus that have yet to be widely studied, leading to safer and more effective treatment regimens.

ACKNOWLEDGEMENTS

Declared none.

CONFLICT OF INTEREST

The authors confirm that this chapter contents have no conflict of interest.

REFERENCES

[1] Popkin BM, Gordon-Larsen P. The nutrition transition: worldwide obesity dynamics and their determinants. International journal of obesity and related metabolic disorders. Journal of the International Association for the Study of Obesity 2004 Nov; 28 Suppl 3: S2-9.
[2] Goran MI, Ulijaszek SJ, Ventura EE. High fructose corn syrup and diabetes prevalence: A global perspective. Global Public Health 2013 Jan; 8(1): 55-64.
[3] Monsour HP, Jr., Frenette CT, Wyne K. Fatty liver: a link to cardiovascular disease--its natural history, pathogenesis, and treatment. Methodist DeBakey Cardiovascular Journal 2012 Jul-Sep; 8(3): 21-5.
[4] Poirier P, Eckel RH. Obesity and cardiovascular disease. Current Atherosclerosis Reports 2002 Nov; 4(6): 448-53.
[5] Fabbrini E, Sullivan S, Klein S. Obesity and nonalcoholic fatty liver disease: biochemical, metabolic, and clinical implications. Hepatology 2010 Feb; 51(2): 679-89.
[6] Gendron TF, Zhang YJ, Petrucelli L. Does Obesity-Induced tau Phosphorylation Tip the Scale Toward Dementia? Diabetes 2013 May; 62(5): 1365-6.
[7] Ye J. Mechanisms of insulin resistance in obesity. Frontiers of Medicine 2013 Mar; 7(1): 14-24.
[8] Louie SM, Roberts LS, Nomura DK. Mechanisms linking obesity and cancer. Biochimica et biophysica acta 2013 Mar 5.
[9] McFarlane SI, Banerji M, Sowers JR. Insulin resistance and cardiovascular disease. The Journal of Clinical Endocrinology and Metabolism 2001 Feb; 86(2): 713-8.
[10] Folsom AR, Kushi LH, Anderson KE, *et al.* Associations of general and abdominal obesity with multiple health outcomes in older women: the Iowa Women's Health Study. Archives of Internal Medicine 2000 Jul 24; 160(14): 2117-28.
[11] Reaven GM. Banting lecture 1988. Role of insulin resistance in human disease. Diabetes 1988 Dec; 37(12): 1595-607.
[12] Sowers JR, Sowers PS, Peuler JD. Role of insulin resistance and hyperinsulinemia in development of hypertension and atherosclerosis. The Journal of Laboratory and Clinical Medicine 1994 May; 123(5): 647-52.
[13] Reaven GM, Lithell H, Landsberg L. Hypertension and associated metabolic abnormalities--the role of insulin resistance and the sympathoadrenal system. The New England Journal of Medicine 1996 Feb 8; 334(6): 374-81.
[14] Kern PA, Ranganathan S, Li C, Wood L, Ranganathan G. Adipose tissue tumor necrosis factor and interleukin-6 expression in human obesity and insulin resistance. American Journal of Physiology Endocrinology and Metabolism 2001 May; 280(5): E745-51.
[15] Trayhurn P, Beattie JH. Physiological role of adipose tissue: white adipose tissue as an endocrine and secretory organ. The Proceedings of the Nutrition Society 2001 Aug; 60(3): 329-39.
[16] Boden G, Shulman GI. Free fatty acids in obesity and type 2 diabetes: defining their role in the development of insulin resistance and beta-cell dysfunction. European Journal of Clinical Investigation 2002 Jun; 32 Suppl 3: 14-23.
[17] Robinson C, Tamborlane WV, Maggs DG, *et al.* Effect of insulin on glycerol production in obese adolescents. The American Journal of Physiology 1998 Apr; 274(4 Pt 1): E737-43.
[18] Kissebah AH, Krakower GR. Regional adiposity and morbidity. Physiological reviews 1994 Oct; 74(4): 761-811.
[19] Forouhi NG, Sattar N, McKeigue PM. Relation of C-reactive protein to body fat distribution and features of the metabolic syndrome in Europeans and South Asians. International journal of obesity and related metabolic disorders : Journal of the International Association for the Study of Obesity 2001 Sep; 25(9): 1327-31.
[20] Barzilai N, She L, Liu BQ, *et al.* Surgical removal of visceral fat reverses hepatic insulin resistance. Diabetes 1999 Jan; 48(1): 94-8.
[21] Petersen KF, Dufour S, Befroy D, Lehrke M, Hendler RE, Shulman GI. Reversal of nonalcoholic hepatic steatosis, hepatic insulin resistance, and hyperglycemia by moderate weight reduction in patients with type 2 diabetes. Diabetes 2005 Mar; 54(3): 603-8.

[22] Vanni E, Bugianesi E, Kotronen A, De Minicis S, Yki-Jarvinen H, Svegliati-Baroni G. From the metabolic syndrome to NAFLD or *vice versa*? Digestive and Liver Disease : Official Journal of the Italian Society of Gastroenterology and the Italian Association for the Study of the Liver 2010 May; 42(5): 320-30.

[23] Charlton M. Nonalcoholic fatty liver disease: a review of current understanding and future impact. Clinical gastroenterology and hepatology : the official clinical practice journal of the American Gastroenterological Association 2004 Dec; 2(12): 1048-58.

[24] Masuoka HC, Chalasani N. Nonalcoholic fatty liver disease: an emerging threat to obese and diabetic individuals. Annals of the New York Academy of Sciences 2013 Jan 30.

[25] Kotronen A, Juurinen L, Hakkarainen A, *et al.* Liver fat is increased in type 2 diabetic patients and underestimated by serum alanine aminotransferase compared with equally obese nondiabetic subjects. Diabetes Care 2008 Jan; 31(1): 165-9.

[26] Eguchi Y, Eguchi T, Mizuta T, *et al.* Visceral fat accumulation and insulin resistance are important factors in nonalcoholic fatty liver disease. Journal of Gastroenterology 2006 May; 41(5): 462-9.

[27] Chalasani N, Deeg MA, Crabb DW. Systemic levels of lipid peroxidation and its metabolic and dietary correlates in patients with nonalcoholic steatohepatitis. The American Journal of Gastroenterology 2004 Aug; 99(8): 1497-502.

[28] Perez-Carreras M, Del Hoyo P, Martin MA, *et al.* Defective hepatic mitochondrial respiratory chain in patients with nonalcoholic steatohepatitis. Hepatology 2003 Oct; 38(4): 999-1007.

[29] Promrat K, Kleiner DE, Niemeier HM, *et al.* Randomized controlled trial testing the effects of weight loss on nonalcoholic steatohepatitis. Hepatology 2010 Jan; 51(1): 121-9.

[30] Andersen T, Gluud C, Franzmann MB, Christoffersen P. Hepatic effects of dietary weight loss in morbidly obese subjects. Journal of Hepatology 1991 Mar; 12(2): 224-9. \

[31] Dumas JF, Simard G, Flamment M, Ducluzeau PH, Ritz P. Is skeletal muscle mitochondrial dysfunction a cause or an indirect consequence of insulin resistance in humans? Diabetes & metabolism 2009 Jun; 35(3): 159-67.

[32] Aguer C, Harper ME. Skeletal muscle mitochondrial energetics in obesity and type 2 diabetes mellitus: endocrine aspects. Best Practice & Research Clinical Endocrinology & Metabolism 2012 Dec; 26(6): 805-19.

[33] Turner N, Heilbronn LK. Is mitochondrial dysfunction a cause of insulin resistance? Trends in endocrinology and metabolism: TEM 2008 Nov; 19(9): 324-30.

[34] Sleigh A, Raymond-Barker P, Thackray K, *et al.* Mitochondrial dysfunction in patients with primary congenital insulin resistance. The Journal of Clinical Investigation 2011 Jun; 121(6): 2457-61.

[35] Nair KS, Bigelow ML, Asmann YW, *et al.* Asian Indians have enhanced skeletal muscle mitochondrial capacity to produce ATP in association with severe insulin resistance. Diabetes 2008 May; 57(5): 1166-75.

[36] Chandalia M, Lin P, Seenivasan T, *et al.* Insulin resistance and body fat distribution in South Asian men compared to Caucasian men. PloS one 2007; 2(8): e812.

[37] Weyer C, Foley JE, Bogardus C, Tataranni PA, Pratley RE. Enlarged subcutaneous abdominal adipocyte size, but not obesity itself, predicts type II diabetes independent of insulin resistance. Diabetologia 2000 Dec; 43(12): 1498-506.

[38] Lundgren M, Svensson M, Lindmark S, Renstrom F, Ruge T, Eriksson JW. Fat cell enlargement is an independent marker of insulin resistance and 'hyperleptinaemia'. Diabetologia 2007 Mar; 50(3): 625-33.

[39] Xu H, Barnes GT, Yang Q, *et al.* Chronic inflammation in fat plays a crucial role in the development of obesity-related insulin resistance. The Journal of Clinical Investigation 2003 Dec; 112(12): 1821-30.

[40] Weisberg SP, McCann D, Desai M, Rosenbaum M, Leibel RL, Ferrante AW, Jr. Obesity is associated with macrophage accumulation in adipose tissue. The Journal of Clinical Investigation 2003 Dec; 112(12): 1796-808.

[41] Di Gregorio GB, Yao-Borengasser A, Rasouli N, *et al.* Expression of CD68 and macrophage chemoattractant protein-1 genes in human adipose and muscle tissues: association with cytokine expression, insulin resistance, and reduction by pioglitazone. Diabetes 2005 Aug; 54(8): 2305-13.

[42] Alessi MC, Bastelica D, Morange, *et al.* Plasminogen activator inhibitor 1, transforming growth factor-beta1, and BMI are closely associated in human adipose tissue during morbid obesity. Diabetes 2000 Aug; 49(8): 1374-80.
[43] Loskutoff DJ, Samad F. The adipocyte and hemostatic balance in obesity: studies of PAI-1. Arteriosclerosis, Thrombosis, and Vascular Biology 1998 Jan; 18(1): 1-6.
[44] Marano MA, Moldawer LL, Fong Y, Wei H, Minei J, Yurt R, *et al.* Cachectin/TNF production in experimental burns and Pseudomonas infection. Archives of Surgery 1988 Nov; 123(11): 1383-8.
[45] Beutler B, Cerami A. The biology of cachectin/TNF--a primary mediator of the host response. Annual Review of Immunology 1989; 7: 625-55.
[46] Stovroff MC, Fraker DL, Norton JA. Cachectin activity in the serum of cachectic, tumor-bearing rats. Archives of Surgery 1989 Jan; 124(1): 94-9.
[47] Offner F, Philippe J, Vogelaers D, *et al.* Serum tumor necrosis factor levels in patients with infectious disease and septic shock. The Journal of Laboratory and Clinical Medicine 1990 Jul; 116(1): 100-5. PubMed PMID: 2376691.
[48] Lang CH, Dobrescu C, Bagby GJ. Tumor necrosis factor impairs insulin action on peripheral glucose disposal and hepatic glucose output. Endocrinology 1992 Jan; 130(1): 43-52.
[49] Hotamisligil GS, Murray DL, Choy LN, Spiegelman BM. Tumor necrosis factor alpha inhibits signaling from the insulin receptor. Proceedings of the National Academy of Sciences of the United States of America 1994 May 24; 91(11): 4854-8.
[50] Mehta JL, Saldeen TG, Rand K. Interactive role of infection, inflammation and traditional risk factors in atherosclerosis and coronary artery disease. Journal of the American College of Cardiology 1998 May; 31(6): 1217-25.
[51] Dhurandhar NV. Contribution of pathogens in human obesity. Drug News & Perspectives 2004 Jun; 17(5): 307-13.
[52] Kol A, Sukhova GK, Lichtman AH, Libby P. Chlamydial heat shock protein 60 localizes in human atheroma and regulates macrophage tumor necrosis factor-alpha and matrix metalloproteinase expression. Circulation 1998 Jul 28; 98(4): 300-7.
[53] Desruisseaux MS, Nagajyothi, Trujillo ME, Tanowitz HB, Scherer PE. Adipocyte, adipose tissue, and infectious disease. Infection and Immunity 2007 Mar; 75(3): 1066-78.
[54] dos Santos VM, da Cunha SF, Teixeira Vde P, *et al.* [Frequency of diabetes mellitus and hyperglycemia in chagasic and non-chagasic women]. Revista da Sociedade Brasileira de Medicina Tropical 1999 Sep-Oct; 32(5): 489-96.
[55] Nagajyothi F, Desruisseaux MS, Weiss LM, *et al.* Chagas disease, adipose tissue and the metabolic syndrome. Memorias do Instituto Oswaldo Cruz 2009 Jul; 104 Suppl 1: 219-25.
[56] Padmalayam I, Suto M. Role of Adiponectin in the metabolic syndrome: current perspectives on its modulation as a treatment strategy. Current Pharmaceutical Design 2013 Feb 20.
[57] Yamauchi T, Kadowaki T. Adiponectin receptor as a key player in healthy longevity and obesity-related diseases. Cell metabolism 2013 Feb 5; 17(2): 185-96.
[58] Coll AP, Farooqi IS, O'Rahilly S. The hormonal control of food intake. Cell 2007 Apr 20; 129(2): 251-62.
[59] Ahima RS, Prabakaran D, Mantzoros, *et al.* Role of leptin in the neuroendocrine response to fasting. Nature 1996 Jul 18; 382(6588): 250-2.
[60] Clement K, Vaisse C, Lahlou N, *et al.* A mutation in the human leptin receptor gene causes obesity and pituitary dysfunction. Nature 1998 Mar 26; 392(6674): 398-401.
[61] Ozata M, Ozdemir IC, Licinio J. Human leptin deficiency caused by a missense mutation: multiple endocrine defects, decreased sympathetic tone, and immune system dysfunction indicate new targets for leptin action, greater central than peripheral resistance to the effects of leptin, and spontaneous correction of leptin-mediated defects. The Journal of Clinical Endocrinology and Metabolism 1999 Oct; 84(10): 3686-95.
[62] Farooqi IS, Matarese G, Lord GM, *et al.* Beneficial effects of leptin on obesity, T cell hyporesponsiveness, and neuroendocrine/metabolic dysfunction of human congenital leptin deficiency. The Journal of clinical investigation 2002 Oct; 110(8): 1093-103.
[63] Chehab FF, Lim ME, Lu R. Correction of the sterility defect in homozygous obese female mice by treatment with the human recombinant leptin. Nature Genetics 1996 Mar; 12(3): 318-20.

[64] Farooqi IS, Jebb SA, Langmack G, *et al.* Effects of recombinant leptin therapy in a child with congenital leptin deficiency. The New England Journal of Medicine 1999 Sep 16; 341(12): 879-84.
[65] Heymsfield SB, Greenberg AS, Fujioka K, *et al.* Recombinant leptin for weight loss in obese and lean adults: a randomized, controlled, dose-escalation trial. JAMA : the Journal of the American Medical Association 1999 Oct 27; 282(16): 1568-75.
[66] Halaas JL, Boozer C, Blair-West J, Fidahusein N, Denton DA, Friedman JM. Physiological response to long-term peripheral and central leptin infusion in lean and obese mice. Proceedings of the National Academy of Sciences of the United States of America 1997 Aug 5; 94(16): 8878-83.
[67] Bluher S, Mantzoros CS. Leptin in humans: lessons from translational research. The American journal of clinical nutrition 2009 Mar; 89(3): 991S-7S.
[68] Roth JD, Roland BL, Cole RL, *et al.* Leptin responsiveness restored by amylin agonism in diet-induced obesity: evidence from nonclinical and clinical studies. Proceedings of the National Academy of Sciences of the United States of America 2008 May 20; 105(20): 7257-62.
[69] McGuire S. WHO, World Food Programme, and International Fund for Agricultural Development 2012. The State of Food Insecurity in the World 2012. Economic growth is necessary but not sufficient to accelerate reduction of hunger and malnutrition. Rome, FAO. Advances in Nutrition 2013 Jan; 4(1): 126-7.
[70] van Abeelen AF, Elias SG, Bossuyt PM, *et al.* Famine exposure in the young and the risk of type 2 diabetes in adulthood. Diabetes 2012 Sep; 61(9): 2255-60.
[71] Hugh-Jones P. Diabetes in Jamaica. Lancet 1955 Oct 29; 269(6896): 891-7.
[72] Samal KC, Kanungo A, Sanjeevi CB. Clinicoepidemiological and biochemical profile of malnutrition-modulated diabetes mellitus. Annals of the New York Academy of Sciences 2002 Apr; 958: 131-7.
[73] Mohan V, Farooq S, Deepa M. Prevalence of fibrocalculous pancreatic diabetes in Chennai in South India. JOP : Journal of the Pancreas 2008; 9(4): 489-92.
[74] Savage DB, Murgatroyd PR, Chatterjee VK, O'Rahilly S. Energy expenditure and adaptive responses to an acute hypercaloric fat load in humans with lipodystrophy. The Journal of clinical endocrinology and metabolism 2005 Mar; 90(3): 1446-52.
[75] Shimomura I, Hammer RE, Ikemoto S, Brown MS, Goldstein JL. Leptin reverses insulin resistance and diabetes mellitus in mice with congenital lipodystrophy. Nature 1999 Sep 2; 401(6748): 73-6.
[76] Handelsman Y, Oral EA, Bloomgarden ZT, *et al.* The clinical approach to the detection of lipodystrophy - an AACE consensus statement. Endocrine Practice : Official Journal of the American College of Endocrinology and the American Association of Clinical Endocrinologists 2013 Jan-Feb; 19(1): 107-16.
[77] Mantzoros CS. Leptin in relation to the lipodystrophy-associated metabolic syndrome. Diabetes & Metabolism Journal 2012 Jun; 36(3): 181-9.
[78] Simha V, Garg A. Lipodystrophy: lessons in lipid and energy metabolism. Current opinion in lipidology 2006 Apr; 17(2): 162-9.
[79] Chan JL, Lutz K, Cochran E, *et al.* Clinical effects of long-term metreleptin treatment in patients with lipodystrophy. Endocrine Practice : Official Journal of the American College of Endocrinology and the American Association of Clinical Endocrinologists 2011 Nov-Dec; 17(6): 922-32.
[80] Mayer L, Walsh BT, Pierson RN, Jr., *et al.* Body fat redistribution after weight gain in women with anorexia nervosa. The American Journal of Clinical Nutrition 2005 Jun; 81(6): 1286-91.
[81] Prioletta A, Muscogiuri G, Sorice GP, *et al.* In anorexia nervosa, even a small increase in abdominal fat is responsible for the appearance of insulin resistance. Clinical Endocrinology 2011 Aug; 75(2): 202-6.
[82] Karczewska-Kupczewska M, Straczkowski M, Adamska A, *et al.* Insulin sensitivity, metabolic flexibility, and serum adiponectin concentration in women with anorexia nervosa. Metabolism: Clinical and Experimental 2010 Apr; 59(4): 473-7.
[83] Delporte ML, Brichard SM, Hermans MP, Beguin C, Lambert M. Hyperadiponectinaemia in anorexia nervosa. Clinical Endocrinology 2003 Jan; 58(1): 22-9.
[84] Halleux CM, Takahashi M, Delporte ML, *et al.* Secretion of adiponectin and regulation of apM1 gene expression in human visceral adipose tissue. Biochemical and Biophysical Research cCmmunications 2001 Nov 16; 288(5): 1102-7.

CHAPTER 5

Moving Beyond Metabolic Syndrome: Assessing Diabetes and Cardiometabolic Risk

K. Indulekha[1,2], C.S. Pitchumoni[3] and V. Mohan[*,1,2]

[1]Department of Diabetology & Epidemiology, Madras Diabetes Research Foundation, India; [2]Dr. Mohan's Diabetes Specialities Centre, Chennai - 600086, India; and [3]Department of Gastroenterology, Hepatology, and Clinical Nutrition, Saint Peter's, University Hospital, New Brunswick, NJ 08903, USA

Abstract: Association of metabolic abnormalities including glucose intolerance, hypertension, central obesity and dyslipidemia comprise what is called "Metabolic Syndrome (MS)". It is known that MS is a risk factor for both diabetes and cardiovascular disease (CVD). Non-alcoholic fatty liver disease (NAFLD) has also emerged as an important metabolic disease which is associated with both diabetes and cardiovascular disease. South Asian countries and particularly India have very high prevalence rates of MS and NAFLD. Moreover, the prevalence of type 2 diabetes and premature coronary artery disease is very high. However, the link between MS, NAFLD and CVD are not very well defined. This chapter reviews in detail the association of MS with CVD and also NAFLD and CVD. It also discusses the controversies with MS and highlights current strategies involved in management of MS and NAFLD.

Keywords: Activity, behavior, cardiovascular disease, cardiovascular risk, global health, hepatology, intervention, lifestyle, liver disease, metabolic syndrome, obesity, overweight, south Asians, type 2 diabetes, wellness.

INTRODUCTION

Metabolic abnormalities, which include glucose intolerance, hypertension, central obesity and dyslipidemia, are often referred to as "Metabolic Syndrome (MS)". Health risks associated with MS include diabetes and cardiovascular disease (CVD). Non-alcoholic fatty liver disease (NAFLD) is an associated metabolic abnormality that may play a role in the pathogenesis of diabetes and cardiovascular disease, but little is known about the relationship. South Asian countries and particularly India have very high prevalence rates of MS and

***Corresponding author** V. Mohan: No. 4 Conran Smith Road, Gopalapuram, Chennai - 600 086. India; Tel: 91-44-43968888; Fax: 91-44-28350935, E-mail: drmohans@diabetes.ind.in

Judith Wylie-Rosett & Sunil S. Jhangiani (Eds)

NAFLD. This chapter reviews how MS is related to obesity and the risk for CVD and NAFLD. It also discusses the controversies surrounding MS and highlights current strategies involved in management of MS and NAFLD.

HISTORY OF METABOLIC SYNDROME (MS)

The concept of MS, or insulin resistance syndrome, or 'Syndrome X' as it was once called, was introduced in 1988 by Gerald Reaven in his Banting lecture titled "The role of insulin resistance in human disease". The underlying pathophysiology of metabolic syndrome was elegantly described by Reaven in terms of a string of metabolic abnormalities including hyperinsulinaemia, hypertension, hyperglycemia and dyslipidaemia with the suggestion that insulin resistance was the core defect [1]. It took several years for Reaven to bring in the theme of central adiposity as a critical factor underlying the pathology of the syndrome which was one of the highlights of his Claude Bernard Lecture several years later. Yet, the 'Syndrome X' described by Reaven was imprecise and had several shortcomings when it came to identifying individuals with the syndrome in terms of the number, combination and cut points of the abnormalities constituting the syndrome [2]. Earlier, Kylin [3] and Jean Vague [4] proposed the association between diabetes, atherosclerosis, central adiposity and gout during the 1920s and 1940s respectively. In 1985, Michaela Modan [5] proposed hyperinsulinemia as the major connecting link between glucose intolerance, obesity and hypertension. 'Syndrome X' has now come to be referred to as the Metabolic syndrome (MS). The original definition of MS included hyperinsulinemia, impaired glucose tolerance, hypertriglyceridemia, reduced HDL cholesterol and hypertension. More expanded definitions have been proposed over the past two decades with the inclusion of alternative traits like prothrombotic state, microalbuminuria and central obesity as components of metabolic syndrome. The existence of various definitions has led to considerable ambiguity and the question of whether MS should be considered as a specific entity at all has arisen. Yet, in its defense, MS has, over time, made physicians and patients aware of the interactions between the individual components of the syndrome and the benefits of lifestyle modifications in its management.

DEFINITIONS OF MS

Current Criteria for MS

Several definitions of MS have been put forth by different organizations like the World Health Organization (WHO) (1999) [6], International Diabetes Federation

(IDF) (2005) [7], the U.S. National Cholesterol Education Program and the Adult Treatment Panel III (NCEP- ATP III) (2001) [8], and the European Group for the Study of Insulin Resistance (EGIR) (1999) [9]. The definitions are summarized in Table **1**.

Table 1. Different criteria for metabolic syndrome.

Components of MS	IDF Consensus (2005)	NCEP ATP III Criteria (2001)	WHO Criteria (1999)	EGIR (1999)
Obesity/Abdominal obesity	Waist circumference ≥ 90 cm (M), ≥ 80 cm (F)-South Asians	Waist circumference ≥ 102 cm (M), ≥ 88 cm (F)	Body mass index (BMI) ≥ 30 kg/m^2 and/or waist-to-hip ratio > 0.90 (M), > 0.85 (F)	Waist circumference ≥ 94 cm (M)), ≥ 80 cm (F)
Blood pressure	> 130 / >85 mm Hg or on medication	> 130 / >85 mm Hg or on medication	≥ 140 / ≥ 90 mm Hg or on medication	≥140/90 mm Hg or on medication
Fasting glucose	≥ 100 mg/dl or pre-existing DM	≥ 110 mg/dl or on medication	Diabetes, impaired glucose tolerance (IGT) or insulin resistance	IGT or Impaired Fasting Glucose (IFG) but not diabetes
Triglycerides	≥ 150 mg/dl	≥ 150 mg/dl	≥ 150 mg/dl	TG ≥ 177 mg/dl and/or HDL-C
HDL Cholesterol	< 40 mg/dl (M), < 50 mg/dl (f)	< 40 mg/dl (M), < 50 mg/dl (F)	Not in criteria	< 39 mg/dl or treated for dyslipidemia
Insulin-resistance	Not in criteria	Not in criteria	glucose uptake below the lowest quartile under hyperinsulinemic, euglycemic conditions	Plasma insulin > 75th percentile
Microalbuminuria	Not in criteria	Not in criteria	Urinary albumin excretion rate ≥20 μg/min or albumin:creatinine ratio ≥30 mg/g	Not in criteria
Metabolic syndrome-definition	Obesity plus two of the other criteria	At least three risk factors	Diabetes, impaired glucose tolerance or insulin resistance plus any two or more risk factors	Insulin resistance plus any two of the other risk factors

Apart from the above major definitions there also exist other definitions with minor variations. For instance, in 2004, the NCEP definition was revised as rNCEP definition by lowering the threshold for fasting glucose to ≥ 100 mg/dl according to the American Diabetes Association (ADA) criteria for impaired fasting glucose (IFG) [9]. Also the South Asian modified (SAM)-NCEP definition has been introduced for the South Asian ethnic group [10].

MS - GLOBAL OVERVIEW

It is difficult to compare the published data on the prevalence of MS in different populations because they differ widely in terms of sample selection, study design, the definition of MS used as well as the age and gender structure of the population. The prevalence of MS in a Chinese population was reported to be 33.7% [11]. Using different definitions, Pakistan showed prevalence ranging from 18-46% comparable to other south Asian nations [12]. Azizi *et al.* based a study in Iran using ATP III definitions and found MS to be prevalent in 30.1% of the population [13]. A study carried out in several geographical regions of Turkey, showed that 27% of males and 38.6% of females had metabolic syndrome by the ATP III criteria [14].

Ireland reported a prevalence of 25% by WHO criteria and 20.7% by ATP III criteria in a survey population recruited from a primary care setting [15]. In the United States, native Americans in the age group of 45-49 showed a prevalence of 50.1% whereas Mexican Americans showed a prevalence of 29% in men and 32.8% in women and among non-Hispanic whites, 23% had MS [16, 17]. The estimated prevalence of MS in a Canadian population was 19.1% [18].

MS in Asian Indians

The prevalence of MS in the south Asian population is high. With the development of MS in the south Asian population, there are many potential risk factors including decreased physical activity, urbanization, high carbohydrate intake, lower intake of w-3 PUFAs, high fat intake and increased life expectancy [19].

Using the ATP III definition (modified for waist circumference as appropriate for Indians), the prevalence of MS has been found to be 41.1% [20]. In another study which used the EGIR definition, the prevalence was reported to be 11.2% in the same population [21]. A study from south India has estimated the prevalence of MS to be 25.8% by the IDF criteria, 23.2% by the WHO criteria and 18.3% by the NCEP ATP III criteria [22]. Moreover the conventional risk factors comprising the metabolic syndrome are highly prevalent in Asian Indians. It has been shown that the prevalence of abdominal obesity is 31.4%; hypertension 55.4%; low HDL 65.5% and raised fasting glucose 26.7% [23-25]. However, the prevalence of MS in a rural area population was found to be as low as 5% in central India [26] compared to an urban area population, where about one third of individuals have MS [23]. The high prevalence of MS in Asian Indians could be attributed to the higher prevalence of insulin resistance [27]. Even in younger populations the prevalence of insulin resistance has been shown to be fourfold higher than that of other ethnic groups [28]. Moreover, Asian Indians show very low levels of HDL compared to other populations which could increase their risk of MS [29]. The levels of LDL and atherogenic small dense LDL have also been reported to be higher among the south Asians [30].

The overall prevalence of MS among the expatriate south Asian population was shown to vary between 21% to 46%. Tan *et al.* [31] have shown that the prevalence of MS in Asian Indians according to NCEP-ATP III criteria was 13.1% in males and 11% in females whereas the modified NCEP-ATP criteria was estimated the prevalence to be 20.9% in males and 15.5% females living in Singapore. In another study done by Tillin *et al.* [32] using WHO criteria, the prevalence of MS in South Asians was determined to be 46% in males and 31% in females. By NCEP-ATP III criteria the prevalence was 29% in males and 32% in females living in London [32]. Hence there is a wide variation in the prevalence of MS in expatriate south Asians according to the degree of urbanization, socio-economic factors and patterns of life style.

MANAGEMENT OF THE RISK FACTORS

Abdominal Obesity

In individuals with MS and abdominal obesity, the first priority is to reduce body weight by means of increasing their physical activity and decreasing their caloric intake [33]. See Fig. (**1**) for the components and causes of metabolic syndrome. The Chennai Urban Population Study (CUPS), an epidemiological study conducted on a south Indian population has shown that the prevalence of MS increased with decrease in physical activity [34]. Radhika *et al.* in a population of urban Asian Indians have shown that the consumption of refined grains was associated with insulin resistance and metabolic syndrome [35]. The initial target of weight reduction could be set to bring about a reduction of about 8- 10% from the original weight in a time span of one year which translates to bringing about a decrease of about 500 calories per day [33]. Attainment of the required amount of weight loss would greatly reduce the severity of most of the metabolic parameters. Obesity could also be managed by means of drugs, but the currently available options are not desirable [36]. In selective cases, bariatric surgery may offer a treatment option [37].

Elevated Blood Pressure

The specific treatment goal for elevated blood pressure in subjects with MS should stress on lifestyle changes. Mild elevations in blood pressure could be adequately managed by control of body weight *via* increased physical activity and by the consumption of a diet rich in fresh fruits and vegetables, and low in salt and fatty foods [38]. Apart from diet and physical activity, angiotensin-converting enzyme (ACE) inhibitors or angiotensin receptor blockers are currently preferred.

Elevated Fasting Glucose

Ford *et al.* (2008) had compared the association between MS and the incidence of diabetes after a follow up period of 6 years using various criteria used for MS [39]. It was found that the hazard ratio by the NCEP definition was 4.6 while that of the IDF definition was 4.5. Among the various components of MS, abdominal obesity and hyperglycemia were most strongly associated with incidence of diabetes [39]. In a population of Pima Indians, hyperinsulinemia, body size, blood pressure, and lipid metabolism had been shown to be more closely related to the incidence of diabetes. Hence, in patients with MS, implementing effective weight reduction or increased physical activity would delay the onset of frank diabetes. Oral hypoglycemic agents like metformin, acarbose or glitazones are conventionally recommended by physicians for the treatment of type 2 diabetes.

Atherogenic Dyslipidemia

Dyslipidemia in south Asians characterized by high circulating levels of apolipoprotein B, lipoprotein a and lower levels of Apo A1 and HDL cholesterol predisposes this population to higher risk of diabetes, metabolic syndrome and coronary heart disease [40]. Controlling LDL-C is the major target of lipid lowering therapy and the next target is the elevated triglyceride levels. Apart from these major targets, an elevated level of apolipoprotein B is also important in lipid lowering therapy [41].

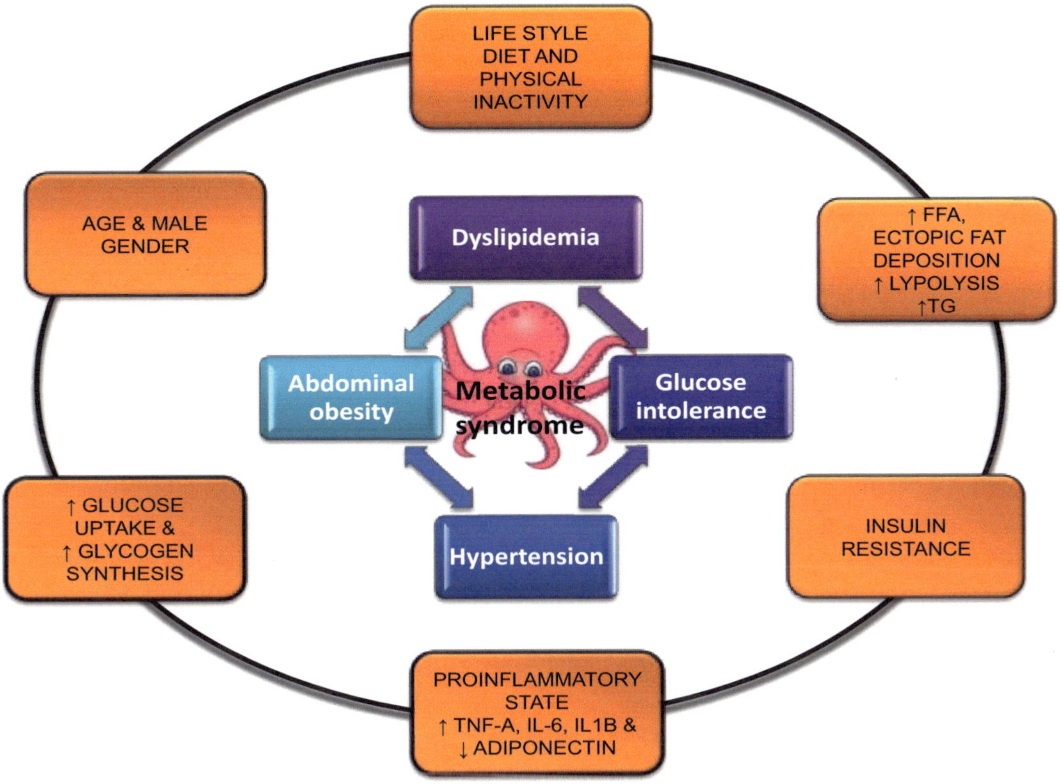

Fig. (1). Components and causes of metabolic syndrome.

Inflammation is a biological response elicited by the tissues to pathogens or cellular stress like high blood glucose/lipids or damaged cells [42]. Persistent inflammation also called chronic inflammation features the migration of macrophages to the site of injury and obesity, an integral component of MS has been shown to be associated with chronic low grade inflammation [43]. We have shown that MS is characterized by the reduced levels of the adiponectin, an anti-inflammatory and anti-atherogenic adipocytokine secreted by the adipose tissue [44]. Moreover MS also shows increased levels of inflammatory markers like high sensitivity C-reactive protein (hs-CRP), tumor necrosis factor-alpha (TNF-a) [45] and atherogenic markers like vascular cell adhesion protein 1 (VCAM), soluble P-selectin and CD40 ligand (CD40L) [46] and Angiopoitein-2 [47]. Also, inflammatory mediators secreted by immune cells such as cytokines Th-1 and Th-2 were also increased in subjects with MS [48]. Intimal media thickness (a surrogate marker for sub-clinical atherosclerosis) has also been found to be associated with metabolic syndrome and glucose intolerance in Asian Indians [49].

MS AND DIABETES

MS and Cardiovascular Vascular Disease (CVD)

A number of longitudinal studies have ascribed the cardiovascular risk associated with MS [50-54]. Meta analysis studies have shown that metabolic syndrome is associated with a higher cardiovascular risk in women when compared to men. After an 8 year follow up, it was shown that the MS group had a 17.9% incidence as against 4.9% in the non-MS group [55]. In subjects without Type 2 DM, it was shown that in MS group, the incidence of CVD was 10.2% and the non-MS group showed an incidence of 4.9% [56]. Among Japanese men, the CVD prevalence was 12.3% in the MS group compared to 6.5% in the non-MS group [57]. In patients without diabetes, the incidence of myocardial infarction after a follow up of 10 years was found to be 5.8% in the MS group and 2.9% in the non-MS group [58]. In a general population, the incidence of MI was found to be 9.1% in the MS group compared to 5.7% in the non- MS group after a follow up of 6 years [59].

Irrespective of the definition used, MS was noted to be associated with an increased risk of CVD mortality. In non-obese men, the CVD mortality in the MS group after a follow up of 10 years was found to be 1.99% compared to 0.53% in the non-MS group [60]. Also, in the general population, the MS group showed a higher CVD mortality of 7.3% compared to 2.4% in the non-MS group [61]. According to the revised NCEP definition for MS, the CVD mortality in the MS group was found to be 7.5% *vs* 3.9% in the non-MS group [62].

CONTROVERSIES AND UTILITY OF MS

Controversies Regarding the Metabolic Syndrome

Due to the existence of various criteria for metabolic syndrome, there are concerns over the etiology of the syndrome itself. Every combination of the proposed risk factors could impart a different degree of risk for the occurrence of CVD [63]. Also the risk for the occurrence of CVD due to MS appears to be equal to that of the sum of its components. Further, other CVD risk factors, such as inflammatory markers, are not included as components of MS [45]. Hence MS would not account for the actual underlying CVD risk that an individual is subjected to. Though insulin resistance has been widely accepted as a causative factor in the pathogenesis of MS, it is likely that insulin resistance could be just another demonstration of an underlying causative factor. Even if MS is identified, the patient is treated only for its individual components. There is no unifying treatment strategy for MS as a whole and this might raise questions about the utility of diagnosing MS [64]. Further, it communicates to the patients that they have a disease even if they do not have one and hence detracts from the need to prioritize treatment based on benefits, risks and cost.

Utility of the Diagnosis Of Metabolic Syndrome

Irrespective of the question of a common etiology underlying the components of MS, identification of MS clearly recognizes individuals at heightened risk for diabetes and cardiovascular diseases [58, 59, 65]. The recommendations proposed by NCEP-ATPIII clearly state that there is a dire need for emphasizing life style interventions to combat the CVD risk factors [66]. Hence diagnosis of MS leads to enhanced treatment strategies. Also conducting research on MS could throw light on the pathophysiological mechanisms that link insulin resistance and CVD risk factors (Fig. **2**). Apart from predicting CVD risk in patients with diabetes, individuals who do not have diabetes can also be assessed for their CVD risk. MS as a risk factor for NAFLD, steatohepatitis, cirrhosis, and as an independent risk factor for CVD warrants a discussion of the topic below.

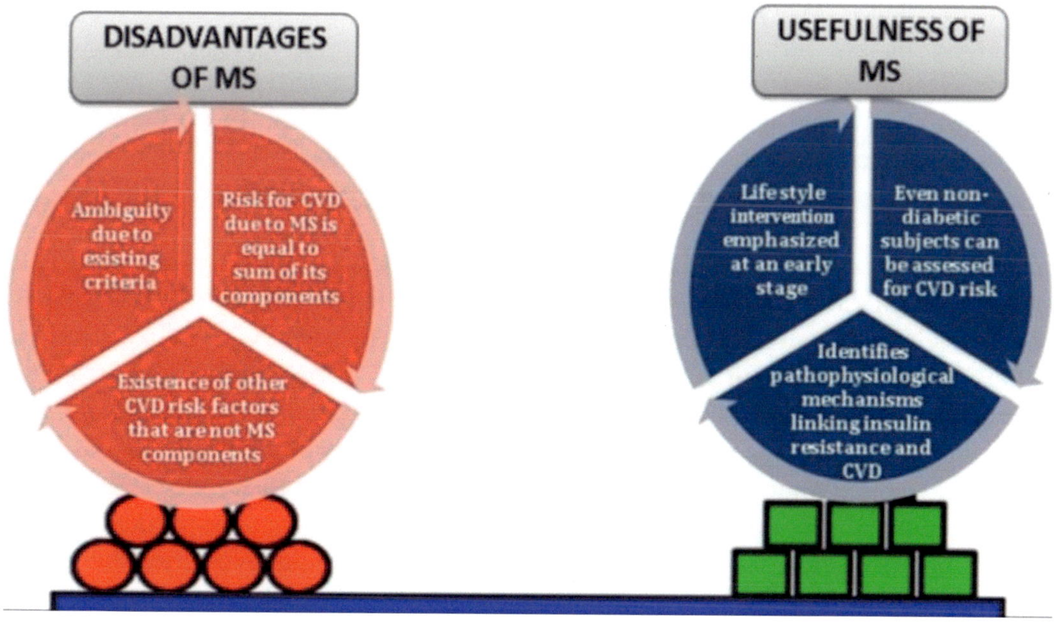

Fig. (2). Disadvantages and usefulness of metabolic syndrome.

NON-ALCOHOLIC FATTY LIVER DISEASE (NAFLD)

It is a spectrum of liver pathology seen in persons without significant alcohol consumption that includes four stages i) simple steatosis or non alcoholic fatty liver (NAFLD), ii) steatosis with inflammatory cells (Non alcoholic steatohepatitis or NASH) and iii) fibrosis with cirrhosis also referred as cryptogenic cirrhosis which may be rarely complicated by iv) hepatoma (see also CHAPTER 7, From Fatty Liver to Cirrhosis: The Toll Rises!). The diagnosis and management of NAFLD is well reviewed recently by three leading professional societies of Gastroenterology in the US, the American Association of Liver Diseases (AASLD), the American College of Gastroenterology (ACG) and the American Gastroenterological Association (AGA) [67]. NAFLD mostly occurs in association with other features of MS although it may be seen in non-diabetics or prediabetics as well.

DIAGNOSIS OF NAFLD AND NASH

NAFLD is often a diagnosis of exclusion on the basis of the following:

- There is evidence of steatosis in the liver noted in histology or in an imaging study
- There is no other cause for steatosis (hepatitis C, B, medications, autoimmune hepatitis, hemochromatosis and malnutrition) and there is no significant alcohol consumption. Although the definition of non-alcoholism or "significant alcohol consumption" is debatable, the threshold has been set as 20g/day for men and 10g/day for women recently [68].

Further in a large, well-characterized population with biopsy-proven NAFLD, modest alcohol consumption was associated with lesser degree of severity as determined by lower odds of the key features that comprise a diagnosis of steatohepatitis, as well as fibrosis. NAFLD is most often clinically silent and hence the prevalence markedly underestimated. The diagnosis is often incidental. A routine liver chemistry or an imaging study such as abdominal ultrasound may pick up the hepatic abnormality. Patients are often noted to have a greater increase in serum levels of alanine amino transferase (ALT) than aspartate amino transferase (AST). The levels are typically elevated less than five times the upper limit of normal, with AST /ALT ratio being less than one except when the disease has progressed to cirrhosis. An initial abdominal ultrasound or CT scan of abdomen will reveal increased echogenicity. Other non-invasive tests such as fibroscan would help in the assessment of liver stiffness. Liver biopsy is expensive, not practical in most patients and is associated with some degree of risk and should be considered only in selected few patients who have competing etiological factors for fatty liver and or in those at risk for advanced fibrosis [67].

The following histologic diagnostic criteria based on the US Pathology Committee system's recommendation suggests semi quantitative estimation of four features a) steatosis, b) lobular inflammation c) hepatocyte ballooning and d) fibrosis [69]. Significant steatosis is defined as fat accumulation in more than 5% of hepatocytes. NASH is diagnosed histologically when there is associated necroinflammation, hepatocyte ballooning and inflammatory infiltrates with or without fibrosis. NAFLD activity score is a term (NAS) that denotes an unweighted composite of steatosis, inflammation and ballooning. NAS is a useful tool to assess the progress in liver histology in clinical trials. A new marker is a serum fragmented Cytokeratin 18 level that reflects the histologic activity score of NASH [70].

PATHOGENESIS OF NAFLD

NAFLD is closely associated with MS and in particular with insulin resistance (IR). IR increases hepatic free fatty acid flux by inhibiting lipolysis and increasing *de novo* lipogenesis. Apoptosis and oxidative stress contribute to disease progression. A two hit or multiple hit hypothesis suggests initial accumulation of fat in the liver that leads to a second hit in some by free fatty acids, cytokines and oxidative stress. An imbalance between pro inflammatory TNF-alpha and adiponectin is a major pathogenetic factor. TNF-alpha is pro-apoptotic and recruits inflammatory cells and promotes insulin resistance. Adiponectin stimulates oxidation, inhibits fatty acid uptake, and decreases insulin resistance [66].

DIABETES AND NAFLD

The prevalence of NAFLD was found to increase in parallel with the severity of glucose intolerance. Kim *et al.* reported an independent association between moderate/ severe NAFLD and incident diabetes compared to patients with mild NAFLD [71]. Elevation in the levels of aminotransferases in the plasma has been shown to increase the risk of type 2 diabetes [72]. Diabetic patients were also found to have almost an 80% increase in intrahepatic fat content than their non-diabetic counterparts [73]. Reports also show that diabetes and insulin resistance are significantly associated with ectopic fat deposition in the liver and hepatic steatosis and hepatic insulin resistance often occur in conjunction. In animal models, it has been shown that insulin resistance is the major pathogenic factor in the initiation and progression of steatohepatitis *via* increases in lipogenic, inflammatory and fibrogenic genes [74]. However, whether hepatic triglyceride accumulation causes insulin resistance or vice versa and the mechanistic pathways involved are not yet clear [75].

CORONARY ARTERY DISEASE AND NAFLD

The overall health risks of patients with NASH are not confined to the liver. There is growing evidence that NAFLD increases the risk for coronary artery disease (CAD) [76-78]. NAFLD may be a mediator of CAD and not just a marker. The 10-year risk of all-cause mortality, fatal and non-fatal CVD and CAD events in relation to elevated ALT was assessed in 1439 subjects participating in the Hoorn Study, using Cox survival analysis. The predictive value of ALT for coronary events, seemed independent of traditional risk factors [77]. The severity of histological abnormality in the liver was noted to be closely associated with markers of early atherosclerosis such as greater carotid artery wall thickness and lower endothelial flow mediated vasodilatation.

As a component of MS, NAFLD is logically expected to be associated with CVD, but NAFLD as a predictor of CVD is rather surprising [79]. Earlier cross sectional studies have demonstrated associations between NAFLD and intima-media thickness and/or plaques of carotid artery as measures of early atherosclerosis [70]. However, whether the observation is an epiphenomenon is to be studied further [68]. In a recent study Targher *et al.* found that CVD is the leading cause of death in patients with advanced NAFLD [80].

TREATMENT OF NAFLD

Treatment options are available only for the manifestations of the components of MS as the syndrome does not have a known single cause. Modification of life style such as bringing about weight loss *via* administration of a healthy diet and increasing physical activity is the first treatment option. When more than one abnormality is present, a more aggressive approach may be considered. The strongly established association between NAFLD and MS does indeed suggest NAFLD is the hepatic manifestation of MS. Also, more mechanistic insights into how lipid overload in MS leads to fibrogenesis and extracellular matrix deposition in the pathogenesis and progression of NAFLD should be ascertained by future studies so that more aggressive treatment strategies could be formulated to combat MS and NAFLD. NAFLD also impacts vascular physiology leading to increased risk of cardiovascular diseases. Irrespective of the definitions used to define MS, obesity and insulin resistance are the major features that play an important role in the pathogenesis of MS, CVD and NAFLD. Hence, in a population like Asian Indians, which is at high risk for insulin resistance and higher body fat percentage, health care workers could use MS and NAFLD to identify patients who are at high risk for diabetes and cardiovascular disease and thus help to decrease morbidity and mortality due to these conditions.

CONCLUSION

Treatment options address the components of MS rather that the syndrome per se. Because the pathogenesis is poorly understood, the treatment focuses on weight management. Modification of life style to achieve weight loss that focuses on a healthy diet and on increasing physical activity is the foundation of treatment. When multiple abnormalities are present, a more aggressive approach may be needed to treat each risk factor separately.

ACKNOWLEDGEMENTS

Declared none.

CONFLICT OF INTEREST

The authors confirm that this chapter contents have no conflict of interest.

REFERENCES

[1] Reaven GM. Banting lecture 1988. Role of insulin resistance in human disease. Diabetes 1988; 37: 1595-607.

[2] Reaven GM. The fourth musketeer - from Alexandre Dumas to Claude Bernard. Diabetologia 1995; 38: 3-13.

[3] Kylin E. Studien über das Hypertonie-Hyperglykämie-Hyperurika miesyndrom. Zentralblatt für Innere Medizin 1923; 44: 105-27.

[4] Vague J. The degree of masculine differentiation of obesities: a factor determining predisposition to diabetes, atherosclerosis, gout, and uric calculous disease. Am J Clin Nutr 1956; 4: 20-34.

[5] Modan M, Halkin H, Almog S *et al.* Hyperinsulinemia. A link between hypertension obesity and glucose intolerance. J Clin Invest 1985; 75: 809-17.

[6] World Health Organisation. Definition Diagnosis and Classification of Diabetes Mellitus and its Complications. Geneva: World Health Organization 1999.

[7] Grundy SM, Brewer HB Jr, Cleeman JI, Smith SC Jr, Lenfant C; National Heart, Lung, and Blood Institute; American Heart Association. Definition of metabolic syndrome: report of the National

Heart, Lung, and Blood Institute/American heart Association conference on scientific issues related to definition. Arterioscler Thromb Vasc Biol 2004; 24: e13-8.

[8] Alberti KG, Zimmet P, Shaw J; IDF Epidemiology Task Force Consensus Group. The metabolic syndrome--a new worldwide definition. Lancet 2005; 366: 1059-62.

[9] Grundy SM, Brewer HB Jr, Cleeman JI, Smith SC Jr, Lenfant C; American Heart Association; National Heart, Lung, and Blood Institute. Definition of metabolic syndrome: Report of the National Heart, Lung, and Blood Institute/American heart Association conference on scientific issues related to definition. Circulation 2004: 27; 109: 433-8.

[10] Grundy SM, Cleeman JI, Daniels SR, *et al.* American Heart Association; National Heart, Lung, and Blood Institute. Diagnosis and management of the metabolic syndrome: an American Heart Association/National Heart, Lung, and Blood Institute Scientific Statement. Circulation 2005; 112: 2735-52.

[11] Ruan X, Jin J, Hua L, Liu Y, Wang J, Liu S. The prevalence of metabolic syndrome in Chinese postmenopausal women and the optimum body composition indices to predict it. Menopause 2010; 17: 566-70.

[12] Basit A, Shera AS. Prevalence of metabolic syndrome in Pakistan. Metab Syndr Relat Disord 2008; 6: 171-5.

[13] Azizi F, Salehi P, Etemadi A, Zahedi-Asl S. Prevalence of metabolic syndrome in an urban population: Tehran Lipid and Glucose Study. Diab Res Clin Pract 2003; 61: 29-37.

[14] Onat A, Ceyhan K, Basar O, Erer B, Toprak S, Sansoy V. Metabolic syndrome: major impact on coronary risk in a population with low cholesterol levels—a prospective and cross-sectional evaluation. Atherosclerosis 2002; 165: 285-92.

[15] Villegas R, Perry IJ, Creagh D, Hinchion R, O'Halloran D. Prevalence of the metabolic syndrome in middle-aged men and women. Diab Care 2003; 26: 3198-9.

[16] Resnick HE. Metabolic syndrome in American Indians. Diab Care 2002; 25: 1246-7.

[17] Meigs JB, Wilson PW, Nathan DM, D'Agostino Sr RB, Williams K, Haffner SM. Prevalence and characteristics of the metabolic syndrome in the San Antonio Heart and Framingham Offspring Studies. Diabetes 2003; 52: 2160-7.

[18] Riediger ND, Clara I. Prevalence of metabolic syndrome in the Canadian adult population. CMAJ 2011; 183: E1127-34.

[19] Eapen D, Kalra GL, Merchant N, Arora A, Khan BV. Metabolic syndrome and cardiovascular disease in South Asians. Vasc Health Risk Manag 2009; 5: 731-43.

[20] Ramachandran A, Snehalatha C, Satyavani K, Sivasankari S, Vijay V. Metabolic syndrome in urban Asian Indian adults—a population study using modified ATP III criteria. Diab Res Clin Pract 2003; 60: 199-204.

[21] Deepa R, Shanthirani CS, Premalatha G, Sastry NG, Mohan V. Prevalence of insulin resistance syndrome in a selected south Indian population—the Chennai urban population study 7 (CUPS-7). Indian J Med Res 2002; 115: 118-27.

[22] Deepa M, Farooq S, Datta M, Deepa R, Mohan V. Prevalence of metabolic syndrome using WHO, ATPIII and IDF definitions in Asian Indians: the Chennai Urban Rural Epidemiology Study (CURES-34). Diabetes Metab Res Rev 2007; 23: 127-34.

[23] Misra A, Khurana L. Obesity and the metabolic syndrome in developing countries. J Clin Endocrinol Metab 2008; 93(11 Suppl 1): S9-30.

[24] Das M, Pal S, Ghosh A. Prevalence of cardiovascular disease risk factors by habitat: a study on adult Asian Indians in West Bengal, India. Anthropol Anz 2011; 68: 253-64.

[25] Kanjilal S, Shanker J, Rao VS, *et al.* Prevalence and component analysis of metabolic syndrome: an Indian atherosclerosis research study perspective. Vasc Health Risk Manag 2008; 4: 189-97.

[26] Kamble P, Deshmukh PR, Garg N. Metabolic syndrome in adult population of rural Wardha, central India. Indian J Med Res 2010; 132: 701-5.

[27] Romeo GR, Lee J, Shoelson SE. Metabolic syndrome, insulin resistance, and roles of inflammation - mechanisms and therapeutic targets. Arterioscler Thromb Vasc Biol 2012; 32: 1771-6.

[28] Petersen KF, Dufour S, Feng J, *et al.* Increased prevalence of insulin resistance and nonalcoholic fatty liver disease in Asian-Indian men. Proc Natl Acad Sci U S A 2006; 103: 18273-7.

[29] Misra A, Luthra K, Vikram NK. Dyslipidemia in Asian Indians: determinants and significance. J Assoc Physicians India 2004; 52: 137-42.

[30] Walldius G, Junger, I. The apoB/apo A-1 ratio- a new predictor of fatal stroke, myocardial infarction and other ischaemic diseases- stronger than LDL and lipid ratios. Atherosclerosis 2006; 7(Suppl): 468.

[31] Tan CE, Ma S, Wai D, Chew SK, Tai ES. Can we apply the National Cholesterol Education Program Adult Treatment Panel definition of the metabolic syndrome to Asians? Diab care 2004; 27: 1182-6.

[32] Tillin T, Forouhi N, Johnston DG, McKeigue PM, Chaturvedi N, Godsland IF. Metabolic syndrome and coronary heart disease in South Asians, African-Caribbeans and white Europeans: a UK population-based cross-sectional study. Diabetologia 2005; 48: 649-56.

[33] Clinical Guidelines on the Identification, Evaluation, and Treatment of Overweight and Obesity in Adults—the Evidence Report. National Institutes of Health. Obes Res 1998; 6(suppl 2): 51S-209S.

[34] Mohan V, Gokulakrishnan R, Deepa R, Shanthirani CS, Datta M. Association of physical inactivity with components of metabolic syndrome and coronary artery disease-the Chennai Urban Population Study (CUPS 15). Diabet Med.2005; 22: 1206-11.

[35] Radhika G, Dam RMV, Sudha V, Ganesan A, Mohan V. Refined Grain Consumption and the metabolic syndrome in urban Asian Indians-Chennai Urbam Rural Epidemiology Study (CURES-57). Metabolism Clinical and Experimental 2009; 58: 675-681.

[36] Klein S, Burke LE, Bray GA, *et al*; American Heart Association Council on Nutrition, Physical Activity, and Metabolism; American College of Cardiology Foundation. Clinical implications of obesity with specific focus on cardiovascular disease: a statement for professionals from the American Heart Association Council on Nutrition, Physical Activity, and Metabolism: endorsed by the American College of Cardiology Foundation. Circulation 2004; 110: 2952-67.

[37] Schigt A, Gerdes VE, Cense HA, *et al*. Bariatric surgery is an effective treatment for morbid obesity. Neth J Med 2013; 71: 4-9.

[38] Chobanian AV, Bakris GL, Black HR, *et al*. National Heart, Lung, and Blood Institute Joint National Committee on Prevention, Detection, Evaluation, and Treatment of High Blood Pressure; National High Blood Pressure Education Program Coordinating Committee. The Seventh Report of the Joint National Committee on Prevention, Detection, Evaluation, and Treatment of High Blood Pressure: the JNC 7 report. JAMA 2003; 289: 2560-72.

[39] Ford ES, Schulze MB, Pischon T, Bergmann MM, Joost HG, Boeing H. Metabolic syndrome and risk of incident diabetes: findings from the European Prospective Investigation into Cancer and Nutrition-Potsdam Study. Cardiovasc Diabetol 2008; 7: 35.

[40] Enas EA, Mohan V, Deepa M, Farooq S, Pazhoor S, Chennikkara H. The Metabolic Syndrome and Dslipidemia Among Asian Indians: A population with high rates of Diabetes and Premature Coronary Artery Disease. J Cardiometab Syndr 2007; 4: 267-75.

[41] National Cholesterol Education Program (NCEP) Expert Panel on Detection, Evaluation, and Treatment of High Blood Cholesterol in Adults (Adult Treatment Panel III). Third Report of the National Cholesterol Education Program (NCEP) Expert Panel on Detection, Evaluation, and Treatment of High Blood Cholesterol in Adults (Adult Treatment Panel III) final report. Circulation 2002; 106: 3143-421.

[42] Ferrero-Miliani L, Nielsen OH, Andersen PS, Girardin SE. Chronic inflammation: importance of NOD2 and NALP3 in interleukin-1beta generation. Clin Exp Immunol 2007; 147: 227-35.

[43] Bastard JP, Maachi M, Lagathu C, *et al*. Recent advances in the relationship between obesity, inflammation, and insulin resistance. Eur Cytokine Netw 2006; 17: 4-12.

[44] Mohan V, Deepa R, Pradeepa R, Vimaleswaran KS, Anjana M, Velmurugan K, Radha K. Association of low adiponectin levels with the metabolic syndrome-the Chennai Urban Rural Epidemiology Study (CURES - 4). Metabolism 2005; 54: 476-81.

[45] Indulekha K, Surendar J, Mohan V. High sensitive C-Reactive Protein, Tumor necrosis factor-alpha, interleukin-6 and vascular cell adhesion molecule levels in Asian Indians with metabolic syndrome and insulin resistance (CURES-105). J Diabetes Sci Technol 2011; 5: 982-8

[46] Gokulakrishnan K, Deepa R, Mohan V, Gross MD. Soluble P-selectin and CD40L levels in subjects with prediabetes, diabetes mellitus and metabolic syndrome-the Chennai Urban Epidemiology Study. (CURES-16). Metabolism 2006; 55: 237-42

[47] Anuradha S, Mohan V, Gokulakrishnan K, Dixit M. Angiopoietin-2 levels in glucose intolerance, hypertension, and metabolic syndrome in Asian Indians (Chennai Urban Rural Epidemiology Study-74). Metabolism 2010. 59: 774-9

[48] Surendar J, Mohan V, Rao MM, Babu S, Aravindhan V. Increased Levels of Both Th1 and Th2 Cytokines in Subjects with Metabolic Syndrome (CURES-103). Diabetes Technol Ther 2011; 13: 477-82.
[49] Mohan V, Gokulakrishnan K, Sandeep S, Srivastava BK, Ravikumar R, Deepa R. Intimal media thickness, glucose intolerance and metabolic syndrome in Asian Indians-the Chennai Urban Rural Epidemiology Study (CURES-22). Diabet Med 2006; 23: 845-50.
[50] Laaksonen DE, Lakka HM, Niskanen LK, Kaplan GA, Salonen JT, Lakka TA. Metabolic syndrome and development of diabetes mellitus: application and validation of recently suggested definitions of the metabolic syndrome in a prospective cohort study. Am J Epidemiol 2002; 156: 1070-7.
[51] Hanson RL, Imperatore G, Bennett PH, Knowler WC. Components of the "metabolic syndrome" and incidence of type 2 diabetes. Diabetes 2002; 51: 3120-7.
[52] Lorenzo C, Okoloise M, Williams K, Stern MP, Haffner SM. The metabolic syndrome as predictor of type 2 diabetes: the San Antonio heart study. Diab care 2003; 26: 3153-9.
[53] Ford ES, Li C, Sattar N. Metabolic syndrome and incident diabetes: current state of the evidence. Diab care 2008; 31: 1898-904.
[54] Ley SH, Harris SB, Mamakeesick M, *et al.* Metabolic syndrome and its components as predictors of incident type 2 diabetes mellitus in an Aboriginal community. CMAJ 2009; 180: 617-24.
[55] Wilson PW, D'Agostino RB, Parise H, Sullivan L, Meigs JB. Metabolic syndrome as a precursor of cardiovascular disease and type 2 diabetes mellitus. Circulation 2005; 112: 3066-72.
[56] Ingelsson E, Sullivan LM, Murabito JM, *et al.* Prevalence and prognostic impact of subclinical cardiovascular disease in individuals with the metabolic syndrome and diabetes. Diabetes 2007; 56: 1718-26.
[57] Kokubo Y, Okamura T, Yoshimasa Y, *et al.* Impact of metabolic syndrome components on the incidence of cardiovascular disease in a general urban Japanese population: the Suita study. Hypertens Res 2008; 31: 2027-35.
[58] Nilsson PM, Engström G, Hedblad B. The metabolic syndrome and incidence of cardiovascular disease in non-diabetic subjects--a population-based study comparing three different definitions. Diabet Med 2007; 24: 464-72.
[59] Butler J, Rodondi N, Zhu Y, *et al.* Health ABC Study. Metabolic syndrome and the risk of cardiovascular disease in older adults. J Am Coll Cardiol 2006; 47: 1595-602.
[60] Katzmarzyk PT, Janssen I, Ross R, Church TS, Blair SN. The importance of waist circumference in the definition of metabolic syndrome: prospective analyses of mortality in men. Diab care 2006; 29: 404-9.
[61] Monami M, Lamanna C, Balzi D, *et al.* Metabolic syndrome and cardiovascular mortality in older type 2 diabetic patients: a longitudinal study. J Gerontol A Biol Sci Med Sci 2008; 63: 646-9.
[62] Noto D, Barbagallo CM, Cefalù AB, *et al.* The metabolic syndrome predicts cardiovascular events in subjects with normal fasting glucose: results of a 15 years follow-up in a Mediterranean population. Atherosclerosis 2008; 197: 147-53.
[63] Kahn R. Metabolic syndrome: Is it a syndrome? Does it matter? Circulation 2007; 115: 1806-10.
[64] Grundy SM: Does a diagnosis of metabolic syndrome have value in clinical practice? Am J Clin Nutr 2006, 83: 1248-51.
[65] Holvoet P, Kritchevsky SB, Tracy RP, *et al.* The metabolic syndrome, circulating oxidized LDL, and risk of myocardial infarction in well-functioning elderly people in the health, aging, and body composition cohort. Diabetes 2004; 53: 1068-73.
[66] Grundy SM, Brewer HB Jr, Cleeman JI, Smith SC Jr, Lenfant C; National Heart, Lung, and Blood Institute; American Heart Association. Definition of metabolic syndrome: report of the National Heart, Lung, and Blood Institute/American heart Association conference on scientific issues related to definition. Arterioscler Thromb Vasc Biol 2004; 24: e13-8.
[67] Chalasani N, Younossi Z, Lavine JE, *et al.* "The Diagnosis and Management of Non-alcoholic Fatty Liver Disease: Practice Guideline by the American Gastroenterological Association, American Association for the Study of Liver Diseases, and American College of Gastroenterology". Gastroenterology 2012; 142: 1592-1609.
[68] Kim CH, Younossi ZM. American Gastroenterological Association; American Association for the Study of Liver Diseases; American College of Gastroenterology. Nonalcoholic fatty liver disease: A manifestation of the metabolic syndrome Cleveland Clinic Journal of Medicine 2008; 75: 721-28.

[69] Kleiner DE, Brunt EM, Van Natta M, *et al.* Nonalcoholic Steatohepatitis Clinical Research Network. Nonalcoholic Steatohepatitis. Clinical Research Network. Hepatology 2005; 41: 1313-21.

[70] Strnad P, Paschke S, Jang KH, Ku NO. Keratins: markers and modulators of liver disease. Curr Opin Gastroenterol 2012; 28: 209-16.

[71] Kim CH, Park JY, Lee KU, Kim JH, Kim HK. Fatty liver is an independent risk factor for the development of type 2 diabetes in Korean adults. Diabet Med 2008; 25: 476-481.

[72] Hanley AJ, Williams K, Festa A, *et al.* Insulin resistance atherosclerosis study. Elevations in markers of liver injury and risk of type 2 diabetes: the insulin resistance atherosclerosis study. Diabetes 2004; 53: 2623-32.

[73] Kotronen A, Juurinen L, Hakkarainen A, *et al.* Liver fat is increased in type 2 diabetic patients and underestimated by serum alanine aminotransferase compared with equally obese nondiabetic subjects. Diabetes Care 2008; 31: 165-169.

[74] Takamura T, Misu H, Ota T, Kaneko S. Fatty liver as a consequence and cause of insulin resistance: lessons from type 2 diabetic liver. Endocr J 2012; 59: 745-63.

[75] Postic C, Girard J. Contribution of *de novo* fatty acid synthesis to hepatic steatosis and insulin resistance: lessons from genetically engineered mice. J Clin Invest 2008; 118: 829-838.

[76] Wong VW, Wong GL, Yip GW, *et al.* Coronary artery disease and cardiovascular outcomes in patients with non-alcoholic fatty liver disease. Gut 2011; 60: 1721-7.

[77] Schindhelm RK, Dekker JM, Nijpels G, *et al.* Alanine aminotransferase predicts coronary heart disease events: a 10-year follow-up of the Hoorn Study. Atherosclerosis 2007; 191: 391-6.

[78] Targher G, Marra F, Marchesini G. Increased risk of cardiovascular disease in non-alcoholic fatty liver disease: causal effect or epiphenomenon. Diabetologia 2008; 51: 1947-53.

[79] Hamaguchi M, Kojima T, Takeda N, *et al.* Nonalcoholic fatty liver disease is a novel predictor of cardiovascular disease. World J Gastroenterol 2007; 13: 1579-84.

[80] Targher G, Day CP, Bonora E. Risk of cardiovascular disease in patients with nonalcoholic fatty liver disease. N Engl J Med 2010; 30; 363: 1341-50

CHAPTER 6

Diabetes Mellitus: Is it Type 1 or Type 2? It May Not Be So Easy

Jason C. Baker*

Weill Cornell Medical Associates. 211 E 80th St, New York, NY 10075, USA

Abstract: Type 1 diabetes arises from the autoimmune-mediated destruction of the pancreatic beta cells leading to a state of insulin deficiency. Type 1 diabetes is estimated to represent 5-10% of all the cases of diabetes, with an incidence that is rising across the globe at a rate of 3-5% annually. The cause of type 1 diabetes is uncertain, although it is believed that both a genetic predisposition and an environmental trigger(s) are necessary for the development of the disease. Treatment of type 1 diabetes requires insulin therapy, along with healthy diet and exercise habits. The amylin analogue Symlin is also approved for use in conjunction with insulin, and metformin and incretin mimetics are also being investigated. Insulin use requires close monitoring of blood sugar levels, with studies indicating that the best control in type 1 diabetes is seen in patients who monitor their blood sugar more frequently. Potential complications from type 1 diabetes include microvascular, macrovascular and psychological complications. Such complications are more severe in resource poor populations, often located in the developing world, which have inadequate access to consistent insulin and testing supplies. With adequate management of glucose levels, many such complications can be prevented. There is currently no cure for type 1 diabetes, although immunotherapy agents (including anti-CD3 mAb, CTLA-4 Ig, and anti-DC20) hold promise. Transplantation, including that of the whole pancreas, islet cells or stem cells, holds promise but issues exist with all modalities, which limits the cohort of patients for whom they may be appropriate.

Keywords: Behavior, blood glucose, diabetes, endocrinology, exercise, fatty liver, fitness, global health, health status, insulin resistance, lifestyle, macrovascular disease, microvascular disease, nephropathy, nutrition, obesity, overweight, pancreas, retinopathy, risk, weight, wellness.

INTRODUCTION

"Type 1 diabetes, previously referred to as insulin-dependent diabetes mellitus (IDDM) or juvenile-onset diabetes, results from the autoimmune-mediated

***Corresponding author Jason Baker:** Weill Cornell Medical Associates. 211 E 80th St, New York, NY 10075, USA; Tel: (646) 962-7300; Fax: (646) 962-0409; E-mail: jcb2007@med.cornell.edu

Judith Wylie-Rosett & Sunil S. Jhangiani (Eds)

destruction of pancreatic beta cells, which leads to a state of insulin deficiency" [1]. "To survive, people with type 1 diabetes must take exogenous insulin although many people with type 2 diabetes are treated with insulin. Typically, Type 1 diabetes strikes children and young adults, although type 1 diabetes can occur at any age. In adults, type 1 diabetes accounts for about 5 percent of all diagnosed cases of diabetes. Other types of diabetes (aside from type 2) are attributed to specific genetic conditions such as maturity-onset diabetes of youth (MODY), surgery, infections, medications, pancreatic disease, and other illnesses. These types of diabetes account for 1 to 5 percent of all diagnosed cases."[1]

TYPE 1 *VERSUS* TYPE 2 DIABETES

Diagnostic Perspective

The distinction between type 1 and type 2 diabetes is frequently difficult to assess, particularly in regions of the world which are unable to test for autoimmune markers associated with type 1 diabetes and where a diagnosis is frequently made clinically and not confirmed biochemically. The growing global waistline stemming from the obesity epidemic has resulted in overweight and even obese people with type 1 diabetes, so the adage that thin and young equated to a clinical diagnosis of type 1 diabetes does not always hold true. "Additionally, it becomes more difficult to diagnose type 1 diabetes in adults since many people with type 2 diabetes also receive insulin therapy. Furthermore, type 1 diabetes in an adult may mimic type 2 diabetes at diagnosis with a slow deterioration in metabolic control and insulin production. This form, called latent autoimmune diabetes mellitus in adults (LADA), represents a slowly progressive form of type 1 diabetes. Both genetic and environmental triggers have been associated with this autoimmune process resulting in type 1 diabetes, although no single cause has been consistently shown to be either protective or to confer increased risk. Overall, males and females appear to be equally affected" [2, 3].

Diagnosis most typically occurs in the pubertal years for both the sexes with studies [4, 5] suggesting the highest increase in incidence is in the <14 years of age group. However, recent studies demonstrate that diagnosis up to the age of 30 or 35 years has become more common [6-11]. From these more recent studies it appears that the incidence in older age groups is lower than that seen in the 0-14 year age range, confirming an incidence peak around puberty. An increased male to female sex ratio is also seen in these studies suggesting that the incidence tends to decrease thereafter for females but remains relatively elevated for males until they reach 35 years of age.

Epidemiological Perspective

In the United States, there are roughly 3 million people who suffer from Type 1 diabetes, which accounts for an estimated 5-10% of all the cases of diabetes; 85% of people living with type 1 diabetes are adults [12]. "Over 30,000 new cases are diagnosed annually, translating into roughly 80 new cases daily according to the Juvenile Diabetes Research Foundation (JDRF) [12, 13]. In the United States, Non-Hispanic white youth had the highest rate of new cases of Type 1 diabetes [14]. The data regarding the global distribution of type 1 diabetes is difficult to determine primarily because of the lack of a centralized database and reliance on a clinical diagnosis rather than screening tests" [14]. Much of the data on type 1 diabetes incidence comes from childhood diabetes (<14 years of age), with an unknown number of adults with type 1. The global distribution of type 1 diabetes is widely variable, which in part may be due to different distributions of risk genes, environmental exposures and methodological problems. According to the International Diabetes Federation (IDF), there are an estimated 440,000 global cases of Type 1 diabetes in children aged 0-14 years, with 70,000 new cases diagnosed annually [15]. The incidence of Type 1 diabetes is growing by 3-5% annually, particularly in populations previously viewed as having a lower incidence (such as China and Japan) [16] and Central and Eastern Europe [17-19].

"Annual incidence varies widely, from 0.61 cases per 100,000 people in China, to 41.4 cases per 100,000 people in Finland [16]. These wide variations in type 1 diabetes incidence rates have been noted between both genetically similar populations, such as Iceland and Norway, and adjacent countries with differing lifestyles such as Estonia and Finland. The incidence in mainland Italy (8.4 cases per 100,000 population) is much lower than the Island of Sardinia (36.9 cases per 100,000 population), while Crete has a lower rate than mainland Greece [20], and Newfoundland has a higher rate than other parts of Canada" [21]. Such variations suggest a role of environmental factors in the development of type 1 diabetes [15, 16]. Another confounder in assessing the global incidence of type 1 diabetes is that incidence data frequently covers only one small part of a large country where marked variability in genetic and environmental exposures likely exists [22]. Examples include India, where incidence data were largely attained from studies performed in Madras, and in Russia where data were attained largely from a small dataset from Karelia. In such large countries, one sees marked variability in both risk gene distribution and environmental exposures (climate, *etc.*).

Small data sets resulting from both a lack of published data as well as high mortality rates are often problematic in calculating type 1 incidence. In particular, this is an issue in sub-Saharan Africa, where mortality among children with diabetes is reported to be high [23, 24] and from which there is a paucity of published data. "Many countries report that incidence rates have more than doubled in the last 20 years [25]. The cause for this marked rise in incidence is unclear, but it may be due to the increased inheritance of genes associated with Type 1 diabetes, environmental triggers and the increased identification of cases due to improved diagnostic technique and disease surveillance.

Etiology

Mounting evidence supports a genetic component for type 1 diabetes. For example, while the risk of developing type 1 diabetes in the general population is roughly 0.4%, the frequency of diabetes developing in children with a mother who has type 1 diabetes is 2-3% and 5-6% if the father has type 1 diabetes. The risk rises to almost 30% if both the parents are diabetic. The inheritance of human leukocyte antigen (HLA) class II molecules DR3 and DR4 is strongly associated with type 1 diabetes. More than 90% of non-Hispanic whites with type 1 diabetes express one or both of these molecules in comparison to 50-60% in the general population" [26-28]. However, despite an identical genetic profile, approximately 50% of monozygotic twins are discordant for type 1 diabetes, suggesting that other non-genetically determined factors also influence susceptibility to disease [29].

Environmental factors often associated with type 1 diabetes include infections, diet and geography. Other risk factors include enteroviral infection in pregnant females, older maternal ages (39-42 years), blood group incompatibility, C-section, increased birth weight, pre- eclampsia, early introduction to cow's milk proteins and closer proximity to the equator [30-34]. "Population-based case-control studies suggest protective factors, including a longer duration of breast feeding [35], vitamin D supplementation [36, 37], pre-school day care [38] and atopic diseases" [39].

Viral infections have been linked to the development of type 1 diabetes and are thought to initiate or modify an autoimmune process leading to destruction of insulin-producing beta cells located in the pancreas, possibly *via* molecular mimicry, in which part of the virus antigen resembles that of the beta cell. Potential culprit viruses include the enteroviruses (Coxsackie and echovirus), rubella virus, mumps virus, rotavirus, parvovirus and cytomegalovirus [33, 34]. These viruses are the subjects of continued experimental and clinical studies aimed at defining their roles in the pathogenesis of type 1 diabetes. "Outbreaks of Coxsackie virus, mumps virus and congenital rubella virus have been associated with an increased incidence of type 1 diabetes. One study suggests that enteroviral infection during pregnancy results in an increased risk for type 1 diabetes mellitus in the offspring [33, 34]. Nonetheless, incidence of type 1 diabetes is highest in areas where the overall burden of infectious disease is lowest, which suggests the involvement of other risk factors" [33]. One theory explaining this is the hygiene hypothesis [40], by which children and infants in modern and more sterile environments are less exposed to viruses and bacteria that help the immune system to mature, which may increase their subsequent risk for type 1 diabetes.

Various dietary factors have been associated with increased risk for type 1 diabetes. Some studies suggest that breast fed infants have a lower risk for type 1 diabetes, whereas infants with earlier introduction to cow's milk (which contains proteins that have antigenic similarities to islet cell antigens) have a higher incidence of type 1 diabetes [32]. Animal models suggest that nitrosamines, chemicals found in smoked foods and some water supplies, have been shown to cause type 1 diabetes although evidence in humans is lacking [34]. "Studies suggest that a higher incidence of type 1 diabetes in childhood is associated with greater estimates of general wealth such as GDP" [41]. This suggests that greater wealth, and concurrent lifestyle habits like higher calorie intake, may increase the risk for development of type 1 diabetes.

"Wealth is a determinant of both birth weight and childhood growth. While autoimmune mechanisms are considered to be responsible for the beta cell destruction leading to type 1 diabetes, overload factors resulting from an excessive calorie intake may accelerate this process [42-44]. Studies suggest that high birth weight, an increased height, weight, weight for height and body mass index (BMI) are risk factors for type 1 diabetes"[45-49]. Obesity is associated with high growth hormone levels and an increased number of fat cells, which can both lead to insulin resistance and beta-cell overload and possibly trigger an autoimmune attack.

PHARMACOLOGICAL ISSUES

The obesity epidemic may not only contribute to the increasing incidence of type 1 diabetes, but also complicate the treatment of people with type 1 diabetes.

People with type 1 diabetes require a careful balance of insulin, diet and exercise to manage their condition successfully, along with frequent monitoring of blood sugar levels. Being overweight or obese will increases insulin requirements. Instead of simple increment in insulin dose, other treatments may be considered to enhance insulin action and limit side effects such as weight gain. These treatments include the use of oral hypoglycemic agents like metformin (off-label) [50], symlin, and incretin mimetics such as liraglutide (Victoza) [51]. "Symlin is an injectable synthetic form of amylin, a molecule normally co-secreted with insulin, which helps blunt postprandial hyperglycemia. Symlin use with insulin may therefore result in a lower insulin dose and concurrent weight loss [52, 53]. Currently, symlin is only approved for use as a separate injection with meals. Studies suggest an association of an increased incidence of type 1 diabetes with an increased distance from the equator.

Lower vitamin D levels may partially explain such an association, as reduced exposure to ultraviolet (UV) light and lower vitamin D levels are more commonly found in people residing in higher latitudes and have been associated with an increased risk of type 1 diabetes [34]. Furthermore, vitamin D supplements may provide protection against the development of type 1 diabetes. Meta-analysis of data from our European studies indicated that children taking vitamin D supplements had a 29% reduction in the risk of developing type 1 diabetes when compared to their peers who were not taking such supplements" [37]. The precise mechanism by which vitamin D supplementation may protect against type 1 diabetes is uncertain, but the identification of receptors for the active form of vitamin D in both immune cells and β cells has led to the suggestion of vitamin D mediated immune modulation.

MORBIDITY AND MORTALITY

"Morbidity and mortality data on type 1 diabetes are shocking, particularly in the developing world. Studies suggest that globally, people living with type 1 diabetes have a mortality rate up to three and a half times than that of the general population with mortality rates directly correlated to the access to healthcare resources" [54, 55]. In the developed world, mortality data varies by geographical location as there is a 10-fold variation in death from Type 1 diabetes globally: lowest rates are found in Western Europe and Canada, and the highest rates are found in Japan, Eastern Europe and Russia. In the developing world mortality rates are even more striking; survival after diagnosis in many African countries is quite poor. "Studies suggest that a person requiring insulin will on average live for 11 years in Zambia, 30 months in Mali and 12 months in Mozambique" [56-58]. Much of the mortality comes from death secondary to hypoglycemia. Authors suggest that the lack of access to health care providers and facilities, and the lack of medications and diabetes testing supplies, contribute significantly to the poor survival among so many in the developing world. Microvascular disease (nephropathy, retinopathy, and neuropathy) continues to be a significant contributor to morbidity associated with type 1 diabetes. Little is known about the prevalence of type 1 diabetes complications in the developing world, so most epidemiologic data come from developed countries.

The most common microvascular complication of type 1 diabetes is diabetic nephropathy, which affects roughly 15-40% patients, with a peak incidence after 15-20 year diabetes duration [59]. Diabetic retinopathy represents the leading cause of vision loss in working age people in the developed countries [60]. In the U.S., diabetic retinopathy results in approximately 10,000 new cases of blindness every year [61]. Both nephropathy and neuropathy are associated with an increased risk for cardiovascular disease. Studies suggest that the incidence of diabetic neuropathy varies between 7 to 57% [62]. Type 1 diabetes is associated with a 10-fold increase in macrovascular disease (heart attack and stroke) as compared with an age-matched non-diabetic population [63, 64]. "Studies suggest that type 1 diabetes patients of any age have a higher mortality from ischemic heart disease when compared to the general population. Additionally, observational studies have shown that the cerebrovascular mortality rate is also elevated at all ages in patients with type 1 diabetes" [65].

"The Diabetes Control and Complications Trial/Epidemiology of Diabetes Interventions and Complications Study (DCCT/EDIC) showed that during the 17 years of prospective analysis, intensive treatment of type 1 diabetes (including lower HbA1c) was associated with a 42% risk reduction in all cardiovascular events and a 57% reduction in the risk of nonfatal MI, stroke, or death from CVD" [66]. The most effective way to avoid both macrovascular and microvascular complications seems to be *via* tight early control soon after diagnosis. Studies suggest "metabolic memory", through which benefits on the heart, eyes, kidneys and nerves persist after 7 years of tight control despite later less stringent control, may be responsible for this protective benefit of early tight control [67]. There is a direct correlation between the risk of microvascular disease with both HbA1c value and the level of glycemic variability [68]. Therefore, the combination of early and persistently tight control of type 1 diabetes is the best method to prevent adverse outcomes related to the disease.

In the U.S., studies demonstrate that diabetes-related mortality seems to be improving, given the evidence that newly diagnosed individuals have better survival compared to those diagnosed previously, independent of the age of diagnosis [54, 56]. The authors conclude that such improvement in mortality likely results from better access to healthcare, better management of co-morbid conditions, and better overall glucose control and monitoring [54, 56].

Mental health issues also contribute to morbidity and mortality in type 1 diabetes. Body image disorders are more common among type 1 diabetics, including eating disorders such as binge eating and "diabulimia" [69, 70]. Studies suggest that females with type 1 diabetes are nearly twice as likely to develop an eating disorder such as bulimia nervosa and anorexia nervosa compared to peers without diabetes [69]. Other studies suggest that nearly half of adolescent females with type 1 diabetes skip insulin injections to prevent weight gain and have higher rates of diabetes-related complications, such as nephropathy and are at a threefold risk of premature death [69, 70]. Depression is also more common in diabetes with depression rates twice as those compared to individuals without diabetes [70, 71]. Depression rates are similar in both type 1 and type 2 diabetes, but are higher in women. Studies suggest that adults with type 1 diabetes and depression are more likely to be single, have less income and poor healthcare follow-up, and are twice as likely to seek primary care through emergency room visits [71].

RESEARCH ISSUES

Many research efforts are underway to find a cure for type 1 diabetes, both in terms of prevention and disease modulation [71-77]. Studies are underway, evaluating disease prevention following administration of agents, such as oral insulin, GAD protein, vitamin D, omega-3 fatty acids and docosahexaenoic acid (DHA) to patients at high risk for developing Type 1 diabetes" [71-72]. "Research is ongoing regarding immunological manipulation in at risk and newly diagnosed type 1 diabetes patients, using agents such as Anti-CD3 mAb (Teplizumab) for Prevention Of Diabetes In Relatives At Risk For Type 1 Diabetes Mellitus, CTLA-4 Ig (Abatacept), Anti IL- 1Beta (Canakinumab) and anti-CD20 (Rituximab), with hopes of prolonging c-peptide production *via* altering the immune system and stopping the destruction of beta cells" [71-73].

Transplantation, including that of the whole pancreas, islet cells or stem cells, is promising but problems exist with all methods, which limits the patients for whom they may be appropriate. Anti-rejection medications that are needed after transplantation are frequently poorly tolerated by patients and are also frequently toxic to the transplanted beta cells, which often results in transplant failure. While islet and stem cell transplants carry less surgical risk and require smaller doses of frequently toxic immuno-suppressive agents, they have not yet resulted in long-term benefits: all patients, who did not require supplemental insulin therapy following transplantation, experienced a subsequent decline in c-peptide levels and an increase in insulin requirements [75]. More research is needed before such treatments can be more widely recommended.

CONCLUSION

To survive, people with type 1 diabetes must take exogenous insulin although many people with type 2 diabetes are treated with insulin. Typically, Type 1 diabetes strikes children and young adults, although type 1 diabetes can occur at any age. Access to advances in treatment for type 1 diabetes is a problem in many areas of the world, which is accompanied by excess morbidity and mortality. However, with globalization the increased risk for type 2 diabetes posed a public health challenge.

ACKNOWLEDGEMENTS

Declared none.

CONFLICT OF INTEREST

Dr. Baker has served as a speaker for Lilly/Medtronic and as an advisor for Ambio Health.

REFERENCES

[1] Kahn R, Weir G, King G, Jacobson A, Smith R, Moses A. Joslin's Diabetes Mellitus, 14th ed. Lippincott Williams & Wilkins, 2005; p. 342-345.

[2] Brekke HK, Ludvigsson JF, van Odijk J, Ludvigsson J. Breastfeeding and introduction of solid foods in Swedish Infants: the all Babies in Southeast Sweden Study. Br J Nutr 2005; 94:377-382.

[3] Wahlberg J, Vaarala O, Ludvigsson J. Dietary risk factors for the emergence of type 1 Diabetes-related autoantibodies in 21 2-year- old Swedish children. Br J Nutr 2006; 95:603-608.

[4] Pundziute-Lyckå A, Dahlquist G, Nyström L, *et al.* The incidence of Type I diabetes has not increased but shifted to a younger age at diagnosis in the 0-34 years group in Sweden 1983-1998. Diabetologia 2002; 45(6): 783-791.

[5] Weets I, De Leeuw IH, Du Caju MV, *et al.* The incidence of type 1 diabetes in the age group 0-39 years has not increased in Antwerp (Belgium) between 1989 and 2000: evidence for earlier disease manifestation. Diabetes Care 2002; 25(5): 840-846.

[6] Joner G, Sovik O. The incidence of type 1 (insulin-dependent) diabetes mellitus 15-29 years in Norway 1978-1982. Diabetologia 1991; 34(4): 271-274.

[7] Blohme G, Nystrom L, Arnqvist HJ, *et al.* Male predominance of type 1 (insulin-dependent) diabetes mellitus in young adults: results from a 5-year prospective nationwide study of the 15-34-year age group in Sweden. Diabetologia 1992; 35(1): 56-62.

[8] Bruno G, Merletti F, Vuolo A, *et al.* Sex differences in incidence of IDDM in age-group 15-29 yr. Higher risk in males in Province of Turin, Italy. Diabetes Care 1993; 16(1):133-136.

[9] Roglic G, Pavlic-Renar I, Sestan-Crnek S, *et al.* Incidence of IDDM during 1988-1992 in Zagreb, Croatia. Diabetologia 1995; 38(5): 550-554.

[10] Feltbower RG, McKinney PA, Parslow RC, Stephenson CR, Bodansky HJ. Type 1 diabetes in Yorkshire, UK: time trends in 0-14 and 15-29-year-olds, age at onset and age-period-cohort modelling. Diabet Med 2003; 20(6): 437-441.

[11] Kyvik KO, Nystrom L, Gorus F, *et al.* The epidemiology of type 1 diabetes mellitus is not the same in young adults as in children. Diabetologia 2004; 47(3): 377-384.

[12] National Institute of Diabetes and Digestive Kidney Diseases (NIDDK): National diabetes information Clearinghouse [updated 2013 Sep, cited 2014 March 28]. Available from: http://diabetes.niddk.nih.gov/dm/pubs/statistics/index.htm#i_youngpeople

[13] Juvenile Diabetes Research Foundation (JDRF): Statistics: JDRF and Diabetes [updated 2014, cited 2014 March 28]. Available from: http://jdrf.org/about-jdrf/fact-sheets/jdrf-and-diabetes-statistics/

[14] Dabelea D. Incidence of diabetes in youth in the United States. JAMA 2007; 297(24):2716-2724.

[15] Soltesz G, Patterson CC, Dahlquist G. Worldwide childhood type 1 diabetes incidence - what can we learn from epidemiology?. Pediatr Diabetes 2007; Oct;8 Suppl 6:6-14.36.

[16] Onkamo P, Väänänen S, Karvonen M, Tuomilehto J. Worldwide increase in incidence of type I diabetes: the analysis of the data on published incidence trends. Diabetologia 1999; 42:1395-1403.

[17] Tuomilehto J, Virtala E, Karvonen M, *et al.* Increase in incidence of insulin-dependent diabetes mellitus among children in Finland. Int J Epidemiol 1995; 24(5): 984-992.

[18] Gardner SG, Bingley PJ, Sawtell PA, Weeks S, Gale EA. Rising incidence of insulin dependent diabetes in children aged under 5 years in the Oxford region: time trend analysis. The Bart's-Oxford Study Group. BMJ 1997; 315(7110): 713-717.

[19] Dahlquist G, Mustonen L. Analysis of 20 years of prospective registration of childhood onset diabetes time trends and birth cohort effects. Swedish Childhood Diabetes Study Group. Acta Paediatr 2000; 89(10): 1231-1237.

[20] Mamoulakis D, Galanakis E, Bicouvarakis S, Paraskakis E, Sbyrakis S. Epidemiology of childhood type 1 diabetes in Crete, 1990-2001. Acta Paediatr 2003; 92(6): 737-739.

[21] Newhook LA, Curtis J, Hagerty D. High incidence of childhood type 1 diabetes in the Avalon Peninsula, Newfoundland, Canada. Diabetes Care 2004; 27(4): 885-888.

[22] International Diabetes Federation (IDF): Diabetes atlas discussion. [homepage on the Internet]. c1994. Available from http://da3.diabetesatlas.org/index9efa.html

[23] Castle WM, Wicks AC. A follow-up of 93 newly diagnosed African diabetics for 6 years. Diabetologia 1980; 18(2): 121-123.

[24] Makame MH. Childhood diabetes, insulin, and Africa. DERI (Diabetes Epidemiology Research International) Study Group. Diabet Med 1992; 9(6): 571-573.

[25] Amos AF, McCarty DJ, Zimmet P. The rising global burden of diabetes and its complications: estimates and projections to the year 2010. Diabet Med 1997;14(suppl 5):S1-S85 1997;14:S7-S85.

[26] Felner EI, Klitz W, Ham M, Lazaro AM, Stastny P, Dupont B. Genetic interaction among three genomic regions creates distinct contributions to early- and late-onset type 1 diabetes mellitus. Pediatr Diabetes. Dec 2005;6(4):213-220.

[27] Kyvik KO, Green A, Beck-Nielsen H. Concordance rates of insulin dependent diabetes mellitus: a population based study of young Danish twins. BMJ 1995;311, 913-917.

[28] Patterson CC, Carson DJ, Hadden DR. Epidemiology of childhood IDDM in Northern Ireland 1989-1994: low incidence in areas with highest population density and most household crowding. Northern Ireland Diabetes Study Group. Diabetologia 1996; 39(9):1063-1069.

[29] Kaprio J, Tuomilehto J, Koskenvuo M. Concordance for type 1 (insulin-dependent) and type 2 (non-insulin-dependent) diabetes mellitus in a population based cohort of twins in Finland. Diabetologia 1993; 35:1060-1067.

[30] National Institute of Diabetes and Digestive Kidney Diseases (NIDDK): Diabetes Statistics.c1999 [updated 2013 March, cited 2014 March 28]. Available from: http://diabetes.niddk.nih.gov/dm/pubs/america/contents.aspx
[31] National Institute of Diabetes and Digestive Kidney Diseases (NIDDK): Diabetes Statistics.c2011 [updated 2013 Sep, cited 2014 March 28]. Available from: http://www.niddk.nih.gov/health-information/health-statistics/Pages/default.aspx#cat:diabetes
[32] Scott FW. Cow milk and insulin-dependent diabetes mellitus: is there a relationship? Am J Clin Nutr 1990; 51:489-491.
[33] Wagenknecht LE, Roseman JM, Herman WH. Increased incidence of insulin-dependent diabetes mellitus following an epidemic of Coxsackievirus B5. Am J Epidemiol 1991; 133:1024-1031.
[34] Dorman J, McCarthy B, O'Leary L, Koehler A. National Institute of Diabetes and Digestive Kidney Diseases (NIDDK): Risk Factors for Insulin-Dependent Diabetes.c1999 [cited 2014 March 28]. Available from: http://diabetes.niddk.nih.gov/dm/pubs/america/pdf/chapter8.pdf
[35] Akerblom HK, Vaarala O, Hyoty H, Ilonen J, Knip M. Environmental factors in the etiology of type 1 diabetes. Am J Med Genet 2002; 115(1): 18-29.
[36] EURODIAB Substudy 2 Study Group Vitamin D supplement in early childhood and risk for Type I (insulin-dependent) diabetes mellitus.. Diabetologia 1999; 42(1): 51-54.
[37] Zipitis CS, Akobeng AK. Vitamin D Supplementation in early Childhood and Risk of Type 1 Diabetes: a Systematic Review and Meta-Analysis. Archives of Disease in Childhood 2008; 93:512-517.
[38] EURODIAB Substudy 2 Study Group Infections and vaccinations as risk factors for childhood type I (insulin-dependent) diabetes mellitus: a multicentre case-control investigation.. Diabetologia 2000; 43(1): 47-53.
[39] EURODIAB Substudy 2 Study Group Decreased prevalence of atopic diseases in children with diabetes.. J Pediatr 2000; 137(4): 470-474.
[40] Okada H, Kuhn C, Feillet F, Bach JF. The 'hygiene hypothesis' for autoimmune and allergic diseases: an update. Clin Exp Immunol 2010 April; 160(1): 1-9.
[41] Patterson CC, Dahlquist G, Soltesz G, Green A. Is childhood-onset type 1 diabetes a wealth-related disease? An ecological analysis of European incidence rates. Diabetologia 2001; 44 Suppl 3: B9-16.
[42] Bjork E, Kampe O, Karlsson FA, *et al.* Glucose regulation of the autoantigen GAD65 in human pancreatic islets. J Clin Endocrinol Metab 1992; 75(6): 1574-1576.
[43] Mandrup-Poulsen T. The role of interleukin-1 in the pathogenesis of IDDM. Diabetologia 1996; 39(9): 1005-1029.
[44] Pipeleers D, Hoorens A, Marichal-Pipeleers M, Van de Casteele M, Bouwens L, Ling Z. Role of pancreatic beta-cells in the process of beta-cell death. Diabetes 2001; 50 Suppl 1: S52-S57.
[45] Blom L, Persson LA, Dahlquist G. A high linear growth is associated with an increased risk of childhood diabetes mellitus. Diabetologia 1992; 35(6): 528-533.
[46] Dahlquist G, Bennich SS, Kallen B. Intrauterine growth pattern and risk of childhood onset insulin dependent (type 1) diabetes: population based case-control study. BMJ 1996; 313(7066): 1174-1177.
[47] Stene LC, Magnus P, Lie RT, Sovik O, Joner G. Birth weight and childhood onset type 1 diabetes: population based cohort study. BMJ 2001; 322(7291): 889-892.
[48] Hypponen E, Virtanen SM, Kenward MG, Knip M, Akerblom HK. Obesity, increased linear growth, and risk of type 1 diabetes in children. Diabetes Care 2000; 23(12): 1755-1760.
[49] EURODIAB Substudy 2 Study Group Rapid early growth is associated with increased risk of childhood type 1 diabetes in various European populations. Diabetes Care 2002; 25(10): 1755-1760.
[50] Gomez R, Mokhashi MH, Rao J, *et al.* "Metformin adjunctive therapy with insulin improves glycemic control in patients with type 1 diabetes mellitus: a pilot study." J Pediatr Endocrinol Metab 2002 Sep-Oct;15(8):1147-51.
[51] American Diabetes Association (ADA): 93rd Annual Meeting & Expo of the Endocrine Society, ENDO 2011.c2011 [updated 2011 June, cited 2014 March 28]. Available from: http://professional.diabetes.org/CongressReport_Display.aspx?CID=84488
[52] Karl D, Philis-Tsimikas A, Darsow T, *et al.* Pramlintide as an adjunct to insulin in patients with type 2 diabetes in a clinical practice setting reduced A1C, postprandial glucose excursions, and weight. Diabetes Technol Ther 2007;9(2):191-199.

[53] Holman RR, Thome KI, Farmer AJ, *et al.* Addition of biphasic, prandial, or basal insulin to oral therapy in type 2 diabetes. N Engl J Med 2007;357(17):1716-1730.
[54] Mäkinen VP, Forsblom C, Thorn LM. Metabolic Phenotypes, Vascular Complications, and Premature Deaths in a Population of 4,197 Patients With Type 1 Diabetes. Diabetes 2008; 57(9): 2480-2487.
[55] National Institute of Diabetes and Digestive and Kidney Diseases (NIDDK). Diabetes Statistics. c2011 [updated 2013 Sep, cited 2014 March 28]. Available from: http://diabetes.niddk.nih.gov/dm/pubs/statistics/index.aspx
[56] World Health Organization (WHO): Facts and figures about diabetes. [cited 2014 March 28]. Available at www.who.int/diabetes.
[57] Diabetes Atlas, third edition, International Diabetes Federation: Diabetes Atlas, third edition.c2008 [updated 2008, cited 2014 March 28]. Available from: http://da3.diabetesatlas.org/index3eec.html
[58] Azevedo M, Alla S. Diabetes in Sub-Saharan Africa: Kenya, Mali, Mozambique, Nigeria, South Africa and Zambia. Int J Diabetes Dev Ctries 2008; 28(4): 101-108.
[59] Gross JL, de Azevedo MJ, Silveiro SP, Canani LH, Caramori ML, Zelmanovitz T. Diabetic nephropathy: diagnosis, prevention, and treatment. Diabetes Care 2005; 28:164-176.
[60] Ciulla TA, Amador AG, Zinman B. Diabetic retinopathy and diabetic macular edema: pathophysiology, screening, and novel therapies. Diabetes Care 2003; 26:2653-2664.
[61] Fong DS, Aiello LP, Ferris FL 3rd, Klein R: Diabetic retinopathy. Diabetes Care 2004; 27:2540 - 2553.
[62] Trotta D, Verrotti A, Salladini C, Chiarelli F. Diabetic neuropathy in children and adolescents. Pediatr Diabetes 2004; 5:44-57.
[63] Laing SP, Swerdlow AJ, Slater SD. Mortality from heart disease in a cohort of 23,000 patients with insulin-treated diabetes.Diabetologia 2003; 46(6):760-765.
[64] Dorman JS, Laporte RE, Kuller LH, *et al.* The Pittsburgh insulin-dependent diabetes mellitus (IDDM) morbidity and mortality study. Mortality results. Diabetes 1984; 33(3):271-276.
[65] Laing SP, Swerdlow AJ, Carpenter LM, *et al.* Mortality from cerebrovascular disease in a cohort of 23 000 patients with insulin-treated diabetes. Stroke 2003; 34:418-421.
[66] Nathan DM, Cleary PA, Backlund JY, *et al.* Intensive diabetes treatment and cardiovascular disease in patients with type 1 diabetes. N Engl J Med 2005; 353:2643 2653.
[67] Lind M, Odén A, Fahlén M, Eliasson B. The shape of the metabolic memory of HbA1c: re-analysing the DCCT with respect to time-dependent effects. Diabetologia 2010; 53(6):1093.
[68] Kilpatrick E, Rigby A, Atkin S. The Effect of Glucose Variability on the Risk of Microvascular Complications in Type 1 Diabetes. Diabetes Care 2006; 29(7):1486-1490.
[69] Mannucci E, Rotella F, Ricca V, Moretti S, Placidi GF, Rotella CM. Eating disorders in patients with type 1 diabetes: a meta-analysis. J Endocrinol Invest 2005; 28(5):417.
[70] Rydall A, Rodin G, Olmsted M, Devenyi R, Daneman D. Disordered Eating Behavior and Microvascular Complications in Young Women with Insulin-Dependent Diabetes Mellitus. New England Journal of Medicine 1997; 336(26):1849-1854.
[71] Anderson RJ, Freedland KE, Clouse RE, Lustman PJ. The prevalence of comorbid depression in adults with diabetes: a meta-analysis. Diabetes Care 2001; 24(6):1069-1078.
[72] National Institute of Diabetes and Digestive and Kidney Diseases (NIDDK): Type 1 Diabetes (T1D) Research.c1999 [updated 2012 May, cited 2014 March 28]. Available from: www.t1diabetes.nih.gov
[73] Type 1 Diabetes TrialNet.c2014 [cited 2014 March 28]. Available from: www.diabetestrialnet.org
[74] Couri CE, Oliveira MC, Stracieri AB. C-Peptide Levels and Insulin Independence Following Autologous Nonmyeloablative Hematopoietic Stem Cell Transplantation in Newly Diagnosed Type 1 Diabetes Mellitus. JAMA 2009; 301(15):1573-1579.
[75] Knowler W, Barrett-Connor E, Fowler S, *et al.* Reduction in the Incidence of type 2 Diabetes With Lifestyle Intervention or Metformin. NEJM 2002;346:393-403.
[76] Serreze DV, DiLorenzo TP. The good turned ugly: Immunopathogenic basis for diabetogenic CD8+ T cells in NOD mice. Immunol. Rev 2005; 204:250-263.
[77] Baker J. Public Health in the 21st Century, Diabetes Mellitus: Challenges for the 21st Century. Santa Barbara: Praeger Publishing, 2010; p. 29-53.

CHAPTER 7

From Fatty Liver to Cirrhosis: The Toll Rises!

Harmit S. Kalia* **and Allan W. Wolkoff**

Division of Gastroenterology and Liver Diseases, Marion Bessin Liver Research Center Albert Einstein College of Medicine and Montefiore Medical Center, Bronx, NY, USA

Abstract: Obesity is a growing epidemic affecting many races and nations. This rise is a major risk factor for many diseases including cardiovascular disease (CVD), diabetes mellitus (DM), certain malignancies and non-alcoholic fatty liver disease (NAFLD). NAFLD is now the most common cause of chronic liver disease in the US and many developed nations. Coexistence of DM and NAFLD can lead to progressive liver disease although mortality is usually due to CVD. The majority of NAFLD patients do not have progressive disease and liver biopsy is required to diagnose those individuals with non-alcoholic steatohepatitis (NASH) which can advance to cirrhosis and its complications. Several dietary, environmental and genetic factors may be important for the development of steatosis and progression of NASH. Although there have been several important observations regarding the pathophysiology of NASH, our understanding remains incomplete. Evaluation of NAFLD should include an assessment of contributory disorders such as metabolic syndrome and evaluation to rule out other causes of liver disease. The management of NAFLD is challenging as there is no effective drug therapy, and although lifestyle modification is often prescribed, clinical efficacy is usually low.

Keywords: Activity, behavior, diet, drug therapy, global health, health status, health, hepatic enzymes, lifestyle, liver, management, metabolic syndrome, non-alcoholic fatty liver disease, non-alcoholic steatohepatitis, nutrition, obesity, overweight, prevention, wellness.

INTRODUCTION

Non-alcoholic fatty liver disease (NAFLD) has become the most common cause of chronic liver disease in the U.S. and many developed nations. Having both diabetes and NAFLD is associated with progressive liver disease as well as cardiovascular disease. This chapter discusses NAFLD and the potential for progression to non-alcoholic steatohepatitis (NASH), which can advance to cirrhosis and its complications. The dietary, environmental and genetic factors

***Corresponding author Harmit S. Kalia:** 1180 Morris Park Ave, 2nd Floor, Bronx, NY 10461, USA; Tel: (347) 498-2421; Fax: (718) 239-6912; E-mail: HKalia@Montefiore.org

Judith Wylie-Rosett & Sunil S. Jhangiani (Eds)

associated with the development of steatosis and NASH are addressed. The chapter also addresses evaluation of NAFLD including assessment of contributory disorders such as metabolic syndrome and evaluation to rule out other causes of liver disease. The challenges related to the management of NAFLD are discussed.

OBESITY AS THE UNDERLYING PROBLEM

Obesity is a global epidemic that has been increasing since the 1970's. In 2008, it was estimated that there were about 1.4 billion overweight and obese adults (defined as BMI >25) in the world. Increased production and lower cost of food has fueled the higher energy intake and subsequent weight gain [1]. Liver metabolism may play a role in the effects of weight gain in increasing risk for diseases that include diabetes, cardiovascular diseases and various cancers. It is projected that obesity trends will continue to intensify and therefore add to morbidity and mortality in the approaching years [1]. Compared to normal weight individuals, obese patients have a reduction of life expectancy by about 7 years [2], which may involve the effects of weight gain on the liver.

This global problem is an inadvertent consequence of modernization that has led to a sedentary lifestyle and high caloric consumption [3]. And surprisingly, in certain parts of Africa, obesity has begun to afflict more children than malnutrition [4]. There is a marked disparity as to how obesity is viewed around the globe. In the context of body image, the slim body is preferred in the USA while in other parts of the world being overweight is desirable as it is thought to emulate wealth and prosperity [4].

Obesity is impacting longevity, quality-of-life, productivity and burdening health care systems globally. In the USA, the obesity epidemic may increase liver disease in addition to its projected increase in cases of diabetes, coronary artery disease (CAD), stroke and cancer, which are likely to cost approximately $66 billion/year [5]. The economic costs of obesity and related disorders have resulted in novel approaches in several European nations. Hungary has started to tax foods containing high salt and sugar with the goal of using the extra funds to offset their overly indebted health care system [6].

NAFLD AND DIABETES

According to the World Health Organization (WHO), an estimated 347 million people worldwide have diabetes. This global epidemic of diabetes is due to rapid increases in overweight, obesity and physical inactivity [7]. Type 2 Diabetes

Mellitus (T2DM) is associated with insulin resistance (IR) at multiple levels including skeletal muscle, liver and adipose tissue. IR precedes Type 2 DM and based on one study in which patients with NAFLD were screened for IR with glucose tolerance test, 85% of them had pre-diabetes [8]. It is therefore important to screen patients with NAFLD for DM [8]. Insulin resistance at the hepatic level prevents increase in hepatic gluconeogenesis and is associated with NAFLD, diminished insulin clearance and peripheral hyperinsulinemia [9]. Also, DM along with obesity, age, advanced fibrosis, cirrhosis, and iron deposition are potential risk factors for the development of hepatocellular carcinoma (HCC) [10]. The risk of HCC in individuals with DM has been found to be reduced in those taking statins [11]. Although randomized controlled trials are needed to evaluate the benefit of statins in NAFLD, this class of medication should be considered to improve the metabolic lipid profile of this patient population.

NAFLD AND CARDIOVASCULAR DISEASE

Cardiovascular disease is the leading cause of death in patients with NAFLD [12]. There are many mechanisms that accelerate the premature cardiovascular disease in this patient population including hypertension, hyperglycemia and dyslipidemia [13]. This is not surprising as CVD and NAFLD share the same risk factors of metabolic syndrome *i.e.*, abdominal obesity, dyslipidemia, hypertension and insulin resistance [14]. NAFLD has been shown to be an independent risk factor for the development and progression of cardiovascular disease causing fatal and non-fatal cardiac events [15-18].

NAFLD AND DIETARY FACTORS

There have been several reports of dietary factors influencing the development of NASH. One report showed that patients with NASH consumed a diet rich in saturated fatty acid and less polyunsaturated fatty acids (PUFA), fiber, and antioxidant vitamins C and E when compared with controls [19]. Another study found that NASH patients had lower carbohydrate consumption and higher intake of omega-6 (n-6) fatty acids along with a high omega-6/omega-3 (n-6/n-3) ratio as compared to controls [20]. In addition, high consumption of soft drinks and of meat has been associated with increased risk for NAFLD, while a higher intake of fish rich in omega-3 fatty acids has been shown to have a protective effect [21]. Fructose, commonly found in soft drinks, like other components of a hyper-caloric diet, tends to add to visceral adiposity as well as an increase in hepatic lipid accumulation and progression to NASH [22]. Consumption of processed food products that are high in fat, salt and sugar content (including soft drinks) is on the rise in high-income and middle income countries. Globally, this industry is subject to few regulations, and it has been suggested that durable public health policies and education are required [23].

Dietary factors that may be protective in NAFLD include moderate coffee consumption, which has been associated with reduction in fibrosis risk in patients with NASH. This observation has been attributed to the antioxidant effect of coffee and not from its content of caffeine [24]. Evidence has also been presented suggesting that moderate alcohol use may have a protective effect on development of NAFLD. In a cross-sectional population study, subjects who consumed one drink of alcohol daily had a lower prevalence of suspected NAFLD than those who did not drink [25]. A protective role of alcohol has also been demonstrated in patients with biopsy proven NAFLD in whom consumption of up to 2 drinks per day reduced the risk of NASH by 50% [26]. A meta-analysis also validated this decreased risk of steatohepatitis in patients with NAFLD who are moderate alcohol drinkers [27]. Alcohol may have a cardioprotective benefit in this population and others but the challenge for clinicians is to counsel patients on the harmful effects of heavy alcohol use and to consider the role of moderate alcohol use in some patients only after assessing the risks *vs* benefits.

EPIDEMIOLOGY

Prevalence of NAFLD

Most studies have used ultrasound imaging to determine the prevalence of NAFLD. Some studies have added aspartate aminotransferase (AST) and alanine aminotransferase (ALT) determinations to characterize NAFLD but for the most part, use of these tests as well as liver biopsies have been limited to studies in high risk populations. These studies have shown that NAFLD is a growing problem worldwide. Table **1** shows the prevalence of NAFLD in diverse sub-populations and although rates vary from population to population, the percentages are indeed quite alarming. Obesity, diabetes, hyperlipidemia, older age and non-Caucasian race are risk factors that have been associated with development of NAFLD. In the USA, the prevalence of chronic liver disease has been stable for all etiologies except for NAFLD which has been increasing [28]. An ethnic predisposition for occurrence of NAFLD has been noted in non-Caucasian populations. Hispanics, in particular, have an increased disease burden and severity compared to other ethnic groups. One study demonstrated that Hispanic patients with NAFLD were more likely to have advanced hepatic fibrosis than Caucasians [29]. In the Dallas

Heart Study of 2000 patients, steatosis was found in 45% of Hispanics, but in only 33% and 24% of Caucasians and African Americans, respectively [30, 31]. In the European DIONYSOS study, occurrence of NAFLD was a function of BMI, occurring in 25% of individuals with BMI <25, 67% with BMI of 25-29 and 91% of persons with BMI > 30 [32]. The prevalence increases in those with risk factors such as metabolic syndrome (also see CHAPTER 5: Moving Beyond Metabolic Syndrome).

Table 1. Prevalence of NAFLD (Adapted from [33]).

Sub-Populations	Prevalence of NAFLD
Asia	9.3-29.5%
China (general population)	12.9-28.9%
Europe	4.7-46%
Israel (general population)	30%
Japan (general population)	13-29%
United States (general population) African Americans Caucasians Hispanics	31% 24% 33% 45%
Patient with diabetes	40 - 69.5%
Patients undergoing bariatric surgery	33.8-99%

Natural History

As described above, NAFLD is an increasingly common chronic liver disorder with worldwide distribution that parallels the global rise in diabetes, obesity and metabolic syndrome [34]. This has the potential to become a major health problem in developed countries. In 2008, it was estimated that there were at least 1.46 billion overweight and obese adults and 170 million obese children worldwide [34]. With obesity and NAFLD on the rise, it is not surprising that among patients with NAFLD, liver disease is the third leading cause of death after cardiovascular disease and malignancy [35]. NAFLD represents a broad spectrum of disorders ranging from simple steatosis to non-alcoholic steatohepatitis (NASH) with cirrhosis and liver failure [36]. Simple steatosis usually has a benign outcome [37] but can progress in approximately 10% of patients to NASH with development of fibrosis [10, 38, 39]. NASH has a high risk of progression into advanced fibrosis, cirrhosis and its complications [40, 41]. It is important to note that regression of fibrosis (pre-cirrhosis) has been described following bariatric surgery [42]. Based on a long term Swedish study, the impact of NAFLD on mortality is remarkable with increased risk of death in patients with NASH compared to the general population [43]. Progression to HCC is well established in patients with NAFLD with advanced fibrosis and cirrhosis and the relative risk appears to be less than due to viral and alcoholic liver cirrhosis but will be overshadowed by the rising rates of NAFLD [44]. It is worrisome to note that HCC has been reported in non-cirrhotic NASH patients [45] and this will continue to be a growing concern as the prevalence of NAFLD rises and indications for HCC surveillance of this population will need to be reconsidered.

PATHOPHYSIOLOGY

In 1998, it was suggested that steatosis followed by oxidative stress, named the "two-hit" model, explained the progression from simple steatosis to steatohepatitis [46]. With over a decade of research since that time, it is now thought that parallel insults from the gut and adipose tissue may contribute to liver inflammation [47]. A detailed explanation of the pathophysiology of NAFLD is beyond the scope of this chapter. In brief, obesity, T2DM and metabolic syndrome create adipose tissue expansion and an environment of high free fatty acid entry into the liver. This in turn increases apolipoprotein B secretion and a dysregulation of insulin (insulin resistance) to suppress VLDL secretion, which in turn leads to lower HDL levels and higher LDL state. This along with a low plasma adiponectin levels (adipocyte-derived hormone that functions in energy homeostasis), may contribute to hepatic steatosis [48]. Several factors, including dietary (fructose, PUFA), interactions between host genetics and environment; immune activity, inflammation, cell injury and cell death are implicated in leading from simple steatosis to NASH [49]. Despite considerable ongoing research in this area, it is the sheer complexity and gaps in knowledge that has not allowed us to fully elucidate the mechanism of liver injury and why some patients do and others do not have progression of disease.

Genetics

There has been a lot of interest regarding genetic factors contributing to the onset of NAFLD and disease progression. NAFLD is most likely a disorder of multifactorial etiology. This has made identification of genetic influences a complicated undertaking. However, observations with twins; family aggregation and variable susceptibilities in different ethnicities have suggested that NAFLD has a genetic component. Several candidate gene and genomic wide association studies have identified multiple genetic modifiers for NAFLD and PNPLA3 is the most validated (Table **2**).

Table 2. Relevant candidate genes in NAFLD (Adapted from [50]).

Gene	Function	Mutation
PNPLA3	It encodes a protein that is a triaclglycerol lipase that mediates triacyglycerol hydrolysis in adipocytes	A single nucleotide mutation has shown to increase the hepatic triacylglyceride concentration.
GCKR	Regulates glucokinase activity which controls glucose metabolism	A single nucleotide polymorphism (SNP) may increase glucose uptake in the liver
PEMT	Catalyses synthesis of phosphatidylcholine, required for VLDL production.	Mutation linked to NAFLD
SCDC	Codes for a protein that binds to the superoxide byproducts of oxidative phosphorylation and converts them to hydrogen peroxide and oxygen, as a protective measure against cell damage.	A SNP in this gene has been associated with hepatic fibrosis in NAFLD
KLF6	Codes for a transcription factor found on satellite cells	A SNP has been associated with milder fibrosis in some NAFLD cohorts
ATGR1	Codes for a receptor that is expressed on the surface of hepatic stellate cell (HSC)	A genetic variation in this gene can play a role in progression of fibrosis in NAFLD

Histology

NAFLD- is an encompassing term that includes a spectrum of histologic findings from simple steatosis through steatohepatitis progressing from mild fibrosis to cirrhosis (Fig. **1**). The steatosis is macro-vesicular, involving > 5% of the liver and often found in zone 3 although it may be panacinar. Microscopic examination of the liver in NASH may have an appearance identical to that seen in alcoholic steatohepatitis with findings of steatosis, characteristic hepatocyte ballooning (cell injury), and zone 3 lobular inflammation (consisting of lymphocytes, with some eosinophils and neutrophils) [51]. A common finding in NASH is apoptotic bodies, which are remains of hepatocytes after programmed cell death. Other histological findings associated with NASH include Mallory-Denk bodies (MDB), megamitochondria, glycogenated nuclei and iron deposition. Fibrosis can be found with steatosis alone but usually is present with steatohepatitis, often perisinusoidal in zone 3. Early on, the fibrosis is in a "chicken wire" pattern due to deposition of perisinusoidal deposition of fibers. This feature along with steatosis, ballooning, MDB may disappear by the time advanced fibrosis or cirrhosis ensues [51, 52].

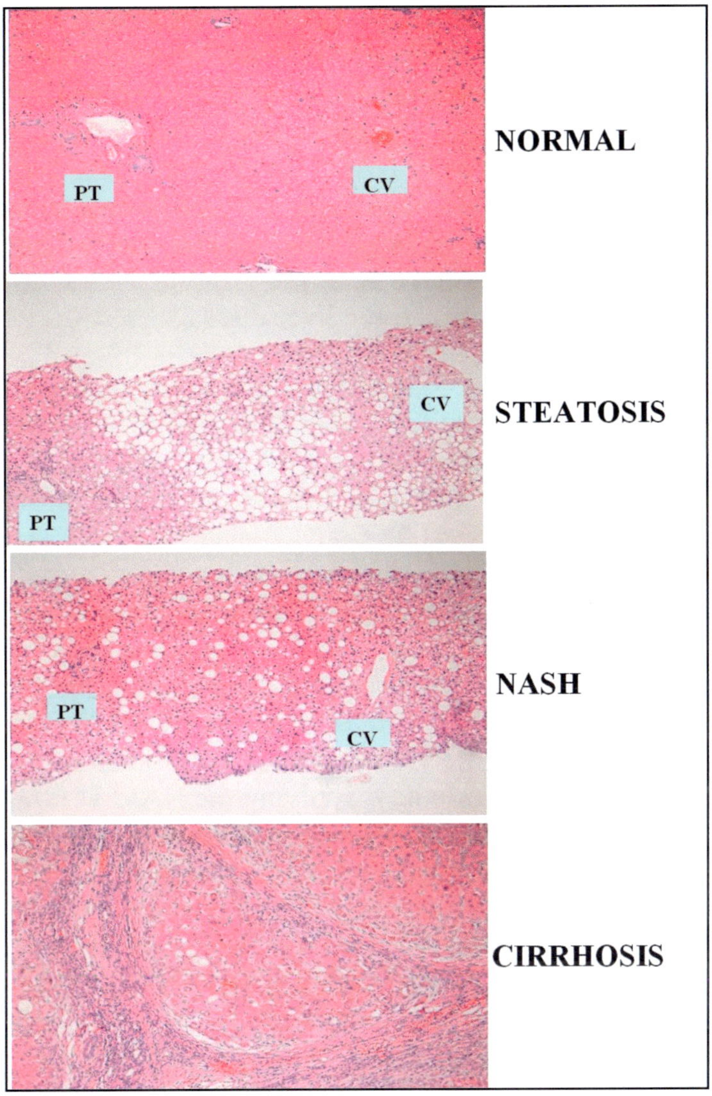

Fig. (1). Histology of normal liver and the NAFLD spectrum (Steatosis, NASH and Cirrhosis). Steatosis: Macrovescicular and occupying > 60% of the field. NASH: showing lobular inflammation. Cirrhosis: cirrhotic nodule. PT: Portal Triad; CV: Central Vein. Courtesy of Katherine Sun, MD, PhD, Montefiore Medical Center, Bronx NY.

ASSESSING FIBROSIS IN NAFLD

The gold standard to assess fibrosis in liver disease is liver biopsy but the procedure is invasive, not without risks and relatively expensive. Furthermore, the fact that histologic lesions of NASH are unevenly distributed within the liver can result in misdiagnosis and inaccurate staging [53]. The risk of fibrosis in NAFLD patients with elevated liver enzymes increases with increasing severity of metabolic conditions such as diabetes mellitus, hypertension, and visceral obesity [54]. Furthermore, in a systematic analysis, presence of inflammation on the initial liver biopsy and age were independently linked with progression to advanced fibrosis in patients with NASH [55]. Therefore, patients with the aforementioned risk factors should be evaluated with a liver biopsy. In an attempt to replace liver biopsy with less invasive tests, several scoring systems based on clinical or laboratory parameters have been proposed to assess advanced fibrosis in patients with NAFLD and other chronic liver diseases [56-60].

Although there are many non-invasive tests (biomarkers and prediction scores) that have been evaluated for NAFLD, none is straightforward and accurate for disease staging [61]. Some of these include, AST/ALT ratio, AST to platelet ratio index, BARD (weighted sum of BMI>28=1 point, AST/ALT ratio >0.8=2 points, Diabetes=1 point), FIB-4 (age x AST (IU/l)/platelet count (x 10^9/litre) and NAFLD fibrosis score [62]. One study showed that the diagnostic accuracy of these non-invasive scoring systems was sufficient to exclude advanced fibrosis and avoid liver biopsies approximately 38-69% of the time [62]. NAFLD fibrosis score is the most extensively validated non-invasive scoring system. NAFLD fibrosis = - 1.675 + 0.037 X age (years) + 0.094 X BMI (kg/m$^{2)}$ + 1.13 X IFG/Diabetes (yes =1, no= 2) + 0.99 x AST/ALT ratio -0.013 x platelet (X 10^9/l)- 0.66 X albumin (g/dl) [60]. In one study, applying the NAFLD fibrosis score (age, hyperglycemia, BMI, platelet count, albumin and AST/ALT ratio) had a positive predictive value (PPV) of 90% and liver biopsy was avoided in 75% of a large cohort [60]. A score of > 0.676 was predictive of advanced fibrosis and < 1.455 excluded it [60]. NAFLD fibrosis score was again reinforced as a superior indicator of advanced fibrosis in NAFLD [63]. The NAFLD fibrosis score has been validated in other populations like the Latin [64] Chinese [65] and Japanese [66] populations with reasonable results. It is a supportive tool in identifying patients with advanced fibrosis who would benefit from a liver biopsy. Transient elastography, approved by the Food and Drug Administration in 2013, is another non-invasive modality that can measure liver stiffness at point of care. In a meta-analysis, the pooled sensitivities and specificities for advanced fibrosis like F3 and F4 were 85% and 82%; and 92% and 92%. A modified probe has to be used in obese patients to improve accuracy [67]. Using a combination of different non-invasive methods to improve overall diagnostic accuracy which would eliminate the need for liver biopsy, has been proposed but requires validation [68].

EVALUATION AND MANAGEMENT OF NAFLD

Diagnosing NAFLD usually involves a several step process of evaluation before obtaining a liver biopsy, which is considered the "gold standard" for diagnosis. There are several risk factors associated with NAFLD that should be considered in the evaluation. If patients have persistent elevation in aminotransferases, risk factors for NAFLD and non-invasive markers suggests advanced fibrosis, a liver biopsy is usually indicated. The algorithm for the evaluation of NAFLD is outlined in Fig. (**2**).

Focus on Risk Factors

At the current time, there is no approved drug for the treatment of NASH. The treatment of NAFLD includes focus on improving metabolic risk factors along with managing the liver disease. Lifestyle change including diet modification and weight loss are central in the management of this disease. The American Association for the Study of Liver Diseases (AASLD) has guidelines for management of NAFLD but has not as yet taken a position on the use of alcohol in prevention or treatment [36]. As these patients have metabolic syndrome, lifestyle modification, with weight loss and exercise are important. And, depending on the metabolic derangement in the patient, optimizing the diabetes, hyperlipidemia, and hypertension are imperative [69]. Over the past few years, several therapeutic agents have been studied but their efficacy is not clear. There are several limitations in the studies for NAFLD. As demonstrated in a meta-analysis of randomized trials for treatment of NAFLD, many studies lacked assessment of post-treatment histology. In addition, determinations of liver enzymes in the circulation and hepatic steatosis may not be reliable parameters, as they fluctuate over time and do not follow the course of inflammation and fibrosis. Many trials had a duration of 2 years, from which predicting efficacy may be difficult [70]. Many agents have been studied in the management of NAFLD with many of them showing some beneficial results. Since reviewing all that data is beyond the scope of this chapter, in this section we will review agents that have consistent results and may have some role in management of NAFLD after the provider has carefully considered their risks and benefits and discussed them with the patient.

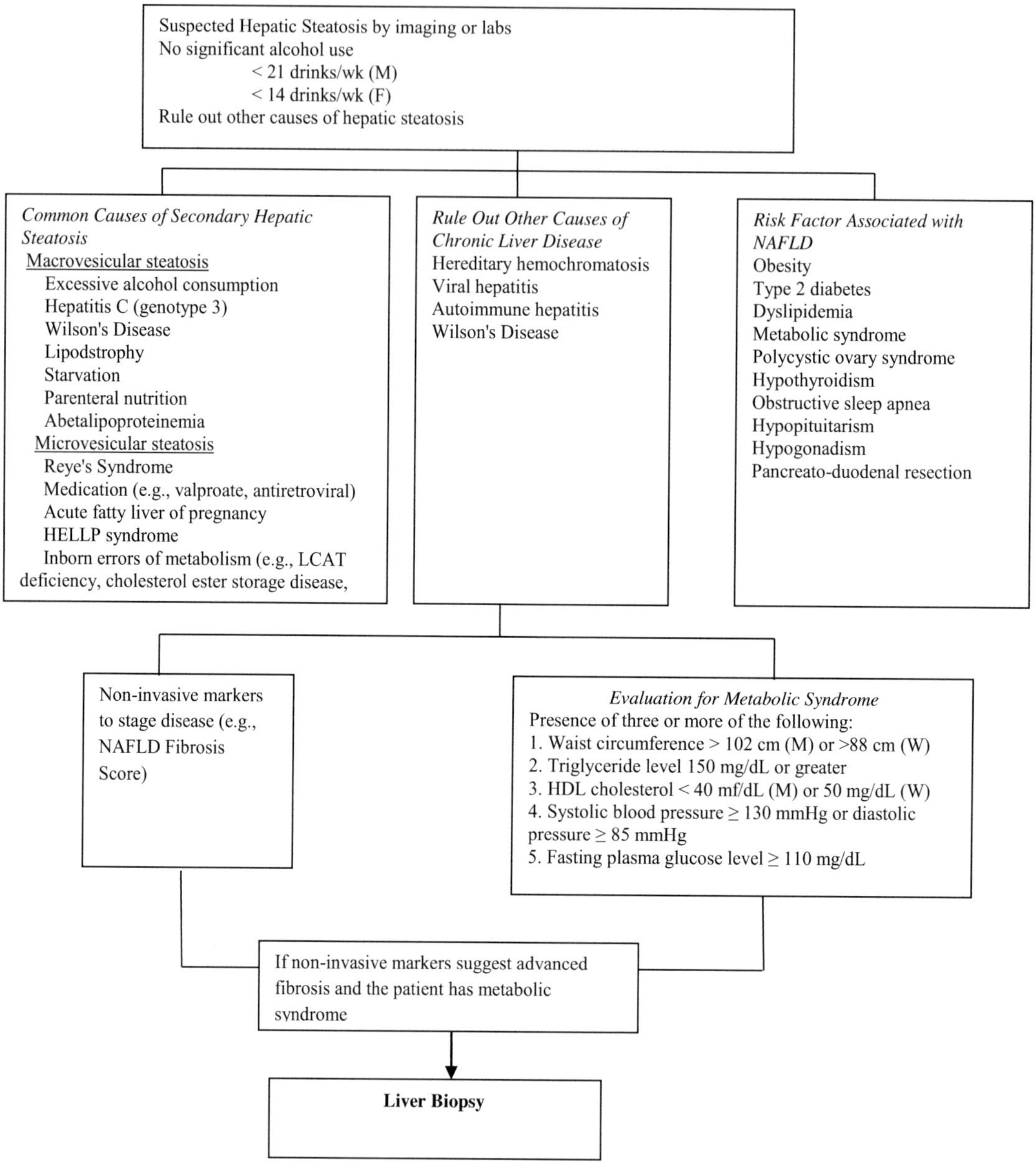

Fig. (2). Evaluation of the NAFLD to assess alcohol and secondary causes (Adapted from the AASLD guidelines [36]).

In a randomized controlled trial on non-diabetic patients with NASH, Vitamin E (antioxidant) showed improvement in NASH greater than Pioglitazone, a peroxisome proliferative-activated receptor (PPAR) gamma agonist. Both agents reduced inflammation and steatosis but not fibrosis [71]. The AASLD guidelines recommend using Vitamin E 800 IU daily in non-diabetics with NASH, but health care providers should acknowledge the concerns of increased mortality [72] and the increased risk of prostate cancer [73] with long term use. Pioglitazone can be used in non-diabetics with NASH, but lacks durability of response [74], may increase risk of bladder cancer [75], heart failure [76] and fractures [77]. Omega 3 fatty acids may reduce triglyceride synthesis in the liver and their use has resulted in some improvement in steatosis. Fish oil (also contains omega 3 fatty acids) can reduce steatosis [78] and is also beneficial for primary and secondary prevention of coronary artery disease [79] but may also increase risk of prostate cancer [80]. Therefore, it is important for the health care practitioner to discuss the long term risks and benefits of these agents with the patient.

There are many other agents being evaluated for the treatment of NASH. One promising agent is obeticholic acid, a semisynthetic derivative of the bile acid chenodeoxycholic acid. It is an agonist of the farnesoid X receptor, which is a nuclear hormone receptor that regulates glucose and lipid metabolism. In a proof of concept, phase 2 study, insulin sensitivity, a marker of liver fibrosis (no histology) and inflammation improved [81]. Larger and long term studies with liver histology are needed to confirm the therapeutic effects for NAFLD, which has a large unmet need for effective, safe treatment [82].

Lifestyle Intervention

Lifestyle intervention with diet modification and exercise has been the universally accepted standard of care in management of NAFLD. In a systematic review of lifestyle interventions, a weight reduction range of 4-14% reduced hepatic steatosis by 35-81%. The studies are heterogeneous and reduction in hepatic steatosis can be attained with exercise without weight change; low calorie diet and exercise and low calorie diet alone. The best lifestyle intervention in patients with NAFLD remains unclear. Although lifestyle interventions reduce hepatic steatosis by redistribution of fat and improvement of insulin sensitivity, their effect on hepatic fibrosis is unclear [83]. Nevertheless, diet modification and exercise should be recommended to these patients with a goal of < 1.6 kg/week as faster weight loss can cause liver injury [84].

Statins

Since NAFLD is considered a hepatic manifestation of metabolic syndrome, many of these patients have concomitant dyslipidemia. Statins are commonly used to treat dyslipidemia in the general population but their role in treating NAFLD is unknown. A Cochrane review found only two trials of statin use in NAFLD that were acceptable for evaluation. Both had high risk bias and did not assess histology, or liver related mortality. Based on these findings, statins were not recommended for use in the treatment of NAFLD and NASH [85]. AASLD Guidelines on NAFLD recommend using statins in NAFLD patients for the following reasons:

1. Cardiovascular disease is the leading cause of death in patients with NAFLD and these patients should have appropriate cardiac risk stratification and treatment with statins if appropriate [36, 86].

2. Patients with NAFLD are not at increased risk of hepatotoxicity with statins as this class of medication has been deemed safe [36].

3. Furthermore, a NHANES III database study of NAFLD patients taking statins for dyslipidemia showed no link between statin use and liver related mortality [87].

Bariatric Surgery

In the past few decades, bariatric surgery has evolved into a safer surgical option for the management of obesity in patients who cannot lose weight with lifestyle modification. The National Institutes of Health (NIH) has published consensus criteria regarding evaluation of obese patients for bariatric surgery [88]. These patients should have a BMI of at least 40 kg/m^2 in the absence of co-morbid conditions or 35 kg/m^2 with a co-morbid condition such as diabetes [88]. The efficacy of bariatric surgery has been remarkable with significant weight loss and improvement of coexisting conditions [88]. Weight recidivism rates are 10-20% [89]. Since NAFLD is considered as a hepatic manifestation of metabolic syndrome, treating it with bariatric surgery would be a logical choice. Unfortunately, although there is improvement in steatosis and inflammation (lobular but not portal) [88], there appears to be little influence on progression of fibrosis [90]. A Cochrane database review in 2010 reported lack of unbiased evidence to support bariatric surgery as a treatment for NASH [91]. The AASLD guidelines recommends that foregut surgery is not contraindicated in an eligible obese patient with fatty liver disease, especially in those who do not have cirrhosis but does not recommend it as treatment specifically for NASH [36].

CONCLUSION

NAFLD is most common cause of liver disease in developed countries and its rise parallels the rise in metabolic syndrome. A proportion of NAFLD is progressive and leads to NASH which has an indolent clinical course to end stage liver disease and its complications like HCC. Cardiovascular disease is major reason for decreased survival in this patient population. Ongoing research efforts in elucidating the pathophysiology and understanding the genetic etiology have been helpful, but far from complete. Making the diagnosis of NASH requires a liver biopsy and once a diagnosis is made, treatment options are limited. Ongoing studies evaluating potential targets for treatment of NASH should be vigorously pursued.

ACKNOWLEDGEMENTS

Declared none.

CONFLICT OF INTEREST

The authors confirm that this chapter contents have no conflict of interest.

REFERENCES

[1] Swinburn BA, Sacks G, Hall KD, *et al.* The global obesity pandemic: shaped by global drivers and local environments. Lancet 2011; 378(9793): 804-14.

[2] Peeters A, Barendregt JJ, Willekens F, Mackenbach JP, Al Mamun A, Bonneux L; NEDCOM, the Netherlands Epidemiology and Demography Compression of Morbidity Research Group. Obesity in adulthood and its consequences for life expectancy: a life-table analysis. Ann Intern Med 2003; 138(1): 24-32.

[3] Gill TP, Antipatis VJ, James WP. The global epidemic of obesity. Asia Pac J Clin Nutr 1999; 8(1): 75-81.

[4] Nonalcoholic fatty liver disease and nonalcoholic steatohepatitis, World Gastroenterology Organisation Global Guidelines - June 2012. c2006-2014 [cited 2014 Mar 18]. Available from: www.worldgastroenterology.org/NAFLD-NASH.html

[5] Wang YC, McPherson K, Marsh T, Gortmaker SL, Brown M. Health and economic burden of the projected obesity trends in the USA and the UK. Lancet 2011; 378(9793): 815-25.

[6] Holt E. Hungary to introduce broad range of fat taxes. Lancet 2011; 378(9793): 755.

[7] World Health Organization. 10 facts about diabetes.c2014 [updated 2013 Oct; cited 2014 Mar 18]. Available from: http://www.who.int/features/factfiles/diabetes/en/index.html

[8] Ortiz-Lopez C, Lomonaco R, Orsak B, *et al.* Prevalence of prediabetes and diabetes and metabolic profile of patients with nonalcoholic fatty liver disease (NAFLD). Diabetes Care 2012; 35(4): 873-8.

[9] Cusi K. Lessons learned from studying families genetically predisposed to type 2 diabetes mellitus. Curr Diab Rep 2009; 9(3): 200-7.
[10] Starley BQ, Calcagno CJ, Harrison SA. Nonalcoholic fatty liver disease and hepatocellular carcinoma: a weighty connection. Hepatology 2010; 51(5): 1820-32.
[11] El-Serag HB, Johnson ML, Hachem C, Morgana RO. Statins are associated with a reduced risk of hepatocellular carcinoma in a large cohort of patients with diabetes. Gastroenterology 2009; 136(5): 1601-8.
[12] Pacana T, Fuchs M. The cardiovascular link to nonalcoholic fatty liver disease: a critical analysis. Clin Liver Dis 2012; 16(3): 599-613.
[13] Lomonaco R, Chen J, Cusi K. An endocrine perspective of nonalcoholic fatty liver disease (NAFLD). Ther Adv Endocrinol Metab 2011; 2(5): 211-25. Assessing Fibrosis in NAFLD
[14] Targher G, Day CP, Bonora E. Risk of cardiovascular disease in patients with nonalcoholic fatty liver disease. N Engl J Med 2010; 363(14): 1341-50.
[15] Hamaguchi M, Kojima T, Takeda N, *et al.* Nonalcoholic fatty liver disease is a novel predictor of cardiovascular disease. World J Gastroenterol 2007; 13(10): 1579-84.
[16] Targher G, Bertolini L, Poli F, Rodella S, Scala L, Tessari R, Zenari L, Falezza G. Nonalcoholic fatty liver disease and risk of future cardiovascular events among type 2 diabetic patients. Diabetes 2005; 54(12): 3541-6.
[17] Targher G, Bertolini L, Rodella S, *et al.* Nonalcoholic fatty liver disease is independently associated with an increased incidence of cardiovascular events in type 2 diabetic patients. Diabetes Care 2007; 30(8): 2119-21.
[18] Haring R, Wallaschofski H, Nauck M, Dörr M, Baumeister SE, Völzke H. Ultrasonographic hepatic steatosis increases prediction of mortality risk from elevated serum gamma-glutamyl transpeptidase levels. Hepatology 2009; 50(5): 1403-11.
[19] Musso G, Gambino R, De Michieli F, *et al.* Dietary habits and their relations to insulin resistance and postprandial lipemia in nonalcoholic steatohepatitis. Hepatology 2003; 37(4): 909-16.
[20] Cortez-Pinto H, Jesus L, Barros H, Lopes C, Moura MC, Camilo ME. How different is the dietary pattern in non-alcoholic steatohepatitis patients? Clin Nutr 2006; 25(5): 816-23.
[21] Zelber-Sagi S, Nitzan-Kaluski D, Goldsmith R, *et al.* Long term nutritional intake and the risk for non-alcoholic fatty liver disease (NAFLD): a population based study. J Hepatol 2007; 47(5): 711-7.
[22] Fan JG, Cao HX. Role of diet and nutritional management in non-alcoholic fatty liver disease. J Gastroenterol Hepatol 2013; 28 Suppl 4: 81-7.
[23] Monteiro CA, Moubarac JC, Cannon G, Ng SW, Popkin B. Ultra-processed products are becoming dominant in the global food system.Obes Rev 2013; 14 Suppl 2: 21-8.
[24] Molloy JW, Calcagno CJ, Williams CD, Jones FJ, Torres DM, Harrison SA. Association of coffee and caffeine consumption with fatty liver disease, nonalcoholic steatohepatitis, and degree of hepatic fibrosis. Hepatology 2012; 55(2): 429-36.
[25] Dunn W, Xu R, Schwimmer JB. Modest wine drinking and decreased prevalence of suspected nonalcoholic fatty liver disease. Hepatology 2008; 47(6): 1947-54.
[26] Dunn W, Sanyal AJ, Brunt EM, *et al.* Modest alcohol consumption is associated with decreased prevalence of steatohepatitis in patients with non-alcoholic fatty liver disease (NAFLD). J Hepatol 2012; 57(2): 384-91.
[27] Sookoian S, Castaño GO, Pirola CJ. Modest alcohol consumption decreases the risk of non-alcoholic fatty liver disease: a meta-analysis of 43175 individuals. Gut 2014; 63(3): 530-2.
[28] Younossi ZM, Stepanova M, Afendy M, *et al.* Changes in the prevalence of the most common causes of chronic liver diseases in the United States from 1988 to 2008. Clin Gastroenterol Hepatol 2011; 9(6): 524-530.
[29] Verma S, Bonacini M, Govindarajan S, *et al.* More advanced hepatic fibrosis in Hispanics with chronic hepatitis C infection: role of patient demographics, hepatic necroinflammation, and steatosis. Am J Gastroenterol 2006; 101: 1817-1823.
[30] Browning JD, Szczepaniak LS, Dobbins R, *et al.* Prevalence of hepatic steatosis in an urban population in the United States; impact of ethnicity. Hepatology 2004; 40: 1387-1395.
[31] Lazo M, Clark JM. The epidemiology of nonalcoholic fatty liver disease: a global perspective. Semin Liver Dis 2008; 28(4): 339-50. doi: 10.1055/s-0028-1091978. Epub 2008 Oct 27.

[32] Bellentani S, Bedogni G, Miglioli L, Tiribelli C, Eur J. The epidemiology of fatty liver. Gastroenterol Hepatol 2004; 16(11): 1087-93.
[33] Lazo M, Clark JM. The epidemiology of nonalcoholic fatty liver disease: a global perspective. Semin Liver Dis 2008; 28(4): 339-50. doi: 10.1055/s-0028-1091978. Epub 2008 Oct 27. Review.
[34] Alberti KG, Zimmet P, Shaw J; IDF Epidemiology Task Force Consensus Group. The metabolic syndrome--a new worldwide definition. Lancet 2005; 366: 1059-62.
[35] Ong JP, Pitts A, Younossi ZM. Increased overall mortality and liver-related mortality in non-alcoholic fatty liver disease. J Hepatol 2008; 49(4): 608-12.
[36] Chalasani N, Younossi Z, Lavine JE, *et al.* The diagnosis and management of non-alcoholic fatty liver disease: practice Guideline by the American Association for the Study of Liver Diseases, American College of Gastroenterology, and the American Gastroenterological Association. Hepatology 2012; 55(6): 2005-23.
[37] Teli MR, James OF, Burt AD, Bennett MK, Day CP. The natural history of nonalcoholic fatty liver: a follow-up study. Hepatology 1995; 22(6): 1714-9.
[38] Pais R, Pascale A, Fedchuck L, Charlotte F, Poynard T, Ratziu V. Progression from isolated steatosis to steatohepatitis and fibrosis in nonalcoholic fatty liver disease. Clin Res Hepatol Gastroenterol 2011; 35(1): 23-8.
[39] Wong VW, Wong GL, Choi PC, *et al.* Disease progression of non-alcoholic fatty liver disease: a prospective study with paired liver biopsies at 3 years. Gut 2010; 59(7): 969-74.
[40] Harrison SA, Torgerson S, Hayashi PH. The natural history of nonalcoholic fatty liver disease: a clinical histopathological study. Am J Gastroenterol 2003; 98(9): 2042-7.
[41] Adams LA, Lymp JF, St Sauver J, *et al.* The natural history of nonalcoholic fatty liver disease: a population-based cohort study. Gastroenterology 2005; 129(1): 113-21.
[42] Weiner RA. Surgical treatment of non-alcoholic steatohepatitis and non-alcoholic fatty liver disease. Dig Dis 2010; 28(1): 274-9.
[43] Söderberg C, Stål P, Askling J, *et al.* Decreased survival of subjects with elevated liver function tests during a 28-year follow-up. Hepatology 2010; 51(2): 595-602.
[44] Vanni E, Bugianesi E. Obesity and liver cancer. Clin Liver Dis 2014; 18(1): 191-203.
[45] K. Yasui, E. Hashimoto, Y. Komorizono, *et al.* Characteristics of patients with nonalcoholic steatohepatitis who develop hepatocellular carcinoma. Clin Gastroenterol Hepatol, 2011; 9(5): 428-33.
[46] Day CP, James OF. Steatohepatitis: a tale of two "hits"? Gastroenterology 1998; 114(4): 842-5.
[47] Tilg H, Moschen AR. Hepatology. Evolution of inflammation in nonalcoholic fatty liver disease: the multiple parallel hits hypothesis. Hepatology 2010; 52(5): 1836-46. http://www.ncbi.nlm.nih.gov/pubmed/21038418 2010; 52(5): 1836-46.
[48] Cusi K. Role of obesity and lipotoxicity in the development of nonalcoholic steatohepatitis: pathophysiology and clinical implications. Gastroenterology 2012; 142(4). 711-725.
[49] Wree A, Broderick L, Canbay A, Hoffman HM, Feldstein AE. From NAFLD to NASH to cirrhosis-new insights into disease mechanisms. Nat Rev Gastroenterol Hepatol 2013; 10(11): 627-36.
[50] Anstee QM, Day CP. The genetics of NAFLD. Nat Rev Gastroenterol Hepatol 2013; 10(11): 645-55.
[51] Kleiner DE, Brunt EM. Nonalcoholic fatty liver disease: pathologic patterns and biopsy evaluation in clinical research. Semin Liver Dis 2012; 32(1): 3-13.
[52] Brunt EM, Tiniakos DG. Histopathology of nonalcoholic fatty liver disease. World J Gastroenterol 2010; 16(42): 5286-96.
[53] Ratziu V, Charlotte F, Heurtier A, *et al.* LIDO Study Group. Sampling variability of liver biopsy in nonalcoholic fatty liver disease. Gastroenterology 2005; 128(7): 1898-906.
[54] Hossain N, Afendy A, Stepanova M, *et al.* Independent predictors of fibrosis in patients with nonalcoholic fatty liver disease. Clin Gastroenterol Hepatol 2009; 7(11): 1224-9.
[55] Argo CK, Northup PG, Al-Osaimi AM, Caldwell SH. Systematic review of risk factors for fibrosis progression in non-alcoholic steatohepatitis. J Hepatol 2009; 51(2): 371-9.
[56] Wai CT, Greenson JK, Fontana RJ, *et al.* A simple noninvasive index can predict both significant fibrosis and cirrhosis in patients with chronic hepatitis C. Hepatology 2003; 38(2): 518-26.
[57] Williams AL, Hoofnagle JH. Ratio of serum aspartate to alanine aminotransferase in chronic hepatitis. Relationship to cirrhosis. Gastroenterology 1988; 95(3): 734-9.

[58] Harrison SA, Oliver D, Arnold HL, Gogia S, Neuschwander-Tetri BA. Development and validation of a simple NAFLD clinical scoring system for identifying patients without advanced disease. Gut 2008; 57(10): 1441-7.
[59] Vallet-Pichard A, Mallet V, Nalpas B, *et al.* FIB-4: an inexpensive and accurate marker of fibrosis in HCV infection. comparison with liver biopsy and fibrotest. Vallet-Pichard A Pol Hepatology 2007; 46(1): 32-6.
[60] Angulo P, Hui JM, Marchesini G, *et al.* The NAFLD fibrosis score: a noninvasive system that identifies liver fibrosis in patients with NAFLD. Hepatology 2007; 45(4): 846-54.
[61] Grandison GA, Angulo P. Can NASH be diagnosed, graded, and staged noninvasively? Clin Liver Dis 2012; 16(3): 567-85.
[62] McPherson S, Stewart SF, Henderson E, Burt AD, Day CP. Simple non-invasive fibrosis scoring systems can reliably exclude advanced fibrosis in patients with non-alcoholic fatty liver disease. Gut 2010; 59(9): 1265-9.
[63] Angulo P, Bugianesi E, Bjornsson ES, *et al.* Simple noninvasive systems predict long-term outcomes of patients with nonalcoholic fatty liver disease. Gastroenterology 2013; 145(4): 782-9.
[64] Pérez-Gutiérrez OZ, Hernández-Rocha C, Candia-Balboa RA, *et al.* Arrese MA, Benítez C, Brizuela-Alcántara DC, Méndez-Sánchez N, Uribe M, Chávez-Tapia NC. Validation study of systems for noninvasive diagnosis of fibrosis in nonalcoholic fatty liver disease in Latin population. Ann Hepatol 2013; 12(3): 416-24.
[65] Wong VW, Wong GL, Chim AM, *et al.* Validation of the NAFLD fibrosis score in a Chinese population with low prevalence of advanced fibrosis. Am J Gastroenterol 2008; 103(7): 1682-8.
[66] Nakano M, Murohisa T, Imai Y, Hiraishi H. Validity of the NAFLD fibrosis score in a Japanese population Nihon Shokakibyo Gakkai Zasshi 2012; 109(5): 751-9.
[67] Kwok R, Tse YK, Wong GL, *et al.* Systematic review with meta-analysis: non-invasive assessment of non-alcoholic fatty liver disease - the role of transient elastography and plasma cytokeratin-18 fragments. Aliment Pharmacol Ther 2014; 39(3): 254-69.
[68] Festi D, Schiumerini R, Marzi L, *et al.* Review article: the diagnosis of non-alcoholic fatty liver disease - availability and accuracy of non-invasive methods. Aliment Pharmacol Ther 2013; 37(4): 392-400.
[69] Lomonaco R, Sunny NE, Bril F, Cusi K. Nonalcoholic fatty liver disease: current issues and novel treatment approaches. Drugs 2013; 73(1): 1-14.
[70] Musso G, Gambino R, Cassader M, Pagano G. A meta-analysis of randomized trials for the treatment of nonalcoholic fatty liver disease. Hepatology 2010; 52(1): 79-104.
[71] Sanyal AJ, Chalasani N, Kowdley KV, *et al.* Pioglitazone, vitamin E, or placebo for nonalcoholic steatohepatitis. N Engl J Med 2010 ; 362(18): 1675-85.
[72] Bjelakovic G, Nikolova D, Gluud LL, Simonetti RG, Gluud C. Antioxidant supplements for prevention of mortality in healthy participants and patients with various diseases. Cochrane Database Syst Rev 2012; 3: CD007176.
[73] Klein EA, Thompson IM Jr, Tangen CM, *et al.* Vitamin E and the risk of prostate cancer: the Selenium and Vitamin E Cancer Prevention Trial (SELECT). JAMA 2011; 306(14): 1549-56.
[74] Lutchman G, Modi A, Kleiner DE, *et al.* The effects of discontinuing pioglitazone in patients with nonalcoholic steatohepatitis. Hepatology 2007; 46(2): 424-9.
[75] Lewis JD, Ferrara A, Peng T, *et al.* Risk of bladder cancer among diabetic patients treated with pioglitazone: interim report of a longitudinal cohort study. Diabetes Care 2011; 34(4): 916-22.
[76] Lincoff AM, Wolski K, Nicholls SJ, Nissen SE. Pioglitazone and risk of cardiovascular events in patients with type 2 diabetes mellitus: a meta-analysis of randomized trials.JAMA 2007; 298(10): 1180-8.
[77] Dormuth CR, Carney G, Carleton B, Bassett K, Wright JM. Thiazolidinediones and fractures in men and women. Arch Intern Med 2009 Aug; 169(15): 1395-402.
[78] Parker HM, Johnson NA, Burdon CA, Cohn JS, O'Connor HT, George J. Omega-3 supplementation and non-alcoholic fatty liver disease: a systematic review and meta-analysis. J Hepatol 2012; 56(4): 944-51.
[79] Roth EM, Harris WS. Fish oil for primary and secondary prevention of coronary heart disease. Curr Atheroscler Rep 2010; 12(1): 66-72.

[80] Brasky TM, Darke AK, Song X, *et al*. Plasma phospholipid fatty acids and prostate cancer risk in the SELECT trial. J Natl Cancer Inst 2013; 105(15): 1132-41.
[81] Mudaliar S, Henry RR, Sanyal AJ, *et al*. Efficacy and safety of the farnesoid X receptor agonist obeticholic acid in patients with type 2 diabetes and nonalcoholic fatty liver disease. Gastroenterology 2013; 145(3): 574-82.
[82] Karpen SJ. Do therapeutic bile acids hit the sweet spot of glucose metabolism in NAFLD? Gastroenterology 2013; 145(3): 508-10.
[83] Thoma C, Day CP, Trenell MI. Lifestyle interventions for the treatment of non-alcoholic fatty liver disease in adults: a systematic review. J Hepatol 2012; 56(1): 255-66.
[84] Luyckx FH, Desaive C, Thiry A, *et al*. Liver abnormalities in severely obese subjects: effect of drastic weight loss after gastroplasty. Int J Obes Relat Metab Disord 1998; 22(3): 222-6.
[85] Eslami L, Merat S, Malekzadeh R, Nasseri-Moghaddam S, Aramin H. Statins for non-alcoholic fatty liver disease and non-alcoholic steatohepatitis. Cochrane Database Syst Rev 2013; 12: CD008623.
[86] Pacana T, Fuchs M. Carotid artery ultrasonography evaluating the intimal thickness may be a way to screen for subclinical cardiovascular disease. The cardiovascular link to nonalcoholic fatty liver disease: a critical analysis. Clin Liver Dis 2012; 16(3): 599-613.
[87] Younoszai Z, Li Z, Stepanova M, Erario M, Cable R, Younossi ZM. Statin use is not associated with liver related mortality. Ann Hepatol 2013; 13(1): 84-90.
[88] Dixon JB. Surgical management of obesity in patients with morbid obesity and nonalcoholic fatty liver disease. Clin Liver Dis 2014 Feb; 18(1): 129-46.
[89] Sheppard CE, Lester EL, Chuck AW, Birch DW1, Karmali S1, de Gara CJ. The Economic Impact of Weight Regain.Gastroenterol Res Pract 2013; 2013: 379564.
[90] Mathurin P, Hollebecque A, Arnalsteen L, *et al*. Prospective study of the long-term effects of bariatric surgery on liver injury in patients without advanced disease. Gastroenterology 2009; 137(2): 532-40.
[91] Chavez-Tapia NC, Tellez-Avila FI, Barrientos-Gutierrez T, Mendez-Sanchez N, Lizardi-Cervera J, Uribe M. Bariatric surgery for non-alcoholic steatohepatitis in obese patients. Cochrane Database Syst Rev 2010; (1): CD007340.

CHAPTER 8

Obesity: Update on Nutrition and Behavioral Strategies

Judith Wylie-Rosett*,[1] and Carlos Marquez[2]

[1]*Albert Einstein College of Medicine, 1300 Morris Park Avenue, Bronx, NY, USA; and* [2]*Ferkauf Graduate School of Psychology, 1165 Morris Park Avenue, Bronx, NY, USA*

Abstract: The global rise in obesity has generated interest in nutrition and behavioral therapies as care processes for managing obesity and related co-morbidities. Growing evidence supports the use of nutritional consultation and intensive behavioral therapy to reduce risk factors associated with obesity. The World Health Organization recommends that the delivery of interventions should be of appropriate intensity and sustained over extended periods of time while noting that even modest changes in risk factor levels may achieve substantial public health benefits. Obesity guidelines provide recommended steps for identifying risk status, matching treatment to risk assessment, and implementing weight loss intervention strategies. A highly collaborative process of care, which focuses on the nutritional and lifestyle management of obesity and selected co-morbidities, is known as medical nutrition therapy (MNT), when provided by a registered dietitian, or as nutrition therapy when provided by other disciplines. Behavioral therapy approaches that focus on collaborative decision making include motivational interviewing and the 5 A's behavioral counseling steps. Motivational interviewing, which includes open-ended questions, reflective listening, affirmation and summarization, helps individuals address their concerns about making lifestyle changes. The 5 A's steps generally include: Ask/**Assess:** ask about/assess behavior and health risk(s); **Advise**: personalize behavior change advice; **Agree**: collaboratively select goals, **Assist**: use behavioral techniques to aid in achieving agreed-upon goals and **Arrange:** schedule follow-up. Training programs can help health professionals develop nutrition and behavioral therapy skills and address bias and discrimination. Weight management approaches and priorities will vary by the risk status and health care settings.

Keywords: 5A's, behavior, diabetes, diet, dietitian, global health, intensive behavioral therapy, medical nutrition therapy, MNT, motivational interviewing, nutrition therapy, obesity, overweight, wellness.

***Corresponding author Judith Wylie-Rosett:** Albert Einstein College of Medicine 1300 Morris Park Avenue, Bronx, NY 10461, USA; Tel: (718) 430-3345; Fax: (718) 430-8634;
E-mail: Judith.wylie-rosett@einstein.yu.edu

INTRODUCTION

A growing number of organizations are developing obesity guidelines to address the global obesity epidemic. These guidelines include recommendations for assessing risk status, matching treatment to risk assessment and implementing weight loss intervention strategies. A highly collaborative process of care, which focuses on the nutritional and lifestyle management of obesity and selected co-morbidities, is known as medical nutrition therapy (MNT), when provided by a registered dietitian, or as nutrition therapy when provided by other disciplines. Behavioral therapy approaches, which focus on collaborative decision making, are discussed. The chapter also provides information about training programs that can help health professionals develop nutrition and behavioral therapy skills. How weight management approach and priorities vary by the risk status and health care settings are also addressed.

GLOBAL PERSPECTIVE

The World Health Organization (WHO) and other health organizations recommend clinical as well as public health strategies to lessen the impact of obesity on the global rise in non-communicable diseases [1-4]. Clinical intervention strategies need to reflect the risk status of the population when most people have a moderate level of risk factors and a smaller number of people have a high level of risk. However, people at moderate risk contribute more to the total burden of noncommunicable diseases than individuals at high risk. Consequently, a comprehensive prevention strategy needs to synergistically blend an approach aimed at reducing risk factors in the general population with the one directed at high-risk individuals. Research evidence supports the use of nutrition and behavioral therapies to reduce cardiometabolic risk markers [5]. The WHO recommends that the delivery of interventions be of appropriate intensity and sustained over extended periods of time. However, it should also note that even modest changes in risk factor levels may have a substantial public health benefit [2].

CLINICAL PRACTICE RECOMMENDATIONS

Clinical practice recommendations and guidelines have been developed to combat the rise in obesity and its co-morbidities using evidence-based criteria [5-14]. Some focus on discipline specific criteria [6, 14], but the approach or care process may be used by other disciplines. The process of care known as medical nutrition therapy (MNT) is specific to counseling provided by a registered dietitian [6], and is referred to as nutrition therapy when provided by other disciplines. Both are highly collaborative processes of care that focus on the nutritional and lifestyle management of obesity and selected co-morbidities. Behavioral therapy approaches, which focus on collaborative decision making with patients such as the 5 A's behavioral counseling steps (Ask/Assess, Advise, Agree, Assist, Arrange), provide a framework for obesity counseling by any health professional [8]. However, in the USA, Medicare coverage for intensive behavioral therapy in treating obesity is restricted to primary care providers who document using the 5's approach [14].

2013 Obesity Guideline-Collaboration of Multiple Organizations in the USA

The 2013 Obesity Guidelines [5] for clinical practice, which were developed by the American College of Cardiology, the American Heart Association and the National Heart, Lung and Blood Institute, involved collaborations with stakeholders and professional organizations. The purpose of the Guidelines [5] was to review the evidence base for assessing cardiovascular risk and making lifestyle modifications to reduce cardiovascular risk in overweight and obese adults. In their review of evidence, the Guidelines Committee found that the nutrition professional providing dietary guidance was usually a registered dietitian. The majority of the studies provided the intervention in university nutrition departments or in hospital medical care settings where access to nutrition professionals was available. The Guidelines [5] noted that trained interventionists in the reviewed studies were usually health professionals (*e.g.*, registered dietitians, psychologists, exercise specialists, health counselors, or professionals in training) who adhered to formal protocols in weight management. Table **1** provides an overview of the 2013 Obesity Guidelines recommendations [5]. The published Guidelines also provide a detailed decision algorithm to help clinicians with assessment and treatment options.

The Guidelines [5] noted that more intensive interventions conducted in academic and clinical research settings achieve more weight loss than less intensive options that may be more accessible. The evidence review found that electronic weight loss programs and telephone delivered weight loss programs with personalized feedback can achieve weight loss. However, the amount of weight loss is usually smaller than with face-to-face interventions. The Guidelines [5] also noted that commercial-based programs, which provide a comprehensive lifestyle intervention, may be considered if there is evidence of safety and efficacy.

Table 1. Overview of 2013 obesity guidelines recommendations [5].

Identifying Patients Who Need to Lose Weight (BMI and Waist Circumference Assessment)
Measure height and weight to calculate BMI at annual visits or more frequently.
Use BMI of 25.0-29.9 kg/m^2 to identify adults at greater CVD risk and ≥ 30 kg/m^2 for elevated risk of mortality from all causes.
Measure waist circumference at annual visits or more frequently in overweight and obese adults.
Advise overweight/obese adults that higher BMI is linked to greater risk of CVD, type 2 diabetes and all-cause mortality.
Advise adults that increasing waist circumference is associated with greater risk of CVD, type 2 diabetes and all-cause mortality.
Matching Treatment Benefits With Risk Profiles (Reduce Body Weight Effect on CVD Risk Factors, Events and Mortality)
Counsel overweight/ obese adults with CVD risk factors (high BP, hyperlipidemia and hyperglycemia), that lifestyle changes that produce even modest but sustained weight loss of 3%-5% produce clinically meaningful health benefits. Advise that greater weight losses produces greater benefits.
Diets for Weight Loss (Dietary Strategies for Weight Loss)
Prescribe a diet to achieve reduced calorie intake for obese/overweight individuals as part of a comprehensive lifestyle intervention. Any of the following methods can be used to reduce food and calorie intake: 1) Prescribe 1,200-1,500 kcal/day for women and 1,500-1,800 kcal/day for men (kcal levels are usually adjusted for the individual's body weight); 2) Prescribe a 500 kcal/day or 750 kcal/day energy deficit or 3) Prescribe one of the evidence-based diets that restricts certain food types (such as high-carbohydrate foods, low-fiber foods or high-fat foods) in order to create an energy deficit by reduced food intake.
Consider the patient's preferences and health status and preferably refer to a nutrition professional* for counseling.
Lifestyle Intervention and Counseling (Comprehensive Lifestyle Intervention)
Refer overweight/obese individuals to a comprehensive lifestyle program that assists participants in adhering to a lower calorie diet and in increasing physical activity through the use of behavioral strategies.
Prescribe (6 months) comprehensive weight loss interventions that are provided in individual or group sessions by a trained interventionist.
Use a very low caloric diet (defined as <800 kcal/day) only in limited circumstances. Counseling should be provided by trained practitioners in a setting where medical monitoring and high intensity lifestyle intervention can be provided. Medical supervision is required to address rapid rate of weight loss and potential health complications.
Recommend long- term comprehensive programs to maintain weight loss.
For weight loss maintenance, prescribe face-to-face or telephone-delivered weight loss maintenance programs that provides regular contact (monthly or more frequent) with a trained interventionist.† Regular contact is needed support engaging in physical activity (*i.e.*, 200-300 minutes/week), monitoring body weight regularly (*i.e.*, weekly or more frequent) and consuming a reduced-calorie diet (needed to maintain lower body weight).
Selecting Patients for Bariatric Surgical Treatment for Obesity
Advise adults with a BMI ≥ 40 kg/m^2 or a BMI ≥ 35 kg/m^2 and obesity-related co-morbid conditions that bariatric surgery may be an appropriate option to improve health and offer referral to an experienced bariatric surgeon for consultation and evaluation. Referral is appropriate if an individual is motivated to lose weight and has not has not achieved health targets using behavioral treatment with or without pharmacotherapy.
Advise patients that choice of a specific bariatric surgical procedure may be affected by patient factors. Consider age, severity of obesity/BMI, co-morbidities, risk of short- and long-term complications, behavioral and psychosocial factors and patient tolerance for risk. Provider factors (surgeon and facility) should also be considered.

The Guidelines [5] included an in-depth review of the evidence regarding bariatric surgery. However, because most research trials use a BMI of $\geq$ 35 kg/m^2 as inclusion criteria, there is insufficient evidence to recommend for or against bariatric surgical procedures for a BMI <35 kg/m^2.

Medical Nutrition Therapy for Obesity

Medical nutrition therapy (MNT) when provided by a registered dietitian (nutrition therapy when provided by other disciplines) is the process of care for assessing and implementing an intervention that addresses individual nutritional needs [6]. Nutrition therapy for obesity addresses energy balance focusing on caloric intake derived from food consumed and energy expenditure from physical activity. Therefore, assessment and intervention with regard to physical activity are integral in the nutrition therapy in overweight and obese individuals. Additionally, the assessment and intervention need to address quality of life issues to address mental health and well being.

The process of care steps for nutrition therapy [6] includes:

1. Performing a comprehensive nutrition assessment determining the nutrition diagnosis.
2. Planning and implementing a nutrition intervention using evidence-based practice guidelines.
3. Monitoring and evaluating an individual's progress over subsequent visits.

Legal Definitions in USA

A variety of health professionals may provide nutrition therapy for obesity. However, the term Medical Nutrition Therapy (MNT) is restricted to and legally defined as the process of care provided by registered dietitians in the USA due to legislation related to Medicare third-party coverage [6, 9]. Other countries have also begun to use the term MNT to describe the unique care processes provided by dietitian. The MNT Medicare benefits include diabetes [6, 7, 9, 10], which is a major obesity co-morbidity, but extending these benefits to obesity and pre-diabetes has been more challenging. However, some private insurers in the USA cover obesity MNT as do the Medicaid and Children's Health Insurance Programs (CHIP) in some states.

MNT is operationally defined as "nutritional diagnostic, therapy, and counseling services for the purpose of disease management, which are furnished by a registered dietitian or nutrition professional [9]". The nutrition counseling component of MNT has been described as "a supportive process to set priorities, establish goals, and create individualized action plans which acknowledge and foster responsibility for self-care [6]". MNT is a component of comprehensive health care that can be utilized to improve health outcomes and quality of life of individuals suffering obesity and related co-morbidities. During an MNT intervention, RDs counsel clients on behavioral and lifestyle changes required to impact long-term eating habits and health. RDs provide MNT and other nutrition services for weight management related to overweight/obesity, bariatric surgery, and eating disorders [6].

MNT Process of Care Criteria

MNT is generally provided as three or more one-on-one consultation sessions, in which the dietitian performs the nutrition assessment, diagnosis, counseling, and other therapy services according to the "MNT Evidence-Based Guide for Practice/Nutrition Protocol" or according to the best available current evidence in the nutrition community [6]. The framework of counseling is standardized and documented as part of the Nutrition Care Process listed in Table **2**.

The nutrition assessment includes a review of laboratory tests, medications, co-morbidities and other conditions noted in the physician referral or by the patient as part of his or her health history, as well as examining the patient's dietary patterns. This information is used to evaluate factors such as the patient's nutritional needs *versus* intake. Standardized coding of nutrition diagnosis provides the foundation for developing a tailored plan and helping the patient attain weight and other goals. Monitoring is an ongoing review process of status in relation to behavioral and clinical goals, which is made during subsequent visits. Evaluation involves adjustment of goals and feedback to the referring physician as well as to the patient.

As part of nutrition monitoring and evaluation, the RD reviews weight changes in relation to lifestyle factors such as dietary intake and physical activity to evaluate the effectiveness of intervention strategies. Nutrition diagnoses and interventions may then be revised based on nutrition-related outcomes.

Table 2. Care process for medical nutrition therapy.

Role of Registered Dietitian (RD)
Nutrition screen/referral
The physician provider sends RD a written referral to provide MNT for obesity or related chronic disease risk *e.g.*, diabetes. The referral includes laboratory test results, medications and other diagnoses.
Nutrition assessment
The RD performs a comprehensive nutrition assessment utilizing Evidenced-Based Nutrition Practice Guideline and Toolkit, as well as the best available current knowledge and evidence, client data, medical record data and other resources.
Nutrition diagnosis
After analyzing assessment data, the RD makes the initial nutrition diagnosis(es) as a patient-oriented statement specific to one problem (P) and one etiology (E). The diagnosis is based on assessment of signs and symptoms (S) and may be written as a combined PES statement *e.g.*, Overweight/obesity (P) related to intake of large portions of sugary beverages (E) resulting in ~500 kcal/day above needs as evidenced by a BMI of 30 kg/m^2 (S) [9].
Nutrition intervention
Intervention counseling is usually guided by the etiology of each problem *e.g.*, large portions of sugary beverages resulting in excessive energy intake. Interventions focus on knowledge, attitudes and behaviors related to the energy intake that exceeds needs.
Nutrition monitoring and evaluation
Monitoring is based on clinical parameters *e.g.*, BMI, cardiometabolic markers (*e.g.*, hemoglobin A1c, lipids and blood pressure) and behavioral goals for food plan/intake, activity and other behavior changes. The RD implements changes to MNT (*e.g.*, patient education goals, nutrition intervention and counseling) in future visits based on outcomes and assessments at each visit.
Nutrition documentation (supports all steps of the Nutrition Care Process)
The RD documents MNT initial assessment, nutrition diagnosis(es) and intervention(s). Documentation is shared with referring physician *via* the patient's health record or consultation report.
Outcome management systems
Based on the analysis and review, the RD: 1) aggregates individual and population outcomes data; 2) analyzes and shares data with quality improvement department/group as indicated and 3) implements improvements to MNT services based on results.

Pan American Health Organization (PAHO) Nutritional Management of Obesity

The Pan American Health Organization (PAHO) [13] describes the process of nutrition therapy in its guide to lower obesity-related risks with emphasis on team care. PAHO has indicated that managing non-communicable disease demands effective allocation of resources. The health team offering nutritional care focuses on managing resources (information, money and materials) to ensure effective and efficient utilization that benefits patients. Table **3** lists the care processes recommended by PAHO for addressing obesity-related risk.

Table 3. Pan American health organization's nutrition management guide for obesity-related risk [13].

Assessment
Health history-explore health factors and/or family history that may influence nutrition status. ***Drug history***-review medications (prescription and over the counter, nutrient supplements, and illegal drugs that may affect nutrition status). ***Socio-economic history***-assess environmental, personal and religious, social and economic factors that can influence food availability, food needs, food intake and nutrient needs and dietary intervention. ***Diet history***-identify possible nutrient imbalances and eating patterns.
Planning *Translating Assessment Findings to Strategies and Activities to Achieve Health Targets*
Purpose of meal planning is: To control weight, blood pressure and/or blood glucose. To ensure that the right types and amounts of food are eaten. To control the specific nutrients as indicated for the targeted disease. To improve overall quality of life. ***The principles which govern meal planning include:*** ***Nutritional adequacy*** – Providing essential nutrients and energy to maintain health. ***Caloric control*** – Managing the amount of energy consumed without over or under-eating. ***Nutrient density*** – Choosing foods that provide more nutrients per calorie. ***Variety and Balance*** – Selecting foods from food groups in proportion to needs. ***Individuality*** – Using the information from the assessment to meet individual needs. ***Flexibility*** – Allowing clients to choose foods within a practical and creative setting.
Implementation
Implementing the Nutritional Care Plan involves providing meal planning and education with follow-up appointments: To involve client and family in setting goals. To ensure that care plan fits into the overall management plan for the client. To develop strategies to achieve goals. To counsel client and significant others. To refer to other members of the health team where appropriate.
A. Coordination
All aspects of Nutritional Care should be communicated to all health care team members to facilitate reinforcement of the nutrition strategies.
B. Evaluation
A. Examine the implementation to determine if the process is achieving targets and desired results including determination of readiness to accept a greater level of self- care. ***Documentation of care should be continuous and serve:*** To establish a written record of the Nutritional Care process. To maintain a strong communication network informing team members of client's status, plans and actions taken. To provide a framework/indication for intervention, re-assessment or follow-up care by the care team. To facilitate continuity of care, thus contributing to accuracy and better quality management. To provide a reference point for evaluating the impact of medical nutrition therapy on medical and clinical outcomes and client's quality of life by linking assessment with goals, intervention and strategies. To provide data for establishing cost-benefit and cost-effectiveness of medical nutrition therapy. To provide information on referral for other services.

(Table 3) contd…..

Nutrition information that should be documented includes:
Evaluation of current diet
Nutrient assessment data
Planned medical nutrition therapy
Counseling and education
Acceptance and tolerance level
Appetite
Planned follow-up
Referrals
Response to therapy
Any data relevant to client's health/nutritional status

BEHAVIORAL THERAPY

Behavioral therapy approaches provide a foundation for addressing obesity within the context of primary care. However, starting the dialogue about obesity is challenging for most primary care providers. Strategies for eliciting a patient's perspective about weight include questions such as: How do you feel about your weight with regard to your health? What do you see as the pros and cons addressing your weight as a health problem? On a scale of 1 to 10 how concerned are you about your weight?

5-A's Framework for Behavioral Therapy

The 5-A's framework for behavior change therapy is an evidence-based approach with applicability to a broad range of health conditions in primary care settings [8, 14-18]. Research suggests that the 5-A's approach is associated with greater patient satisfaction [17, 18] and better weight loss [15, 16] than a more directive approach that does not include shared decision making.

The Canadian Obesity Network has developed 5-A's practice tools to guide primary care practitioners in obesity counseling and management, which are available at: http://www.obesitynetwork.ca/5As

The 5-A's steps developed by Canadian Obesity Network include:

Ask for permission to discuss weight and explore readiness for change.

Assess obesity-related health risk and potential "root causes" of weight gain.

Advise about obesity risks and discuss benefits of treatment options.

Agree on realistic weight-loss expectations and on a SMART (specific, measurable, achievable, rewarding, timely) plan to achieve behavioral goals.

Assist in addressing drivers and barriers. Offer education and resources, refer to provider, and arrange follow-up.

Behavioral counseling based on 5-A's approach is supported by the Centers for Medicare & Medicaid Services (CMS) [14] as a "preventive services" for Medicare recipients who are obese (BMI $\geq$ 30 kg/m^2). Qualified primary care physicians or other primary care practitioners in a primary care setting are to provide the 5-A's counseling. See: http://www.cms.gov/Regulations-and-Guidance/Guidance/Transmittals/downloads/R142NCD.pdf

The CMS 5-A's framework [14] varies slightly from the Canadian approach [8] and includes:

Assess: Ask about/assess behavioral health risk(s) and factors affecting behavior change goals/methods. Assess how behavioral issues are related to health history/status.

Advise: Give clear, specific, and personalized behavior change advice, including information about personal health harms and benefits.

Agree: Collaboratively select appropriate treatment goals and methods based on the patient's interest in and willingness to change the behavior.

Assist: Use behavior change techniques (self-help and/or counseling) to help the patient achieve agreed-upon goals. Techniques focus on acquiring the skills, confidence and supports for behavior change. Assistance may also include adjunctive medical treatments may also be needed.

Arrange: Schedule follow-up contacts (in person or by telephone) to provide ongoing assistance/support and to adjust the treatment plan as needed.

The CMS 5A's Intensive Behavioral Therapy [14] services include:

- One face-to-face visit every week for the first month
- One face-to-face visit every other week for months 2-6

- One face-to-face visit every month for months 7-12 if the beneficiary meets the 3kg (6.6 lbs) weight loss requirement during the first six months.

WEIGHT MANAGEMENT BEHAVIORAL TRAINING

Weight Management Certificate Training

The Commission on Dietetic Registration of the Academy of Nutrition and Dietetics provides behavioral skills training to achieve the Certificate in Adult Weight Management or Childhood & Adolescent Weight Management. Both the adult and child/adolescent training programs are provided online as self-study modules as well being offered in a short-course format several times a year in various American cities. A description of course offerings is available at: http://cdrnet.org/pub/search.cfm?keyword=weight+management+certificate, and questions may be submitted by mail at weightmgmt@eatright.org.

Motivational Interviewing

Training in motivational interviewing related to weight management is not discipline specific. Motivational interviewing focuses on the use of open-ended questions, reflective listening, affirmation, and summarization (ORAS) to address lifestyle change issues [7]. Information about training in the use of motivational interviewing is available through the Motivational Interviewing Network of Trainers (MINT) website at: http://www.motivationalinterviewing.org/motivational-interviewing-training. The MINT website also provides an international listing of trainers and schedule of training events and information regarding qualifications for MINT.

Training Related Weight Bias and Discrimination

Obesity-related stigma and bias are pervasive in society, and many health professionals are unaware of their own biases [19, 20]. The Rudd Center for Food Policy & Obesity provides online training to develop skills for addressing weight bias and stigma at: http://www.uconnruddcenter.org/weight-bias-stigma. The website has training modules and materials that are tailored to specific groups including health professionals, employers, policy makers and individuals who may have encountered weight bias or stigma. Modules include self-assessments to increase the user's awareness of his or her implicit bias. Video clips address communication difficulties and bias as providers discuss the topic of weight with patients who are overweight or obese.

INTERFACE BETWEEN CLINICAL CARE AND POPULATION HEALTH

Public health strategies that can be applied to obesity prevention and treatment through quality improvement efforts is a variety of settings [21]. Developing a collaborative approach to weight management services helps develop health provider competency, empowers patients, and may reduce potential obesity-related bias and discrimination.

CARE SETTING

Ambulatory Care (Out-Patient) Issues

International data [22] suggest that primary care physicians devote the majority of their ambulatory care/out-patient visits to providing care for patients, who are overweight or obese. The International Day for the Evaluation of Abdominal Obesity (IDEA) study [22] involved over 6,000 randomly chosen primary care offices in 63 countries from eleven geographic regions across five continents. Almost 170,000 consecutively recruited adult patients were evaluated to assess how relative body weight and waist circumference were related to CVD and diabetes risk status. The IDEA study [22] found that one half to two thirds of the primary care patients were overweight or obese. Abdominal obesity, measured by waist circumference had a graded relationship with both CVD and diabetes mellitus at all levels of BMI, even in patients with a "normal" BMI. The association between waist circumference and having diagnosed CVD and diabetes was consistent across regions for both men and women even though there was up to 3-fold difference in the frequency of CVD and diabetes mellitus across the regions. Primary care practices in the IDEA study [22] obtained waist circumference, which facilitated identifying cardiometabolic risk in normal weight patients. Obesity screening initiatives needs to address how to integrate waist circumference measurement into the clinical routine of primary care practices.

Cross-sectional data analysis from the National Health and Nutrition Examination Survey (NHANES) [23] in the USA indicate that obesity is not being adequately addressed in primary care. Overweight/obese NHANES participants, whose physician/health professional addressed weight, were 6- to 8-fold more likely report having weight-related health concerns and had a 5- to 8-fold greater desire to lose weight. They also reported twice as many recent attempts to lose weight than obese/overweight NHANES participants who did not have the weight addressed by a care provider. However, between one-third and one-half of overweight and obese NHANES participants were never told that they were overweight or obese. Primary care practices need to develop a systematic approach to assessing and treating overweight and obesity to help prevent the recent favorable trends in cardiovascular morbidity and mortality from being reversed.

In-Patient Issues

In acute care and other in-patients care facilities, obesity is a common co-morbidity. However, co-morbidities may overshadow obesity as a diagnosis except for patients being admitted for bariatric surgery. Assessing nutritional needs of obese hospitalized patients is complex. Bed rest, concomitant conditions as well as treatments have been linked to sarcopenic obesity, a condition for which BMI assessment alone is inadequate [24, 25]. Sarcopenic obesity is generally characterized on the basis of having a relative increase in fat mass and a reduction in lean mass. However, defining sarcopenia based on muscle mass alone and elevated fatness for obesity may not adequately assess the relationship between sarcopenic obesity and impaired physical function. Reduced lean tissue mass, which is primarily reflecting reduced muscle mass, appears clinically important when it is accompanied by low muscle strength or another indicator of reduced physical functioning [24-26].

Nutrition support for the critically ill obese patient is designed to provide sufficient nutrients to facilitate: 1) clinical recovery, 2) minimize risks relative to the inherent metabolic complications associated with obesity, 3) minimize protein loss and 4) achieve net protein anabolism during the recovery phase of the hospitalization [27, 28]. Specific parameters that need to be monitored include: clinical outcomes, nitrogen balance, serum protein response and changes in body weight.

Hospitalized post-bariatric surgery patients need nutrition assessment [29-31], which should include lab tests for potential vitamin and mineral deficiencies with emphasis on iron (*i.e.*, complete blood count with differential, ferritin, iron, total iron binding capacity, and percent of oxygen saturation), folic acid (folate), bone health (25-hydroxyvitamin D, calcium, and parathyroid hormone), and vitamin B12. Although care recommendations include life-time follow-up by a multidisciplinary bariatric care team, patients may be treated elsewhere especially for acute health problems.

System and Resource Issues

The global rise in the prevalence of overweight and obesity is associated with escalating health care costs due weight-related illnesses that pose resource challenges for health care systems. The Academy of Nutrition and Dietetics website at (http://www.eatrightpro.org/resources/research/evidence-based-resources/evidence-analysis-library) provides the Academy's evidence-based review and recommendations for weight management. Utilization of weight management nutrition and behavioral therapy may be limited by service availability *via* the health system or self-referral, third-party payer options and the patient's self-pay willingness/ability. In the USA, registered dietitian referral information is available *via* "Find an Expert" at www.eatright.org. International resources for dietitian referrals are available at: http://eatrightoverseas.org/page/aoda-country-representatives.

The International Confederation of Dietetic Associations (ICDA) is an organization of national associations of Dietitians and Nutritionist that represents national dietetics associations in over 40 countries. The national associations that belong to ICDA represent about 160,000 Dietitians and Nutritionists around the world. Information about national dietetics information is available *via* a website link at http://www.internationaldietetics.org/.

CONCLUSION

Nutrition and behavioral therapies can achieve substantial reductions in the levels of risk factors and in disease outcomes related to obesity. The WHO recommends that the delivery of interventions should be of appropriate intensity and sustained over extended periods of time. Health systems need to expand the nutrition and behavioral therapy services for at-risk individuals. However, even modest changes in risk factor levels will have a substantial public health benefit. Strategies for improving obesity-related outcomes include incorporating weight management into primary care, training health professionals to provide weight management service, issuing clinical guidance for screening and treatment, and avoiding stigmatization of obese people.

ACKNOWLEDGEMENTS

Declared none.

CONFLICT OF INTEREST

The authors confirm that this chapter contents have no conflict of interest.

REFERENCES

[1] World Health Organization. Diet, Nutrition and the Prevention of Chronic Disease. Technical Report 916. Geneva, Switzerland: World Health Organization 2002. [cited 2014 Jan 4] Available from: http://whqlibdoc.who.int/trs/who_trs_916.pdf

[2] World Health Organization. 2008-2013 Action Plan for the Global Strategy for the Prevention and Control of Noncommunicable Diseases. Geneva, Switzerland: World Health Organization; 2008. [cited 2014 Jan 4] Available from: http://www.who.int/nmh/publications/9789241597418/en/.

[3] United States Department of Health and Human Services. The Basics [homepage on the internet]. No date [cited 2013 Jun 5]. Available from: http://healthfinder.gov/prevention/ViewTopicFull.aspx?topicID=25

[4] World Health Organization European Ministerial Conference on Counteracting Obesity: Diet and Physical Activity for Health. c2006 [cited 2013 Jun 5]. Available from http://www.euro.who.int/data/assets/pdf_file/0009/87462/E89567.pdf

[5] Jensen MD, Ryan DH, Apovian CM, *et al.* 2013 AHA/ACC/TOS guideline for the management of overweight and obesity in adults: a report of the American College of Cardiology/American Heart Association Task Force on Practice Guidelines and The Obesity Society. *Circulation.* 2013 [cited 2014 Jan 4] published online 2013 Nov 12. Available at: http://circ.ahajournals.org/content/early/2013/11/11/01.cir.0000437739.71477.ee.citation

[6] Academy of Nutrition and Dietetics. Medical Nutrition Therapy (MNT) [homepage on the internet]. No date [cited 2013 Jun 5]. Available from: http://www.eatright.org/healthprofessionals/content.aspx?id=6877#.UODG1WfdWt8

[7] Christie D, Channon S.The potential for motivational interviewing to improve outcomes in the management of diabetes and obesity in paediatric and adult populations: a clinical review. Diabetes Obes Metab. 2013 [cited 2014 Jan]. [Epub ahead of print].

[8] Canadian Obesity Network. 5As of obesity Management. [cited 2014 Jan 5] Available from: http://www.obesitynetwork.ca/5As

[9] Hager MH. Centers for Medicare & Medicaid Services telehealth coverage of MNT--what ADA members need to know. Journal of the American Dietetic Association. 2006; 106(4): 513-6. Epub 2006/03/29. [cited 2013 Jun 5].

[10] Franz MJ, Powers MA, Leontos C, *et al.* The evidence for medical nutrition therapy for type 1 and type 2 diabetes in adults. Journal of the American Dietetic Association. 2010; 110(12): 1852-89. Epub 2010/11/30. [cited 2013 Jun 5].

[11] American Dietetic Association. Nutritional Diagnosis: A Critical step in the Nutrition Process [homepage on the internet]. c2006 [cited 2013 Jun 5].

[12] Evert AB, Boucher JL, Cypress M, *et al.* Nutrition Therapy Recommendations for the Management of Adults With Diabetes Diabetes Care January 2014 37: S120-S143. [Cited 2014 Jan 5] Available from: http://care.diabetesjournals.org/content/37/Supplement_1/S120.full.pdf+html

[13] Pan American Health Organization. Protocol for the Nutritional Management of Obesity, Diabetes and Hypertension in the Caribbean. [serial online] c2004 [cited 2012 Jun 05]; PAHO publication PAHO/CAR/3.1/01.01. Available from: http://www.worlddiabetesfoundation.org/sites/default/files/Nutrition_Protocol_English.pdf

[14] Intensive behavioral therapy for obesity. ICN 907800 August 2012 [cited 2014 Jan 5] Available from: http://www.physiciansfirst.com/uploads/images/documents/ibtobesity.pdf

[15] Alexander SC, Cox ME, Boling-Turer CL, *et al.* Do the five A's work when physicians counsel about weight loss? Fam Med. 2011 Mar; 43(3): 179-84. [cited 2014 Jan 5] Available from: http://www.ncbi.nlm.nih.gov/pmc/articles/PMC3367376/

[16] Jay MR, Gillespie CC, Schlair SL, *et al.* The impact of primary care resident physician training on patient weight loss at 12 months. Obesity (Silver Spring). 2013 Jan; 21(1): 45-50. [cited 2014 Jan 5] Available from: http://www.ncbi.nlm.nih.gov/pubmed/23505167

[17] Jay M, Schlair S, Caldwell R, Kalet A, Sherman S, Gillespie C. From the patient's perspective: the impact of training on resident physician's obesity counseling. Journal of General Internal Medicine 2010 May; 25(**5**): 415-22. [cited 2014 Jan 5] Available from: http://www.ncbi.nlm.nih.gov/pmc/articles/PMC2855014/

[18] Jay M, Gillespie C, Schlair S, Sherman S, Kalet A. Physicians' use of the 5As in counseling obese patients: is the quality of counseling associated with patients' motivation and intention to lose weight? BMC Health Services Research. 2010 Jun 9; 10: 159. [cited 2014 Jan 5] Available from: http://www.biomedcentral.com/1472-6963/10/159

[19] Sikorski C, Luppa M, Brahler E, Konig HH, Riedel-Heller SG. Obese children, adults and senior citizens in the eyes of the general public: results of a representative study on stigma and causation of obesity. PloS one. 2012; 7(10): e46924. Epub 2012/10/17. [cited 2014 Jan 5] Available from: http://www.plosone.org/article/info%3Adoi%2F10.1371%2Fjournal.pone.0046924

[20] Sikorski C, Riedel C, Luppa M, *et al.* Perception of overweight and obesity from different angles: a qualitative study. Scandinavian Journal of Public Health. 2012; 40(3): 271-7. Epub 2012/05/29. [cited 2013 Jun 5] Available from: https: //www.thieme-connect.com/ejournals/abstract/10.1055/s-0031-1283633

[21] Wylie-Rosett J. The diabetes epidemic: what can we do? Journal of the American Dietetic Association. 2009; 109(7): 1160-2. Epub 2009/06/30. 2013 Jun 5].

[22] Balkau B, Deanfield JE, Despres JP, Bassand JP, Fox KA, Smith SC, Jr., *et al.* International Day for the Evaluation of Abdominal Obesity (IDEA): a study of waist circumference, cardiovascular disease, and diabetes mellitus in 168,000 primary care patients in 63 countries. Circulation. 2007; 116(17): 1942-51. Epub 2007/10/30. [cited 2013 Jun 5] Available from: http://circ.ahajournals.org/content/116/17/1942.full.pdf+html

[23] Post RE, Mainous AG 3rd, Gregorie SH, Knoll ME, Diaz VA, Saxena SK. The influence of physician acknowledgment of patients' weight status on patient perceptions of overweight and obesity in the United States. Arch Intern Med. 2011 Feb 28; 171(4): 316-21. [2014 cited Jan 5] Available from: http://archinte.jamanetwork.com/article.aspx?articleid=226670

[24] Gallagher D, DeLegge M. Body composition (sarcopenia) in obese patients: implications for care in the intensive care unit. JPEN Journal of parenteral and enteral nutrition. 2011; 35(5 Suppl): 21S-8S. Epub 2011/08/03.

[25] Petak S, Barbu CG, Yu EW, Fielding R, Mulligan K, Sabowitz B, Wu CH, Shepherd JA. **The** Official Positions of the International Society for Clinical Densitometry: body composition analysis reporting. Journal of Clinical Densitomertry. 2013 Oct-Dec; 16(4): 508-19. doi: 10.1016/j.jocd.2013.08.018.

[26] McClave SA, Kushner R, Van Way CW, 3rd, Cave M, DeLegge M, Dibaise J *et al.* Nutrition therapy of the severely obese, critically ill patient: summation of conclusions and recommendations. JPEN Journal of Parenteral and Enteral Nutrition. 2011; 35(5 Suppl): 88S-96S. Epub 2011/09/09. [cited 2013 Jun 5] Available from: http://pen.sagepub.com/content/35/5_suppl/88S.long

[27] Dickerson RN, Drover JW. Monitoring nutrition therapy in the critically ill patient with obesity. JPEN Journal of Parenteral and Enteral Nutrition. 2011; 35(5 Suppl): 44S-51S. Epub 2011/08/03. [cited 2013 Jun 5] Available from: http://pen.sagepub.com/content/35/5_suppl/44S.abstract

[28] Kushner RF, Drover JW. Current strategies of critical care assessment and therapy of the obese patient (hypocaloric feeding): what are we doing and what do we need to do? JPEN Journal of parenteral and enteral nutrition. 2011; 35(5 Suppl): 36S-43S. Epub 2011/08/03. [cited 2013 Jun 5] Available from: http://pen.sagepub.com/content/early/2011/07/31/0148607111413776.full.pdf+html?ijkey=/RCT959lg1MIY&keytype=ref&siteid=sppen

[29] Karmali S, Johnson Stoklossa C, Sharma A, Stadnyk J, Christiansen S, Cottreau D, *et al.* Bariatric surgery: a primer. Canadian family physician Medecin de famille canadien. 2010; 56(9): 873-9. Epub 2010/09/16. Available from: http://www.ncbi.nlm.nih.gov/pmc/articles/PMC2939109/pdf/0560873.pdf

[30] Leslie D, Kellogg TA, Ikramuddin S. Bariatric surgery primer for the internist: keys to the surgical consultation. The Medical Clinics of North America. 2007; 91(3): 353-81, x. Epub 2007/05/19. [cited 2013 Jun 5] Available from: http://www.ncbi.nlm.nih.gov/pubmed/17509383

[31] Furtado LC. Nutritional management after Roux-en-Y gastric bypass. British journal of nursing. 2010; 19(7): 428-36. Epub 2010/05/28. Available from: http://www.internurse.com/cgi-bin/go.pl/library/article.cgi?uid=47440; article=BJN_19_7_428_436

Obesity and Disease in an Interconnected World, 2015, 149-162

CHAPTER 9

The Healthy Diet: Easy as 1, 2 and 3

Jeannette M. Beasley* **and Beth A. Conlon**

Department of Epidemiology and Population Health, Albert Einstein College of Medicine, Bronx, NY, USA

Abstract: Inhabitants of Western countries are at an increased risk of energy imbalance, where processed and fast foods are the dominant food supply and the ability to make healthier food choices is clouded by persuasive marketing campaigns and a fast-paced convenience culture. Healthcare professionals and policy makers must take into account the vast behavioral, sociocultural, environmental, and genetic factors that influence dietary behavior and body weight. Food components to reduce include sodium, added sugars, and saturated as well as trans fats. Foods to increase include whole grains, fruits, and vegetables. Achieving these dietary recommendations requires effecting change at the individual, community, and global level.

Keywords: Behavior, carbohydrates, diet, dietary recommendations, fat, food choices, global health, health status, nutrition, obesity, overweight, protein, resting metabolic rate, risk, sodium, sugars, weight management, wellness, whole grains.

INTRODUCTION

There is no shortage of advice regarding ways to achieve a healthy diet available through innumerable channels. In the literature, there are dietary guidelines published by the World Health Organization (WHO) [1], governments (*i.e.* Indian National Institute of Nutrition, (Indian NIN)) [2], and associations (*i.e.* World Cancer Research Fund/American Institute for Cancer Research) [3]. The United States Department of Agriculture operationalized their food guidance system by providing resources for healthy eating encapsulated by the MyPlate symbol (Fig. **1**) [4]. The Academy of Nutrition and Dietetics conducts evidence-based reviews of the literature regarding key topics related to special diets such as meat-restricted or adapted for chronic conditions, including diabetes, hypertension, and chronic kidney disease [5]. In the popular media, it is difficult to turn on the

***Corresponding author Jeannette M. Beasley:** 1300 Morris Park Ave., Belfer Building, Room 1312C, Bronx, NY 10461, USA; Tel: (718) 430-3089; Fax: (718) 430-3076;
E-mail: jeannette.beasley@einstein.yu.edu

Judith Wylie-Rosett & Sunil S. Jhangiani (Eds)

television or open a web browser without hearing something that one should or should not be eating. Each year, thousands of books are published proclaiming to have found the answer to the world's dieting woes.

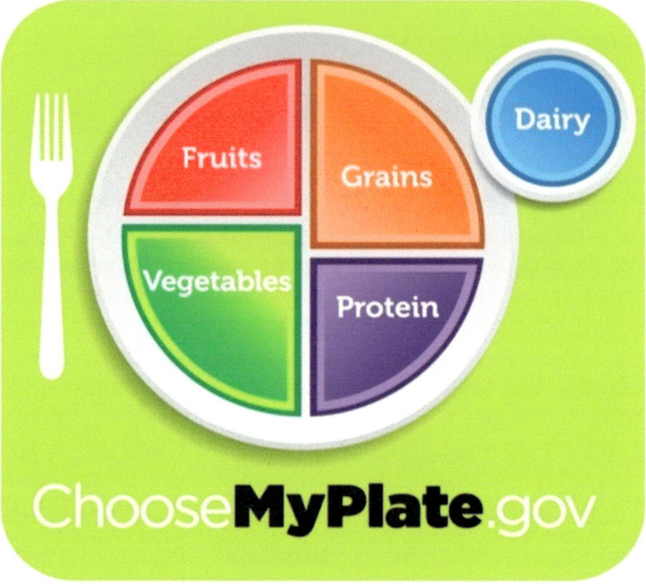

Fig. (1). MyPlate is the United States Department of Agriculture's food guidance system symbol.

Being bombarded with all of this information and several sound bites from different sources can overwhelm the senses and breed frustration and/or confusion. However, in many cases the information is quite similar even if it is packaged slightly differently. Though there are separate dietary guidelines for cardiovascular disease [6] and cancer [7], recommendations are cohesive for many dietary components [8]. The purpose of this chapter is to sift through all of the noise in order to encapsulate the key messages to be conveyed to facilitate achieving a healthy diet.

In reviewing key dietary recommendations published by the WHO [1] as well as two government agencies, India [2] and the United States (US) [9], messages can be classified into three categories: 1) Achieving Energy Balance; 2) Foods and food components to reduce; and 3) Foods and food components to increase. This chapter will compare WHO diet recommendations to those published by India and the US as representative examples of nutrition guidelines in developing and developed countries, and, where possible, discuss successful implementation approaches.

ACHIEVING ENERGY BALANCE

Determining Energy Needs for Weight Maintenance

The simplest explanation for the global obesity epidemic is energy imbalance—individuals consume more calories than they expend, leading to weight gain. However, the obesity epidemic is far more complex than calories-in and calories-out. The food and lifestyle choices made by individuals are shaped by their environment. Inhabitants of Western countries are at an increased risk of energy imbalance, where processed and fast foods are the dominant food supply and the ability to make healthier food choices is clouded by persuasive marketing campaigns and a fast-paced convenience culture. Healthcare professionals and policy makers must take into account the vast behavioral, sociocultural, environmental, and genetic factors that influence dietary behavior and body weight. The 2013 guideline for the Management of Overweight and Obesity provides an evidence-based algorithm for evaluating patients based on BMI and treating patients using behavioral, pharmaceutical, and/or surgical approaches [10].

At the individual level, energy needs for weight maintenance can be estimated using an empirically-derived predictive equation, indirect calorimetry, direct calorimetry, or tracer methods (*e.g.*, doubly labeled water) to measure resting metabolic rate (RMR). RMR represents the energy needed to sustain life and vital physiological functions, accounting for 60-75% of total daily energy expenditure [11]. Calorimetric and tracer methods are more accurate measurements of RMR than predictive equations, but require sophisticated equipment and are costly and time-consuming. Thus, mathematical equations derived from regression analysis of indirect and direct calorimetric measurements in specific population groups are practical alternatives.

The Academy of Nutrition and Dietetics conducted a systematic review [12] in 2005 and identified the four prediction equations that are most commonly used in clinical practice (Table **1**). The Mifflin-St. Jeor equation using actual body weight was found to be the most accurate predictor of RMR, to within 10% measurement accuracy when compared to indirect calorimetry in obese and non-obese subjects. The predictive equations work best for the specific groups of people from whom the equation was developed, and caution and clinical judgment should be exercised whenever applying a predictive formula to an alternative population. The accuracy of energy prediction equations varies with ethnicity and geographic location, as exemplified by studies from Korea [13] and the Netherlands [14].

Table 1. Predictive equations for calculating resting metabolic rate.

Predictive Equation	Calculation	Derived Population
Mifflin-St. Jeor [20]	♀: RMR = 9.99(W) + 6.25(H)-4.92(A) + 5 ♂: RMR = 9.99(W) + 6.25(H)-4.92(A) - 161	- United States - Normal weight, overweight, obese, and morbidly obese men and women ages 19-78 years old (44.5 ±14.1 y) - Race not specified - Poor representation of older adults
Harris Benedict [21]	♀: RMR = 66.47 + 13.75(W) + 5.0(H)-6.755(A) ♂: RMR = 655.1 + 9.563(W) + 1.85(H) = 4.676(A)	-United States - Normal weight white men, ages 16-63 years (27 ±9 y), and normal weight white women, ages 15-74 years (31 ± 14 y) - Year 1907-1917 - Overestimation of energy expenditure is common
Owen [22, 23]	♀: RMR = 879 + 10.2(W) ♂: RMR = 795 + 7.18(W)	- United States -Normal weight, obese, and morbidly obese white, black, Asian men ages 18-82 (38 ± 15.6 y); normal weight, obese, and morbidly obese women ages 18-65 year (35 ± 12 y) -Race not reported for women
WHO/FAO/UNU [24]	♀ 10-18 = 16.6W + 77H + 572 ♀ 18-30 = 15.4W - 27H + 717 ♀ 30-60 = 11.3W + 16H + 901 ♀ >60 = 8.8W + 1 128H-1,071 ♂ 10-18 = 7.4W + 482H + 217 ♂ 18-30 = 13.3W + 334H + 35 ♂ 30-60 = 8.7W -25H + 865 ♂ >60 = 9.2W + 637H -302	-Male and female European military and police recruits ages 19-82 years

Abbreviations: ♀ = Male; ♂ = Female; W=weight in kg; H=height in cm; A=age in years.

Inaccurate use of these equations can lead to undesirable weight changes in individuals, as underestimation would lead to weight loss and overestimation would lead to weight gain among adherent individuals. The Penn State 2003 [15], Swinamer [16], and Ireton-Jones [17] equations are alternatives for critically ill patients. RMR can be used in combination with physical activity level (PAL) coefficients to compute the estimated energy requirement (EER) of individuals [18]. The EER represents the energy intake needed to maintain energy balance in healthy individuals and accounts for energy intake, expenditure, age, sex, weight, height, and physical activity level. The Institute of Medicine (IOM) published prediction equations based on doubly labeled water experiments to establish the Dietary Reference Intakes (DRI) for energy as the EER, in their report Dietary Reference Intakes for Energy, Carbohydrate, Fiber, Fat, Fatty Acids, Cholesterol,

Protein and Amino Acids [19]. EERs are provided for healthy adults and special populations, including infants and young children, and women who are pregnant or lactating. For overweight and obese adults, a formula called total energy expenditure (TEE) replaces the EER. The EERs provide a foundation for determining the macronutrient and micronutrient needs of individuals, as well as facilitate the design of weight management intervention programs.

MACRONUTRIENTS: CARBOHYDRATE, PROTEIN, FAT, AND ALCOHOL

Carbohydrates

The WHO recommends a total daily carbohydrate intake of 55-75% of energy. Carbohydrates provide 4 kcal per gram (16.736 kJ) and provide the largest dietary source of energy for the majority of individuals worldwide. The Dietary Guidelines for Indians (DGIs) report that carbohydrates constitute 70-80% of the average Indian diet, derived from plant foods such as cereals, millets, and pulses. Data from the National Health and Examination Survey (NHANES) 2007-2008 indicated that the average carbohydrate intake in the United States is 47.9% and 50.5% for men and women, respectively [25]. Each of the three guidelines (Table **2**) consistently recommends a moderate intake of carbohydrate (defined as 40-65% total energy); except for the upper limit of the WHO guidelines which are classified as high carbohydrate intake range (>65% total energy) [26]. The Dietary Guidelines for Americans (DGAs) and DGIs highlight how urbanization has increased the consumption of refined carbohydrates that contain less fiber, nutrients, and more added sugars. The quality of carbohydrates plays an important role in the development of diabetes, independent of other metabolic risk factors, and diets high in refined carbohydrates have been attributed to the cause of the globalization of diabetes [27]. Global health efforts are needed to stem the rising intake of processed carbohydrates and simple sugars, and revert consumption patterns back towards historically native plant-based diets rich in whole grains, fruits, vegetables, legumes, nuts, and seeds.

Protein

The WHO recommends a total daily protein intake of 10-15% of energy, which is consistent with the DGIs. The DGAs allot a broader intake range for protein (10-35%). Protein provides 4 kcal per gram (16.736 kJ). In India and many parts of the world, protein-energy malnutrition (PEM) from lack of calories and/or protein

Table 2. Comparison of dietary guidelines from the WHO, the DGIs from the Indian National Institute of Nutrition (Indian NIN), and the DGAs from US Department of Agriculture and Department of Health & Human Services (USA).

	World Health Organization Dietary Guidelines	Dietary Guidelines for Indians (DGIs)	Dietary Guidelines for Americans (DGAs)
Energy balance	Achieve energy balance and a healthy weight	Overeating should be avoided to prevent overweight and obesity.	Maintain calorie balance over time to achieve and sustain a healthy weight.
Carbohydrates	55-75% total; 0-10% Free Sugars 50-70% Complex Carbohydrate 27-40 g Fiber	50-60% total, mostly from complex carbohydrates, low glycemic foods, and fibre rich diet.	45-65% carbohydrate; limit the consumption of foods that contain refined grains, especially refined grain foods that contain solid fats, added sugars, and sodium. Choose foods that provide more dietary fiber.
Protein	10-15% protein	10-15% total; adults should choose low-fat, protein-rich foods such as lean meat, fish, pulses, and low-fat milk.	10-35%; choose a variety of protein foods, which include seafood, lean meat and poultry, eggs, beans and peas, soy products, and unsalted nuts and seeds.
Fat	15-30% Total 0-10% SFA 3-7% PUFA 0-300 mg Cholesterol	20-30% total; use fats and oils in moderation and consume varieties of foods to get good proportion of all fatty acids for optimal health benefits.	20-35%; use oils to replace solid fats where possible.
Alcohol	Not specified; (maybe b/c Recommendations are country-specific. Certain countries prohibit the consumption of alcohol by law.)	Avoid alcohol. Those who drink should limit its intake.	If alcohol is consumed, it should be consumed in moderation—up to one drink for women and two drinks per day for men—and only by adults of legal drinking age.
Sodium	Limit salt (sodium) consumption from all sources and ensure that salt is iodized.	Use salt in moderation/ Restrict salt intake to minimum.	Reduce daily sodium intake to less than 2,300 mg and further reduce intake to 1,500 mg among persons who are 51 and older and those of any age who are African American or have hypertension, diabetes, or chronic kidney disease. The 1,500 mg recommendation applies to about half of the U.S. population, including children, and the majority of adults.

(Table 2) contd…..

	World Health Organization Dietary Guidelines	Dietary Guidelines for Indians (DGIs)	Dietary Guidelines for Americans (DGAs)
Dietary fat and cholesterol	Limit energy intake from total fats and shift fat consumption away from saturated fats to unsaturated fats and towards the elimination of *trans* fatty acids	Ensure moderate use of edible oils and animal foods and less use of ghee/ butter/ vanaspati.	Consume less than 10 percent of calories from saturated fatty acids by replacing them with monounsaturated and polyunsaturated fatty acids. Keep *trans* fatty acid consumption as low as possible by limiting foods that contain synthetic sources of *trans* fats, such as partially hydrogenated oils, and by limiting other solid fats. Reduce the intake of calories from solid fats Consume less than 300 mg per day of dietary cholesterol
Sugars	Limit the intake of free sugars	Minimize the use of processed foods rich in salt, sugar and fats.	Reduce the intake of calories from [added sugars].
Grains	Increase consumption of [whole grains]	N/A	Consume at least half of all grains as whole grains. Increase whole-grain intake by replacing refined grains with whole grains.
Vegetables and Fruits	Increase consumption of fruits and vegetables	Eat plenty of vegetables and fruits.	Increase vegetable and fruit intake.

(from meats, legumes, and other sources) is an important public health concern. In India, PEM is attributed to caloric deficiencies rather than protein deficiencies, with approximately 70% of households facing energy inadequacies. Data from the Food and Agriculture Organization of the United Nations' *The State of Food Insecurity in the World*, 2012, indicate that 870 million people (12.5% of the world's population) face hunger and undernourishment [28]. PEM begins at conception with poor maternal nutrition and extends into later life. Its consequences include severe underweight, stunted growth, micronutrient deficiencies, and increased risk of infectious diseases. Protein intake is typically adequate in Western countries per dietary guidelines; however, high intakes of red meat and high-fat dairy are common sources of protein in the Western Diet, and are attributable to the growing rate of cardiovascular diseases in these countries. The WHO, DGAs, and DGIs are consistent in their recommendation to increase protein intake from lean meats, fish, low-fat dairy, and plant-based sources like legumes, nuts, and seeds.

Fat

The WHO recommends a total daily fat intake of 15-30% of energy, which is approximately consistent with the DGIs (20-30%) and DGAs (20-35%). Fat provides 9 kcal (37.656 kJ) per gram, which is more than twice the amount of carbohydrates and protein; thus, is the densest source of energy. The rapid increase in the energy density of diets since the early 1980s changed the landscape of public health diseases from primarily undernutrition and infectious diseases to primarily obesity and its related non-communicable diseases. The China National Nutrition and Health Survey 2002 showed an increase in overweight and obesity from 14.6% in 1992 to 21.8% in 2002 that paralleled an increase in animal foods from 9.3 to 13%, and percentage in total fat intake from 22.0 to 29.8% [29]. This trend is common throughout developed and developing nations, particularly in urban settings. Vanaspati (*i.e.* hydrogenated vegetable oil) and animal ghee (*i.e.* clarified butter) are staple cooking ingredients throughout India and Southeast Asia, but are extremely high in *trans* and saturated fatty acids, respectively. The DGIs warn against the dangers of indulging in excess fat and highlight the importance to use edible oils and animal fats in moderation and to use less vanaspati, ghee, and butter. The DGAs and WHO also emphasize the importance of increasing intake of fats from oils and plant-based foods and decreasing the intake of solid and animal-based fats. Although a recent systematic review [30] has questioned the adverse effects of saturated fat in heart disease, the American Heart Association continues to support limiting saturated fat intake [6, 31].

Alcohol

The WHO, DGAs, and DGIs are consistent with their recommendation on alcohol—to avoid alcohol, and if it is consumed, it should be consumed in moderation. The DGAs define moderation as no more than one drink per day for women and two drinks per day for men, and only by adults of legal drinking age (21 years in the United States). The WHO warns against the harmful effects of alcohol that burdens many nations worldwide, and discusses its adverse health and social consequences in its report, "Global Status Report on Alcohol and Health 2011" [32]. The report indicated the worldwide per capita consumption of alcoholic beverages in 2005 was 6.13 liters of pure alcohol consumed by every person aged 15 years and older. Alcohol provides 7 kcal per gram (29.288 kJ) but contains little nutrients, contributing excess empty calories to the diet that can result in weight gain if consumed on a regular basis. While many observational studies have reported that drinking certain types of alcohol in moderation, like red wine, may improve cardiovascular health, further research is merited before evidence-based recommendations can be made to use alcohol for these potential benefits.

FOODS AND FOOD COMPONENTS TO REDUCE

Sodium

Each of the three dietary guidelines encourages salt reduction (Table **2**), but recommendations vary from being as generic as minimizing salt intake (WHO) to providing specific targets depending on demographic characteristics (US). The Dietary Approaches to Stop Hypertension (DASH) diet, which in randomized, controlled trials reduced systolic blood pressure by 11.4 mmHg and diastolic blood pressure by 5.5 mmHg compared to a typical US diet [33], has provided us with guidance on how to intervene on diet to lower risk of chronic disease [34]. Resources for adhering to the DASH diet are readily available [35].

Fats (Saturated, Trans)

The guidelines are consistent in encouraging the consumption of less saturated and *trans* fat, though the WHO and US guidelines state this more explicitly than the Indian guidelines, which names commonly consumed fats that are rich in saturated (*i.e.,* ghee) and *trans* (*i.e.* vanaspati) fats. In a meta-analysis of eight randomized controlled trials including 13,614 participants with 1,042 events, replacing saturated fat with polyunsaturated fat reduced the occurrence of coronary heart disease by 19% (95% CI = 5-30%) [36]. Saturated and *trans* fats can often be replaced by fats rich in monounsaturated (*i.e.,* olive oil) or polyunsaturated (*i.e.* canola oil) fatty acids in cooking. A regulation passed in 2006 prohibits New York City food service establishments from using, storing, or serving food that contains partially hydrogenated vegetable oil and has a total of 0.5 grams per serving. To evaluate the impact of the NYC *trans* fat regulation, Angell *et al.* sampled purchases (6969 in 2007 and 7885 in 2009) from 168 lunchtime chain restaurants before and after full implementation of the *trans* fat regulation reporting a decline of 2.4 g (95% CI, -2.8 to -2.0 g; $P < 0.001$) with a slight increase in saturated fat of 0.55 g (95% CI 0.1 to 1.0 g; $P < 0.011$) [37].

Sugars

Added sugars include high fructose corn syrup, white sugar, brown sugar, corn syrup, corn syrup solids, raw sugar, malt syrup, maple syrup, pancake syrup, fructose sweetener, liquid fructose, honey, molasses, anhydrous dextrose, and crystal dextrose. Each guideline contains a statement to limit/minimize/reduce sugar intake. The DGIs specifically mention minimizing the consumption of processed foods. The DGAs indicate the intent of reducing added sugar intake is to reduce caloric intake. Sweetened foods can be replaced with foods that do not contain added sugar. For example, purchasing plain yogurt and adding blueberries rather than consuming blueberry yogurt will reduce intake of added sugars. In the US, the major sources of added sugar are soda, energy drinks, and sports drinks (36% of added sugar intake), grain-based desserts (13%), sugar-sweetened fruit drinks] (10%), dairy-based desserts (6%), and candy (6%) [38-40].

FOODS AND FOOD COMPONENTS TO INCREASE

Whole Grains

The WHO encourages consumption of whole grains as part of a generic statement. The DGIs mention consuming grains during pregnancy and to wash them appropriately to avoid microbial infection. The US guidelines encourage consuming at least half of one's grains as whole grains. A multi-component school-based intervention in Stockholm involving 3,135 boys and girls in grades 1-4 promoted whole-grain over white bread, low-fat dairy products, and eliminated sweets and sweetened drinks along with a promotion of physical activity to at least 30 minutes per day to achieve a decrease in the prevalence of overweight and obesity in the interventions schools by 3.4% ($P<0.05$) compared to an increase of 2.8% in the control schools [41].

Vegetables and Fruits

The guidelines are consistent in their recommendation to increase vegetable and fruit intake. The WHO leaves it to the national dietary guidelines to establish recommendations regarding optimal amounts of vegetable and fruit intake. Preparation methods, growing conditions, supply *versus* demand, and several other country-specific factors impact the ability of citizens to readily consume produce. According to the DGIs, in India, total vegetable production is 30% less than demand. While food availability is greater in the US, on average just 42% of the population meets the recommendation of 1-2 cups depending on calorie needs for fruits and 59% of the population meets the recommendation of 1-4 cups depending on calorie needs for vegetables. Media and educational campaigns promoting vegetable and fruit consumption have been developed and evaluated by the US 5-A-Day for Better Health! Campaign initiated by the National Cancer Institute with collaboration from industry and the federal government in 1991 that was replaced by the "Fruits & Veggies-More Matters campaign in 2007" [42]. International media campaigns have also demonstrated success in increasing public awareness and consumption of fruits and vegetables [43, 44].

CONCLUSION

Recommendations for improving health take into account the vast behavioral, sociocultural, environmental, and genetic factors that influence dietary behavior and body weight. Dietary recommendations focus on reducing intake of sodium, added sugars, and saturated as well as trans fats, which are readily available in the food supply. Alternately, health recommendations focus on increasing intake of whole grains, fruits, and vegetables, which are less readily available. Thus, achieving these dietary recommendations will require effecting change at the individual, community, and global level.

ACKNOWLEDGEMENTS

None declared.

CONFLICT OF INTEREST

The authors confirm that this chapter contents have no conflict of interest.

REFERENCES

[1] World Health Organization. Global Strategy on Diet, Physical Activity and Health 2004 [cited 2015 February 12]. Available from: http://www.who.int/dietphysicalactivity/strategy/eb11344/strategy_english_web.pdf

[2] National Institute of Nutrition Hyderabad. Dietary Guidelines for Indians: A Manual 2011 [cited 2013 January 23, 2013]. Available from: http://www.ninindia.org/DietaryGuidelinesforNINwebsite.pdf.

[3] Wiseman M. The second World Cancer Research Fund/American Institute for Cancer Research expert report. Food, nutrition, physical activity, and the prevention of cancer: a global perspective. The Proceedings of the Nutrition Society 2008; 67(3): 253-6.

[4] United States Department of Agriculture. ChooseMyPlate.gov 2013 [January 28, 2013]. Available from: http://www.choosemyplate.gov/.

[5] Academy of Nutrition and Dietetics: Evidence Analysis Library. Nutrition Guidelines List 2013 [January 16, 2013]. Available from: http://andevidencelibrary.com/category.cfm?cid=14&cat=0

[6] Eckel RH, Jakicic JM, Ard JD, de Jesus JM, Houston Miller N, Hubbard VS, *et al* 2013 AHA/ACC guideline on lifestyle management to reduce cardiovascular risk: a report of the American College of Cardiology/American Heart Association Task Force on Practice Guidelines. Journal of the American College of Cardiology 2014; 63(25 Pt B): 2960-84.

[7] Kushi LH, Doyle C, McCullough M, Rock CL, Demark-Wahnefried W, Bandera EV, *et al.* American Cancer Society Guidelines on nutrition and physical activity for cancer prevention: reducing the risk of cancer with healthy food choices and physical activity. CA: A Cancer Journal for Clinicians 2012; 62(1): 30-67.

[8] Krebs-Smith SM, Kris-Etherton P. How does MyPyramid compare to other population-based recommendations for controlling chronic disease? Journal of the American Dietetic Association 2007; 107(5): 830-7.

[9] U.S. Department of Agriculture, U.S. Department of Health and Human Services. Dietary Guidelines for Americans, 2010. 7 ed. Washington, DC, USA: U.S. Government Printing Office; 2010.

[10] Jensen MD, Ryan DH, Apovian CM, Ard JD, Comuzzie AG, Donato KA, *et al* 2013 AHA/ACC/TOS guideline for the management of overweight and obesity in adults: a report of the American College of Cardiology/American Heart Association Task Force on Practice Guidelines and The Obesity Society. Journal of the American College of Cardiology 2014; 63(25 Pt B): 2985-3023.

[11] RD L. Energy Balance and Body Weight. In: Nelms M, Sucher KP, Long S, editors. Nutrition Therapy and Pathophysiology Belmont, CA: Thomson Brooks/Cole; 2007.

[12] Frankenfield D, Roth-Yousey L, Compher C. Comparison of Predictive Equations for Resting Metabolic Rate in Healthy Nonobese and Obese Adults: A Systematic Review. Journal of the American Dietetic Association 2005; 105(5): 775-89.

[13] Lawrence JC, Lee HM, Kim JH, Kim EK. Variability in results from predicted resting energy needs as compared to measured resting energy expenditure in Korean children. Nutrition Research 2009; 29(11): 777-83.

[14] Weijs PJ. Validity of predictive equations for resting energy expenditure in US and Dutch overweight and obese class I and II adults aged 18-65 y. The American Journal of Clinical Nutrition 2008; 88(4): 959-70

[15] Frankenfield D, Smith JS, Cooney RN. Validation of 2 approaches to predicting resting metabolic rate in critically ill patients. JPEN Journal of Parenteral and Enteral Nutrition 2004; 28(4): 259-64.

[16] Swinamer DL, Grace MG, Hamilton SM, Jones RL, Roberts P, King EG. Predictive equation for assessing energy expenditure in mechanically ventilated critically ill patients. Critical Care Medicine 1990; 18(6): 657-61.

[17] Ireton-Jones CS, Turner WW, Jr., Liepa GU, Baxter CR. Equations for the estimation of energy expenditures in patients with burns with special reference to ventilatory status. The Journal of Burn Care & Rehabilitation 1992; 13(3): 330-3.

[18] Gerrior S, Juan W, Basiotis P. An easy approach to calculating estimated energy requirements. Preventing Chronic Disease 2006; 3(4): A129.

[19] Institute of Medicine, Food and Nutrition Board. Dietary reference intakes for energy, carbohydrate, fiber, fat, fatty acids, cholesterol, protein, and amino acids (macronutrients). Washington, D.C.: National Academy Press; 2005.

[20] Mifflin MD, St Jeor ST, Hill LA, Scott BJ, Daugherty SA, Koh YO. A new predictive equation for resting energy expenditure in healthy individuals. The American Journal of Clinical Nutrition 1990; 51(2): 241-7.

[21] Harris JA, Benedict FG. A Biometric Study of Human Basal Metabolism. Proceedings of the National Academy of Sciences of the United States of America 1918; 4(12): 370-3.

[22] Owen OE, Holup JL, D'Alessio DA, Craig ES, Polansky M, Smalley KJ, *et al.* A reappraisal of the caloric requirements of men. The American Journal of Clinical Nutrition 1987; 46(6): 875-85.

[23] Owen OE, Kavle E, Owen RS, Polansky M, Caprio S, Mozzoli MA, *et al.* A reappraisal of caloric requirements in healthy women. The American Journal of Clinical Nutrition 1986; 44(1): 1-19.

[24] Food and Agriculture Organization, World Health Organization, United Nations University. Energy and protein requirements. Report of a joint FAO/WHO/UNU Expert Consultation. World Health Organization technical report series 1985; 724: 1-206.

[25] Wright JD, Wang CY. Trends in intake of energy and macronutrients in adults from 1999-2000 through 2007-2008. NCHS data brief 2010(49): 1-8.

[26] Wylie-Rosett J, Aebersold K, Conlon B, Isasi CR, Ostrovsky NW. Health Effects of Low-Carbohydrate Diets: Where Should New Research Go? Current Diabetes Reports 2012; 13(2): 271-8.

[27] Hu FB. Globalization of diabetes: the role of diet, lifestyle, and genes. Diabetes Care 2011; 34(6): 1249-57.

[28] Food and Agriculture Organization, World Food Programme, International Fund for Agricultural Development. The State of Food Insecurity in the World 2012. Economic growth is necessary but not sufficient to accelerate reduction of hunger and malnutrition. Rome, 2012.

[29] Wang Y, Mi J, Shan XY, Wang QJ, Ge KY. Is China facing an obesity epidemic and the consequences? The trends in obesity and chronic disease in China. International Journal of Obesity (2005) 2007; 31(1): 177-88.

[30] Chowdhury R, Warnakula S, Kunutsor S, Crowe F, Ward HA, Johnson L, *et al.* Association of dietary, circulating, and supplement fatty acids with coronary risk: a systematic review and meta-analysis. Annals of Internal Medicine 2014; 160(6): 398-406.

[31] American Heart Association. Saturated Fats [September 25, 2014]. Available from: http://www.heart.org/HEARTORG/GettingHealthy/NutritionCenter/HealthyEating/Saturated-Fats_UCM_301110_Article.jsp.

[32] World Health Organization. Global status report on alcohol and health 2011 [January 23, 2013]. Available from: http://www.who.int/substance_abuse/publications/global_alcohol_report/en/.

[33] Appel LJ, Moore TJ, Obarzanek E, Vollmer WM, Svetkey LP, Sacks FM, *et al.* A clinical trial of the effects of dietary patterns on blood pressure. DASH Collaborative Research Group. The New England Journal of Medicine 1997; 336(16): 1117-24.

[34] Appel LJ, Champagne CM, Harsha DW, Cooper LS, Obarzanek E, Elmer PJ, *et al.* Effects of comprehensive lifestyle modification on blood pressure control: main results of the PREMIER clinical trial. JAMA : the Journal of the American Medical Association 2003; 289(16): 2083-93.

[35] National Heart Lung and Blood Insuitute. Your guide to lowering your blood pressure with DASH: DASH eating plan. 2nd ed2006. [cited 2015 February 12].
Available from: https//www.nhlbi.nih.gov/health/resources/heart/hbp-dash-index.htm

[36] Mozaffarian D, Micha R, Wallace S. Effects on coronary heart disease of increasing polyunsaturated fat in place of saturated fat: a systematic review and meta-analysis of randomized controlled trials. PLoS Medicine 2010; 7(3): e1000252.

[37] Angell SY, Cobb LK, Curtis CJ, Konty KJ, Silver LD. Change in trans fatty acid content of fast-food purchases associated with New York City's restaurant regulation: a pre-post study. Annals of Internal Medicine 2012; 157(2): 81-6.

[38] Wang YC, Bleich SN, Gortmaker SL. Increasing caloric contribution from sugar-sweetened beverages and 100% fruit juices among US children and adolescents, 1988-2004. Pediatrics 2008; 121(6): e1604-14.

[39] Kit BK, Fakhouri TH, Park S, Nielsen SJ, Ogden CL. Trends in sugar-sweetened beverage consumption among youth and adults in the United States: 1999-2010. The American Journal of Clinical Nutrition 2013; 98(1): 180-8.

[40] Slining MM, Mathias KC, Popkin BM. Trends in food and beverage sources among US children and adolescents: 1989-2010. J Acad Nutr Diet 2013; 113(12): 1683-94.

[41] Marcus C, Nyberg G, Nordenfelt A, Karpmyr M, Kowalski J, Ekelund U. A 4-year, cluster-randomized, controlled childhood obesity prevention study: STOPP. International Journal of Obesity (2005) 2009; 33(4): 408-17.

[42] Produce for Better Health Foundation. State of the Plate: 2010 Study on America's Consumption of Fruits and Vegetables 2010 [cited 2015 February 12]. Available from: http://www.pbhfoundation.org/pdfs/about/res/pbh_res/stateplate.pdf..

[43] Pomerleau J, Lock K, Knai C, McKee M. Interventions designed to increase adult fruit and vegetable intake can be effective: a systematic review of the literature. The Journal of Nutrition 2005; 135(10): 2486-95.

[44] Woodside JV, Young IS, McKinley MC. Fruits and vegetables: measuring intake and encouraging increased consumption. The Proceedings of the Nutrition Society 2013; 72(2): 236-45.

CHAPTER 10

Regular Physical Activity: A Prescription for Lifelong Health in the Community

Philip Haberstro[*,1], Lynn Rivers[2] and Mary Stottele[3]

[1]Wellness Institute of Greater Buffalo, Buffalo, NY, USA; [2]Department of Physical Therapy, D'Youville College, Buffalo, NY, USA; and [3]AmeriCorps VISTA, Buffalo, NY, USA

Abstract: There is overwhelming evidence for both the individual and societal benefits of a physically active lifestyle on maintaining high quality of life, decreasing the economic burden of sickness care spending, and reducing risk factors associated with non-communicable diseases. A 60 year historical review of the physical activity movement in the United States reveals movement from a focus on physical fitness as a means for readiness to serve in the military, to a dose/response prescription approach to physical activity for all ages, to the current evolution of an active living approach at the community level. There is evidence in many countries of the economic, human, social, and environmental benefits of a physically active community at both the societal level and all age levels: youth, adults, and older adults however a civic engagement process is necessary to develop a more physically active community and thus obtain these incredible benefits. There are ten key steps in the civic change process that any community can utilize to engage its citizens in a more physically active and healthful lifestyle. The steps rely on civic engagement, trust building, and sustaining community support. There are a host of websites and further reading to supplement the reader's knowledge of current physical activity research, movements, and community engagement efforts.

Keywords: Activeville, behavior, exercise, fitness, global health, health, life expectancy, lifestyle choices, nutrition, obesity, overweight, physical activity, physical inactivity, risk, wellness.

INTRODUCTION

There is overwhelming evidence for both the individual and societal benefits of a physically active lifestyle on maintaining high quality of life [1-3], decreasing the economic burden of sickness care spending [4-8], and reducing risk factors associated with non-communicable diseases [9, 10]. Despite this evidence,

***Corresponding author Philip Haberstro:** 65 Niagara Square Room 607 Buffalo, NY 14202, USA; Tel: (716) 851-4052; Fax: (716) 851-4309; Email: wellness@city-Buffalo.org

Judith Wylie-Rosett & Sunil S. Jhangiani (Eds)

communities around the world struggle with increasing rates of obesity and preventable non-communicable diseases. This chapter explores the history of the physical activity movement in the United States, the societal and personal benefits of physical activity, and educates the reader about the civic engagement process that is necessary to develop a more physically active community and thus obtain these incredible benefits.

We will share a brief history of recent physical activity advocacy in the U.S., exploring the trends and actions taken to promote regular physical activity from "military physical readiness" in the 1950's to the development of the first U.S. *National Physical Activity Plan* to the current "Active Living" movement, which aims to reintegrate physical activity into our daily lives. We will then update you on the evidence-based societal benefits of regular physical activity at any stage of life.

The concluding section builds on recent trends in physical activity promotion in the US and the ever-expanding list of societal benefits of a physically active population to provide a practitioner's checklist of "Civic Steps" that document the civic process of action necessary to gain the benefits that come from having a physically active population. We will begin with a dose of "civic physiology 101". We will then walk with you through a checklist of ten important steps that combine marketing, civic duty, trust-building, and community engagement to develop a shared vision and an action plan that create a sustainable community culture capable of achieving a physically active population. The chapter concludes with a list of resources that we believe will be helpful to you and your partners in your ongoing work to improve and maintain regular physical activity behaviors in your community.

In an appendix to the chapter you are going to visit "*Activeville*," U.S.A, a *mythical* community that the US Centers for Disease Control and Prevention (CDC: www.cdc.gov) and the American College of Sports Medicine (ACSM: www.acsm.org) have identified as the American community with the most physically active population (at all life stages) in the United States (U.S.). This outstanding recognition connects both the personal and community enriching benefits that Activeville's citizens and organizations have gained from their high prevalence of regular physical activity, which has consequently strengthened community culture.

RECENT HISTORY OF PHYSICAL ACTIVITY PROMOTION IN THE UNITED STATES (1954-PRESENT)

Before diving into the suggested guidelines for creating a more physically active community, it is important to look at the recent history of physical activity advocacy. This will give a basic understanding of how the medical community has arrived at its current scientific foundation and why we recommend a multi-disciplinary, inter-sector approach for promoting regular physical activity. This will also set the stage for thinking about your own up-and-coming initiatives and use of our proposed strategy to help you achieve your community's physical activity goals.

With the advent of the Industrial Revolution, humankind has witnessed a general decrease in the need for physical activity to accomplish daily tasks. Society has additionally witnessed a concomitant rise in non-communicable diseases, many of which are linked to dietary and activity patterns. In 2009, physical inactivity was identified as the fourth leading risk factor in non-communicable diseases and accounted for more than 3 million preventable deaths [11]. According to data from the World Health Organization (WHO) global health observatory data repository, 31.1% of adults (aged 15 and over) are physically inactive [12]. Additionally, 80.3% of 13-15 year-olds do not achieve the minimum of 60 minutes of moderate to vigorous physical activity per day. Physical activity tends to be less in countries with higher income, and this has been attributed to physical labor-replacing improvements in technology. Additionally, physical activity trends have shifted from occupational labor to leisure activity. Using the United States as an example, it is possible to examine this shift and its implications for improving physical activity among all populations.

Over the past six decades the US's official relationship with physical activity has evolved through four overlapping phases: "Military preparedness" with the President's Council on Youth Fitness; the "Physical Fitness" Movement; the "Physical Activity" Movement; and the current "Active Living" Movement. Importantly, scientific research conducted by governmental, academic, and private institutions has fueled these advances and continues to fuel trends in physical activity policy and promotion. It is important to note that throughout this time, communications, land use patterns, and technology evolved in ways that impacted both population health and physical activity promotion strategies. It is also necessary to distinguish a few concepts before beginning the discussion. As stated, the US's focus has shifted from promoting exercise, to promoting physical activity, and finally to promoting active living. Physical activity is the broadest of these three concepts, encompassing the other two. It is defined as any bodily movement produced by skeletal muscles, which results in energy expenditure [13]. Exercise, on the other hand, is a sub-category of physical activity that describes planned, structured, and repetitive movements that intend to improve or maintain a particular component of physical fitness [13]. Finally, active living is the process of reincorporating physical activity into daily life.

The President's Council on Youth Fitness 1950s-60s

Following World War II, Americans became more accustomed to a less physically active and more luxurious lifestyle, enjoying economic prosperity and an abundance of food, with factory-manufactured food on the rise. As a consequence, studies demonstrated that American youth were becoming "soft" compared with their European counterparts; 56.6% of American youth failed to achieve the minimum physical fitness measures required for health, compared to a failure of only 8.3% of European children [14]. This would become a major "military readiness" issue in the event of another large-scale war [15]. Activities surrounding combat also spurred many institutions to engage in exercise physiology research that directly addressed the concerns of the male-oriented military [14]. In 1954 the American College of Sports Medicine was founded by a group of physical educators and physicians with the intent to research physical activity in ultra-fit individuals in order to better study the influence of physical activity on certain medical disorders of the lungs and heart [16]. The 50s marked a boom in physical activity research, from the components of physical fitness to the physiological and health benefits of exercise [14]. Through this research and the advocacy of people like Dr. Hans Kraus, it increasingly became apparent that in order to achieve physical fitness and the muscle tone that previously came from daily activities and manual labor, citizens would have to actively engage in regular exercise.

In response to the alarming lack of youth physical fitness, President Dwight D. Eisenhower held the President's Conference on the Fitness of American Youth in 1956, which resulted in the recommendations that physical fitness should be popularized among youth; schools should have increased funds, equipment, instructors, and time for physical education; and that research on fitness should discern which kinds of activity and how much is necessary for basic fitness. In addition, President Eisenhower issued Executive Order 10673, establishing the President's Council on Youth Fitness, which he saw as a catalytic agent for establishing action within communities at the grassroots level. President Eisenhower envisioned increased physical activity as a solution to both the military's complaints that recruits were below fitness requirements and to the US's increasing concern with juvenile delinquency. The role of the Council under his presidency was to educate the public about the current state of low youth physical fitness and inspire communities to take action, rather than dictating specific actions or governmental programs. While the Council has adapted throughout the years, it still primarily serves President Eisenhower's vision as a stimulator for community action. Under President Kennedy's leadership, the President's Council on Youth Fitness became the President's Council on Physical Fitness [14]. The group received another name change in 1968 when the word "sport" was added, making the official title the President's Council on Physical Fitness and Sports. Today, in 2013, the Council is titled The President's Council on Fitness, Sport and Nutrition, adding the healthy-eating concept during President Obama's first term in office.

The Physical Fitness Movement and Dr. Kenneth Cooper's "Aerobic Fitness" 1970s-80s

The 1970s marked a shift from focusing on the military readiness and sports performance benefits of physical *exercise* to the health-related benefits of physical *fitness* [14]. Accordingly, organizations such as the American Association for Health, Physical Education, Recreation and Dance (AAHPERD) commissioned the creation of a Health Related Physical Fitness Test. This movement paralleled the ground breaking research and advocacy of Dr. Kenneth Cooper, who promoted physical activity as a means of improving cardiovascular health. Specifically, Dr. Cooper advocated a form of physical activity, which he termed "aerobics," in his 1968 book, *Aerobics*. This was the first time that "aerobic" was used in reference to physical activity. In *Aerobics,* Dr. Cooper offered a point system to quantify different forms of exercise based on the type, duration, and intensity of the aerobic activity and recommended that an individual attain 120 points per month to maintain good cardiovascular and overall health [17]. As a side note, Dr. Cooper's involvement in the evolution of physical activity in the US speaks to an important point about physical activity research; it is multidisciplinary. Dr. Cooper is a medically trained physician, not an exercise scientist or physiologist. The field of exercise research has expanded throughout history to include a whole range of disciplines from psychology to physics to neuroscience and to urban planning, and it will continue to evolve.

Moving back to the science and policies of the 1970s and 80s, experts, based on the scientific knowledge of the day, began to recommend particular physical activity programs or exercise prescriptions to improve physical fitness and health [14]. This period relied on the dose-response model of exercise, in which increased performance was seen as a result of a prescribed dose of exercise, usually with increased dose resulting in increased performance. This emphasized the effects of endurance exercise training on maximal aerobic power. Recommendations usually fell between 20 to 60 minutes of moderate to high-intensity exercise performed three or more times per week in order to achieve maximal increased capacity and disease prevention [18]. Physical fitness was viewed as a resource for "health for all" and not just a national tool for military readiness or sports performance. This approach to the physical health of the American people greatly expanded the market for physical fitness services and products. Title IX of U.S. Federal law (http://www.dol.gov/oasam/regs/statutes/titleix.htm) required equity for women's sports at the high school and collegiate level, opening the doors of sport participation to millions of American girls and young women as part of national policy.

The Physical Activity Movement 1980s-2000s

Beginning in the early 1980s and continuing into the 2000s, public health and advocacy began to shift away from emphasis on being physically *fit via* aerobic exercise and resistance training to simply being physically *active*. The CDC Behavior Risk Factor Surveillance Studies began to quantify physical activity levels in America, and the first ever U.S. "Healthy People" Goals and Objectives for the Nation (released in 1980) had a physical activity target for 1990. The movement was fueled by research that began suggesting that in order to obtain the cardiovascular and substantial health benefits of regular physical activity, a person did not need to participate in highly structured high-intensity aerobic exercise. Major report recommendations began to promote the societal value of moderate physical activity as a valid and sustainable alternative to high intensity exercise and claimed that the health benefits of physical activity are related to the total weekly amount of physical activity performed, not necessarily consecutive aerobic activity [18]. This effectively meant that being physically active throughout the day would lead to the same preventive health benefits as performing a 20-minute bout of higher intensity aerobic activity. In 1995, the CDC and the ACSM released a report that recommended that "Every U.S. adult should perform at least 30 minutes or more of moderate-intensity physical activity on most, preferably all, days of the week". The report also stated that the 30 minutes could be accumulated throughout the day *via* short bouts of activity. About ten years later in 2007, the ACSM and the American Heart Association released a study with new recommendations for physical activity. While the recommendations were basically unchanged from the ones released in 1995, the new set clarified that physical activity should be conducted at a minimum of 30 minutes per day, five days per week and also clarified that the short bouts of physical activity must be of duration of at least ten minutes [9]. The new guidelines also indicated that while the minimum amount is protective for health, performing above the minimum requirements would confer even greater health advantages. Finally, the new requirements incorporated muscle-strengthening activities, as well as aerobic activity, recommending that each adult perform 8-10 muscle-strengthening activities on two or more nonconsecutive days each week using the major muscle groups [9].

Moving back to the late 90s, in 1996 the US Surgeon General released the first ever report on Physical Activity and Health [14]. This book-style report covered the history of physical activity, its conferred physiological and social benefits, patterns of activity in the U.S., and recommendations for national physical activity promotion. This report also marked a greater shift toward incorporating physical activity into the government's health policy agenda. The late 90s also began to see early stage - research to achieve a greater understanding of the economic impact of physical activity on direct and indirect medical spending, the role of the built environment in facilitating physical activity, and the impact of regular physical activity on employee health and productivity, and student health and academic success. The late 1990s also saw the formation of the nonprofit, National Coalition for Promoting Physical Activity (www.ncppa.org).

The Active Living Movement 2000s-Present Day

In the early 2000s the concept of "Active Living" began appearing in the United States, recognized through major institution-led initiatives like Active Living by Design (www.ActiveLivingbydesign.org). First pioneered in North America by Canada, Active Living expanded the previous message of the US "Physical Activity" movement (which was basically to increase regular physical activity throughout the week) by promoting reintegration of physical activity into everyday activities, not simply planned exercise. In previous decades, technology, automobiles, declines in school physical education class time, and urban sprawl had gradually engineered former daily opportunities for physical activity out of our lives, and the Active Living movement aimed to return those opportunities.

The notion of including physical activity in everyday activities automatically adds a structural component to the physical activity discussion that for the most part had gone unnoticed. Successful Active Living requires modifications to the built-environment of a community, including building design, bike lanes in new or rebuilt highways (the Compete Streets concept), increasing accessibility to sidewalks, and mixing land purposes [19]. Active Living is the most comprehensive approach to physical activity promotion to date; it includes the scientific, policy and social components of creating physically active communities, considering issues such as unsafe neighborhoods, food insecurity, and economic disparities. Measures were first directed at wealthy or middle-class communities; however in the second half of the past decade, individuals and organizations have raised awareness for the need for Active Living approaches in underserved urban communities. Such advocacy has raised awareness about socioeconomic constraints with regard to physical activity. This has brought the language of social justice into the conversation regarding chronic disease prevention, obesity reduction, and the societal value of a physically active population on the health, happiness, and economic wellbeing of the American people. Further federal policy initiatives in the mid 2000s saw the release of the first ever National Physical Activity Guidelines (Dept. of Health and Human Services www. health.gov/paguidelines/) and the federal legislation requirement (Dept. of Agriculture) that all school districts that receive federal support develop a district-wide wellness policy. Learning from other nations' experiences, the first ever US National Physical Activity Plan (www.physicalactvityplan.org) was developed through a consortium of public, private, and non-profit agencies to further guide the nation's efforts to be more physically active.

Returning to a global perspective, it can be seen that similar trends are occurring in most developed nations. The need for improved physical activity is apparent, and various countries are undertaking nation-wide health campaigns to increase levels of physical activity and therefore overall health among their citizenry. Findings from the WHO have indicated that one of the most important aspects in promoting a successful campaign to engage citizens in increased physical activity is creating and sustaining partnerships between health agencies, public, non-profit, and private organizations that promote community-based supports and programs [20]. Such civic and social capital building relationships and programs will be discussed further in this chapter.

SOCIETAL BENEFITS OF PHYSICAL ACTIVITY

The physiological health benefits of physical activity for persons throughout life are well established [1, 10, 21-24]. Increasingly, investigators are documenting societal benefits which go beyond individual physical health and include decreased economic burden on public dollars for health care spending [4-8]; improved cognitive learning and academic achievement in children [25, 26]; decreased risk factors for non-communicable diseases (NCDs) in adults and children [9, 10]; increased worker productivity [8, 27]; and improved quality of life and decreased morbidity in older adults [2, 3].

Economic Burden: National Costs of Inactivity

Several countries around the world have examined the economic burden of inactivity and obesity on their national healthcare systems. Canada has taken a lead with respect to tracking the economic burden on the public healthcare system, reporting in 2000 that approximately $2.1 billion, or 2.5% of their total direct healthcare costs, were attributable to physical inactivity and obesity in the previous year [5]. A 10-year follow up study by Katsmarzyk [6] in 2011 focused on the largest province, Ontario, which demonstrated continued increase in the public health burden with physical inactivity and obesity as major contributing factors. Similarly in the late 1990s, the United States reported that 2.4% of US healthcare expenditures were related directly to obesity and physical inactivity [7]; France reported approximately 2% of national healthcare costs [28]; Netherlands reported 4% of national healthcare costs [29]; and Australia reported 2% of national healthcare costs [30]. All direct costs were associated with physical inactivity and obesity, which could have been prevented or minimized with a physically active population.

The World Health Organization (WHO) in 2008 estimated that 36 million of the 57 million global deaths were due primarily to cardiovascular diseases, cancers, chronic respiratory diseases, and diabetes, including 9 million deaths before the age of 60. The United Nations General Assembly is working in close coordination with the WHO to establish policy and member-state partnerships to develop strategies to address two key risk factors for NCDs: physical inactivity and poor nutrition [31, 32].

AGE-RELATED ISSUES

Youth

The WHO reports that in 2010 the number of overweight children under the age of five was estimated to be over 42 million. Close to 35 million of these were living in developing countries. The global rise in childhood obesity and earlier onset of NCDs, such as diabetes and cardiovascular disease, in adolescence and younger children confirms the societal need to address the promotion of physical activity for youth. Overweight and obesity, as well as their related diseases, are largely preventable. Prevention of childhood obesity therefore needs to be a high priority, with physical activity being a key strategy alongside nutrition.

Physical activity for school-aged children is also linked to improved academic performance [25, 26]. Research has demonstrated that physical activity stimulates the generation of new brain cells in areas that support memory [33] and increases executive control functions such as planning, attention, problem solving, and verbal reasoning [34, 35]. In adolescence, physical activity has been linked to improved mental health, bone health, and is associated with long-term benefits of commitment to physical activity in adulthood [36].

Adults

There is clear and consistent evidence that regular physical activity is effective in the primary and secondary prevention of chronic diseases (*e.g.,* cardiovascular disease, diabetes, cancer, osteoporosis, depression) and the risk of premature death [10]. Adults living in urban environments are increasingly limited in pursuing physical activity due to modern urban design and safety issues [20, 37].

In industrialized nations, technological automation and laborsaving innovations in the workplace and at home are removing the need for physical activity in adults. This sedentary lifestyle at both work and home is contributing significantly to the risk factors for obesity and physical inactivity, earlier onset of NCDs in adults, and rising health care costs [21, 38]. The promotion of workplace nutrition and physical activity programs are consistently demonstrating positive effects on controlling employee overweight and obesity [37]. Support and promotion of employer-sponsored physical activity in the workplace could be a key strategy to decreasing the economic burden on society.

Older Adults

In 2010, U.S. direct medical costs due to falls in older adults, inflation adjusted, exceeded $30 billion dollars. This medical care resulted from 2.3 million nonfatal fall injuries, which were treated in emergency departments, and more than 662,000 of these patients were hospitalized [39]. Physical activity programs included in multi-factor programs globally are decreasing the number and risk of falls and are beginning to focus on integrating physical activity into the daily living activities of older adults, rather than traditional group or home exercise programs [40, 41]. Quality of life and cognition in older adults, including frail adults, is shown to improve with increased physical activity, which can contribute significantly to a strong, thriving community as the proportionate number of older adults living in communities continues to climb [42].

HOW TO CREATE COMMUNITY CULTURE CHANGE FOR LIFE-LONG HEALTH

Today, both in the U.S. and worldwide, data demonstrate that we are headed in a very unhealthy direction with the insufficiently physically active, and the overweight/obese now holding a statistical majority in the adult population [31, 32]. What can communities do to reverse this direction and promote life-long health?

In human physiology, movement is the tool that produces healthy bodies. In the "civic physiology" of the US, democracy is the tool for change- "use it or lose it" works for both. Similar to human physiology, in civic physiology, simply being informed about physical activity is not enough to produce results. It is necessary to act on that knowledge in order to obtain valuable results. This section proposes ten essential steps to sustainable community change that will help you act on your knowledge and create real culture change in your community. For a more detailed example of this process, please see the Appendix.

Step 1: Define the Issue

In civic physiology, the term "issue" is used to define a need, challenge, or opportunity that exists within a community. The first step to achieving more active communities is to recognize and gather baseline data on the physical activity level of a community; this sets the stage for justification of community action. However, realizing that a community has unacceptable levels of physical inactivity also involves researching whether existing government entities, nonprofits, or private sector organizations are already addressing this issue, so as to not duplicate existing efforts. If an organization already exists, it may be more fruitful to join forces and strengthen or better organize existing efforts. If not, it is time to convene a community team to address the public health issue of physical activity.

Step 2: Convene a Community Team

While researching the physical activity promotion reality in a community, you are likely to find a variety of people who are interested in the topic. Make note of such people and invite them to be on the team. It is important to make sure that your team is a representation of the wider community, so as to have representation from all fronts. A contemporary form of leadership style known as "servant leadership," in which the initiator of the change process recruits stakeholders to be part of said process, is very useful in a case such as this. This leadership approach greatly enhances the success and sustainability of the community change process by insuring buy-in and shared accountability for results. While convening a community team, four basic groups should be kept in mind.

1. Public Sector Representatives-these stakeholders come from taxpayer-funded institutions, which include public schools, elected officials, government staff, and representatives from any government-sponsored authorities or citizen volunteers on government commissions.

2. Private Sector (business) Representatives

3. Nonprofit Representatives

4. Citizen Stakeholders (including youth /adults/older adults)

After convening the team, it is important to set up a structure for your organization. There should at least be a chair, perhaps a co-chair, and if you have a large group, a formal board of directors should be elected. It is then important to set ground rules for team governance, meeting management procedures, the decision-making processes, and the methods utilized to report progress to your community.

Step 3: Creating a "Mission" Statement

A mission statement is the group's purpose or reason for existence. It is important to formally create, record, and publicize this statement so that throughout the process, the group can focus itself on its initial aim, ensure that all strategies, goals and projects fall under that aim, and perhaps change the aim if work seems to be drifting into another direction. It also serves to give group members a shared sense of purpose and the creation process strengthens relationships between team members fostering social capital. A mission statement should be brief, clear, and easy to communicate, usually one sentence with active verbs. (*i.e.,* Increase physical activity).

Step 4: Documenting your Current Reality

Current reality is defined as the current situation with regard to whatever issue a group decides to tackle, in this case physical activity. This process will involve gaining specific baseline statistics regarding physical activity in a community and sharing those statistics with relevant stakeholders and media outlets. This keeps all individuals starting from the same baseline and provides a metric from which progress can be measured. It is also important to look at communities similar to yours that have both failed and succeeded in promoting physical activity and to learn from their mistakes and successes. Tackling the issue of physical inactivity will require a strategic approach, one that comprehensively utilizes and addresses public policy, the environment, builds the capacity and sustainability of your community team, evidence-based and/or innovative programs, and an ongoing public communication campaign.

Step 5: Create a Shared Vision

A vision statement captures the "desired future" created by the group's mission statement. The vision documents what the group's work should produce; it provides a picture of how the community will look. For the purposes of this chapter, a sample "*shared vision*" might read: "The people of (your community), at all stages of life, enjoy the health, social and economic benefits from living a physically active lifestyle". The visioning process is best done when multiple community stakeholders are invited and work together to create a shared ideal. This creates community buy-in and energizes group efforts and is vital to public and resource support.

Step 6: Create an Action Plan

An action plan is a strategic planning process that will detail goals, priorities for action, timelines, milestones, and budgets/resources. Typically strategic action plans are developed for one to three-year periods and are monitored monthly for progress reporting and revision as necessary. The term *strategic* in this step implies that policy, environment, communication elements and strengthening the capacity of the group are critical components to the action plan along with the evidence based or innovative programs. These elements are essential to create a community culture that supports physical activity through the life span. It is useful to have a written and not just electronic version of an action plan, so that it is physically present with the group and serves as a constant reminder of the work that needs to be done. It will also boost morale as accomplishments are visually added to the document.

Step 7: Implement the Action Plan

After creation of the plan, it is important to create subgroups to achieve each of the established goals and objectives. Again, it is necessary to monitor the progress of the plan monthly and ensure that the proper work is being done. This process phase also offers opportunities to develop new leaders and recruit additional players with specific skill sets that will help with getting each sub group to results.

Step 8: Monitor and Manage the Plan

Monthly or quarterly team meeting with advance agendas for reporting progress, lessons learned and challenges in accomplishing the Action Plan work. Particularly important to the overall success is managing the work (a key leadership task) that goes on between meetings. The how and who of this, needs to be addressed and determined *before* the implementation phase starts. In addition to internal process management of the action plan, it is important to report out to the community that supports the group's efforts and engage them whenever possible in the work. Spokespersons need to be identified and if necessary trained in media relations. It is suggested to invite local media to monthly meetings. Above all, it is important to report to funders on progress (milestones /results /challenges) to ensure continued trust in your work and support in the future.

Step 9: Evaluate the Plan During and After Year One

As it has been previously mentioned, it is important to monitor the plan's progress throughout the year. Additionally, after the first year it is useful to have an external objective party, such as volunteers from non-related agencies, to evaluate the plan's progress and suggest areas that could be improved upon in the coming year. A report should be sent to all stakeholders in the process and actions/adjustments to the Action plan and/or process management made. This "Continuous Quality Improvement" management tactic will facilitate long term progress. Media attention to the year's successes is also helpful in furthering group and community momentum.

Step 10: Celebrate Your Success and Modify the Plan

After the first year of a group's work, it is important to take a step back and celebrate the achievements. This is most easily done by a community event that highlights the past year's progress and perhaps even fundraises for the future. After celebration, the evaluation of the past year's plan should be utilized to create an even stronger and more focused agenda for the following year. This process will be repeated annually as the goal of a more physically active community is being achieved and sustained.

To review, here are listed some advice and key messages from the ten steps just described:

Key Principles for Becoming a Physically Active Community

- Inter-sector (public/private/nonprofit/citizens at the community table) and an inter-disciplinary (environmental/economic/civic/human) approach to the issue.

- Built on a citizen empowerment model, not just expertise. Engaged citizens and partners know the "Current reality"(where we are), where we want to be (Crafted a "Share Vision") and created a comprehensive strategic Action plan to achieve the Shared Vision. (fosters ownership and accountability for results)

- Strategic-most important part; allows you to avoid the fault in most well-intentioned community change efforts of depending solely on education or programs and instead strategically addresses policy, environment, communications and community capacity-building along with programs. (read the WHO Ottawa Charter for Health Promotion)

- Sustainable-critical to real community culture change
- Reflects community values and therefore gains adequate resources to do the work
- Equity: all stakeholders have an equal share of responsibility and benefit
- Action Plan incorporates Integration or infiltration tactic: find opportunities in the community to integrate health promotion into the community (*i.e.* setting up a wellness fair at the local auto show/getting local economic development funds invested in employee health promotion)
- Maintain a firm conviction that local politics are less polluted by money, and therefore real opportunity to create community culture change rests with the local citizens
- Keep in mind other issues may surface throughout your work: gender issues, body image, serving physically challenged populations, school budgets and physical education) Be prepared to address these as you transform your community support for Active Living.

This chapter has taken you through some history, some science, and some practical advice, intending to demonstrate how to learn from the past, use science to support your case, and make use of community and civic engagement to achieve the outcomes you seek for yourself and others. Creating healthy communities and the culture that sustains healthy behaviors is not easy work and takes time and persistence. It took the U.S. five decades to transform from a nation in which 50% of all adults were smokers into one in which only 20% now smoke; however, we still have to fight every day to protect our children from beginning to smoke. The public health war on physical inactivity and poor nutrition has learned much from the tobacco wars. Key among these lessons is the importance and power of grassroots community movements, policy change, and environmental supports to promote a community culture change. Although it is at times a steep uphill battle, civic change truly can begin with the spark and tenacity of one passionate citizen, who envisions a better life for him or herself and the community at large. Please feel free to use any of the resources listed below to get started on this worthwhile process!

ADDITIONAL RESOURCES & LINKS:

National and International Health and Fitness Organizations

President's Council on Fitness, Sport, and Nutrition: www.fitness.gov

Centers for Disease Control and Prevention: http://www.cdc.gov/

American College of Sports Medicine: http://www.acsm.org/

Institute of Medicine: http://www.iom.edu/

World Health Organization: http://www.who.int/en/

WHO Ottawa Charter for Health Promotion: http://www.who.int/healthpromotion/conferences/previous/ottawa/en/

Milestones in Health Promotion: Statements from Global Conferences: http://www.who.int/healthpromotion/milestones.pdf

Trust for America's Health: http://healthyamericans.org/

American Alliance for Health, Physical Education, Recreation, and Dance (AAHPERD): http://www.aahperd.org/

Wellness Council of America (WELCOA): http://www.welcoa.org/

Active Living

Active Living by Design: http://www.activelivingbydesign.org/

Robert Wood Johnson Foundation: Active Living Research Program: http://www.rwjf.org/en/research-publications/find-rwjf-research/2011/07/active-living-research.html

Built Environment

Safe Routes to School: http://www.nhtsa.gov/people/injury/pedbimot/bike/safe-routes-2002/

Physical Activity for Persons with Disabilities

National Center for Physical Activity for Persons with Disabilities: www.ncpad.org

Physical Activity Research

1996 Surgeon General's Report on Physical Activity and Health: http://books.google.com/books?hl=en&lr=&id=sASnZqD4CGUC&oa=fnd&pg=PA3&dq=surgeon+general+health+report+1996+&ots=nfDyT-g9ki&sig=SE2HBP4maJiSx8STz1LfdusJV6Q

"Spark: The Revolutionary New Science of Exercise and the Brain" by John J. Ratey: http://www.sparkpe.org/

Economic Impact of Physical Inactivity and Obesity

"The Long-term Returns of Obesity Prevention Policies" by Alex Brill: http://www.rwjf.org/content/dam/farm/reports/reports/2013/rwjf405694

David Chenoweth's Physical Inactivity Cost Calculator:
http://www.ecu.edu/picostcalc/pdf_file/Methods.pdf

Civic Change Tools and Organizations

Civic Change, Inc.: http://www.civicchange.org/

National Civic League: http://www.nationalcivicleague.org/

Community Visioning and Strategic Planning Handbook: http://www.cpn.org/tools/manuals/Community/pdfs/VSPHandbook.pdf

Community Builders: http://www.communitybuilders.ro/

Community Toolbox from the University of Kansas:
http://ctb.ku.edu/en/help-taking-action

Health Promotion

Health Promotion Advocates: http://healthpromotionadvocates.org/

Institute for Health and Productivity: http://www.ihpm.org/

Health Enhancement Research Organization (HERO): http://www.the-hero.org/

The Guide to Community Preventive Services: http://www.thecommunityguide.org/index.html

Older Adult

American Association for Retired Persons (AARP): http://www.aarp.org/

National Institute on Aging: http://www.nia.nih.gov/

A WORD OF ADVICE

Local nonprofits and Public Health Departments are good resources for physical activity advice and opportunities throughout the lifespan!

APPENDIX

How "Activeville" Became the Most Physically Active Community in the United States!

It is important to note that while Activeville is a fictitious community; its course of action can be replicated in any place in the world. It can be your neighborhood, village, town, city, county, province or congressional district (we like to use government entities because they allow for political accountability within a specific geographical district). Activeville can be North or South, East or West, urban, suburban, or rural. Activeville's path to becoming a more "physically active" community reflects a melding of some very simple community culture change work, coupled with key health promotion action principles developed by the WHO at the 1986 Health Promotion Summit on creating community health, held in Ottawa, Canada.

Several years ago, a small group of people living in Activeville, U.S.A. (they were friends who met regularly to walk together) became aware of the fact that state reports had documented a decline in health status and physical activity levels in Activeville. After several discussions, the group decided to do something about improving their community's health and wellbeing by proactively addressing the level of physical activity. Fortunately for them, one of their group members worked in a nonprofit and understood that by working together to achieve their shared Vision of a physically active community, they would need to go beyond simply raising community awareness of the issue or holding a health fair. They recognized that their small but committed group needed to first educate themselves (and then others) about the issue and better understand "how to create community change" *before* they invested time and finite resources in creating an Activeville Action Plan to improve physical activity levels and wellbeing. They then asked, "What is our path forward?" The answer was not simply gaining a better understanding of human physiology (they all knew, as did most of their neighbors, that regular physical activity was essential for good health), but rather obtaining a better understanding of the "civic physiology" of communities. Learning how Activeville's civil society functioned (or did not) was critical in creating a comprehensive community plan in which a regularly physically active population would come to exist! Their research on community culture change helped them understand that the available scientific data and the health education programs that Activeville offered were not enough to stave off the physical inactivity epidemic and achieve the optimally beneficial level of regular physical activity. They also found that there was no community wide group addressing this issue. They researched culture and strategies to create health in communities and came across the WHO's Ottawa Charter for Health Promotion, which helped them create a comprehensive action plan. Additionally, organizations like the National Civic League (www.NCL.org) helped Activeville residents use democracy to understand and facilitate the community change process that would over time create the culture necessary for becoming America's most physically active community as well as a community with one of the best levels of "civic health" in the nation!

In human physiology, movement is the tool that produces healthy bodies. In the "civic physiology" of the US, democracy is the tool for change-"use it or lose it" works for both. Similar to human physiology, in civic physiology simply being informed about physical activity is not enough to produce results. It is necessary to act on that knowledge in order to obtain valuable results. Here we use the Activeville story to introduce ten essential steps to community change that will help you act on your knowledge and create real change in your community.

You, the reader, are the initial citizen change advocate-you may be a medical or public health professional, a student, a CEO or an elected official. Whatever your position, you have looked at your community either through observation or data, and you have determined that your community population is not regularly physically active, as did one resident of Activeville, which leads to Step 1 of our 10 steps to an Active Community!

Step 1: Define the Issue

One day, a resident of Activeville, let's call her Marilyn, began to suspect that her community was overweight/obese. She observed this while visiting her child's school, taking the bus to work, and even through local media stories. Years of research (see the WHO Reports on Physical Activity or the U.S. Surgeon General's report on Physical Activity and Health (1996)) and common sense informed her that being physically active was part of the solution (along with good nutrition) to many of Activeville's health issues, and she decided to focus on making Activeville more physically active. She first checked with her local mayor's office and Council members; local public health office; school board; Chamber of Commerce; United Way; and older adults' services office to see if there was any existing local commission or group that was working to improve physical activity levels and discovered that there was none.

If you, like Marilyn, have done this, you have demonstrated leadership just by noticing a need or opportunity in your community, which in civic physiology is termed the *issue*. In Activeville's case, the issue was its low levels of physical activity among residents of all ages (and that the issue was not being addressed!). This is how change often starts-someone in the community sees a need to be met or an opportunity to do good and decides to take action. In very simple terms, this is civic leadership coming to life-and throughout the process of getting Activeville moving, leadership will be challenged, frustrated, and rewarded-but through the change process sustained leadership is essential. One must be ready for the journey, since true cultural change is often an outcome of a lengthy and on going civic process. A contemporary form of leadership style known as "servant leadership," in which the initiator of the change process recruits stakeholders to be part of the process, is very useful in a case such as this. This leadership approach greatly enhances the success and sustainability of the community change process because it creates community ownership of the issue and the social capital (trust and reciprocity) to address it.

Step 2: Convening the Activeville Community Team

Convening a team takes us to an important element of civic physiology-understanding who the players are in your community. Through Marilyn's research, she found some effort within individual organizations, but nothing community-wide. She also learned that a number of folks at these different community institutions were *interested* in this issue and wanted to be kept informed of what she learned, so she set up a simple list serve on her home computer and began communicating with others who shared her interest in addressing this community challenge and opportunity!

While making your community team, you, like Marilyn, should keep four key groups in mind. Leave one out, and you do so at the peril of your change initiative. Here are the four groups:

1. Public Sector Representatives-these stakeholders come from taxpayer-funded institutions, which include public schools, elected officials, government staff, and representatives from any government-sponsored authorities or citizen volunteers on government commissions.

2. Private Sector (business) Representatives

3. Nonprofit Representatives

4. Citizen Stakeholders

After convening, the community team elected a chair and co-chair and set the initial ground rules for how the team would govern itself, how the meetings would run, and how the group's decision-making process would occur. The choices for where the group would be housed were multiple. Each scenario (from existing as an informal group to being housed in an existing legal organization; private sector corporation; nonprofit; or public sector entity) offers advantages and options to be considered. Activeville's team, after due deliberation, opted to be housed in a local nonprofit that offered them an office for one year; willingness to assist them in fundraising and act as their fiscal agent; and provide basic insurance coverage. The newly formed Activeville Physical Activity Community Team (now known as APACT) co-chairs, with the approval of their team, developed a budget for the next three years and then went about the community with a very simple one page funding request to raise the resources necessary to fund the work. It took six months to bring the initial funding/investment in but the team made a strong case for the health and economic impact and found interested investors in several foundations, businesses, health insurers and the Mayor. A logo and membership campaign were developed so that a year-to-year operating fund could be established to hire a process facilitator, administrative support person, and sustain fund-raising, with the option for hiring an in-house development person or outsourcing that function. APACT signed a memorandum of understanding with the sponsoring nonprofit and was ready to take the next action step.

Note: It is also quite possible that in your own community a collaboration may already exist to promote physical activity, and you will find yourself, your talents, and energy very welcome with the group since these civic entities constantly need new volunteers.

Step 3: Creating an APACT "Mission" Statement

Next, it was important for the group to formally create a mission statement, which is defined as the group's purpose or reason for existence. A mission statement should be brief, clear, and easy to communicate. Activeville's inter-sector community team chose "Increasing Regular Physical Activity". A local strategic planning firm donated the services of a neutral facilitator to assist the Activeville team in completing this important step of their formation process. A mission statement gave the group a shared "sense of purpose" and the process of creating one had the added benefit of strengthening the "social capital" within the group.

Step 4: Documenting your Current Reality

One of the key components to Activeville's success is that before acting, APACT did their homework and learned where the community was and better understood what the community truly needed. Documenting the community Current Reality-simply put as "knowing where your community is" with regard to a variety of measurable variables (that will form a baseline for progress)—provided all APACT members with a shared understanding of where Activeville was and informed decision-making and priorities for action. They then shared their findings with the local media, community decision makers, and the community at large. This action is very important in any community change process since it raises community awareness of the issue, educates the public, and sets the stage for taking further action.

APACT also looked at other communities that had success, and some that did not, and learned from them. They learned that improving physical activity requires much more than campaigns and slogans; it requires a *strategic approach* that comprehensively utilizes and addresses public policy, capacity building, the environment, evidence-based and/or innovative programs, and an ongoing public communication campaign (such as Be Active Activeville!). Integrating all these elements was essential to both short-term results and sustainable change.

Step 5: Create a Shared Vision

Once APACT understood their community's Current Reality, their next step was to create a shared Vision for physical activity that would guide their work. Creating the Vision statement was intended to provide a picture of how the community would look. To further engage the public in this Visioning effort, a neutral party facilitated several community Vision sessions (this time a planning department professor and his students from a local college did the facilitation). The facilitators also identified zip codes, gender and age ranges at the Visioning meetings to be sure all segments of Activeville's population were represented.

With the Activeville picture now getting much clearer, the community understood its Current Reality and had collectively created a shared Vision for what it wanted its new reality to be. And they were bold. Their Vision was "Activeville is the most physically active community in the United States". Their progress, which they published often, and fun, educational fundraising events won them more volunteers and critical resources from sponsors and grants.

Step 6: Create an Action Plan

Building on a sound civic process and a shared understanding of both the Current Reality and community Vision, it was time to facilitate the creation of a comprehensive strategic action plan. The plan used the health promotion action principles identified in the WHO's Ottawa Charter for Health Promotion, which addresses five key areas: Public Policy, Environment, Community Capacity, Personal Skills, and emphasis on Prevention and Health Promotion over treatment. APACT subcommittees were formed to address physical activity in youth (schools/afterschool), adults (workplaces) and older adults in the home and community). Each subcommittee prepared an initial three-year action plan with first year priorities for action, timelines, milestones, and budget/resources.

Step 7: Implement the APACT Action Plan

APACT members formed a communication team with help from local marketing and public relations professionals, crafted a year-round "Be Active Activeville!" campaign with the subcommittee action plans that targeted youth, adult, and older adult markets with gender and culturally appropriate messages that promoted the benefits and opportunities of leading a physically active lifestyle. They held a major community-wide press conference and special event to launch the implementation of the plan.

Step 8: Monitor and Manage the Plan

It was important for APACT to monitor and manage the actions, while reporting regularly to themselves, the public, and sponsors. Monthly meetings of APACT were held, open to the public and televised on the local public access TV channel. School Physical education programs AND afterschool resources were strengthened-An Activeville wide workplace health promotion survey was completed and a quality of the program assessment followed by trainings to improve at work physical activity opportunities was successfully implemented serving employer of all sizes and from all sectors. An across the Activeville older adults falls prevention initiative with help from local first responders and a strong focus on improving physical activity for older adults through faith based, community center and the local PBS channel had a measurable impact on falls. Reporters from the local print and electronic media were invited to the meetings and they regularly contributed articles and stories about APACT's work. The APACT website included a Facebook and Twitter account for promoting activities and meetings and soliciting sponsors, donations, and feedback. Milestones that were identified in the action plans were reviewed, and the well-managed monthly meetings kept the team on track and allowed for adjustments to planned actions. Funders, members and sponsors were also kept informed of progress, challenges, lessons learned and resources were extended for the full three year Action plan.

Step 9: Evaluate the APACT Plan During and After Year One

The Activeville plan for evaluation included both the process (how efficient and effective the plan was) and the outcomes achieved in Activeville that supported or actually fostered improvements in levels of physical activity. Outside agencies (Department of Public Health and area colleges) were recruited to evaluate the process, document outcomes and report on health, economic, civic impacts. Quarterly progress reports were made to APACT members and funders. An annual report was sent to all stakeholders and the media, which included recommendations for the coming year.

Step 10: Celebrate Your Success and Modify the Plan

After one year, the APACT team hosted a community picnic and walk to celebrate their successes, share their stories and to get ready for year two of the action plan. The APACT change process continued to recycle itself year after year and become institutionalized in the Activeville community culture for the young, the working age, the retired, and those with special needs. As part of this recycling process, capacity building training provided ongoing personnel skills enhancement, leadership renewal/development and APACT organizational sustainability, growth and national recognition as an ALL AMERICA CITY by the National Civic League.

Summary of Activeville's 10 Steps to becoming the most physically active community

1. Define the issue in the community: improving levels of physical activity

2. Convene a team: inter-sector/inter-disciplinary team, elect co-chairs, and start identifying and raising resources to address the issue and sustain the project

3. Create a Mission Statement: "Increasing regular physical activity"

4. Document Current Reality: what physical activity looks like in community

5. Create a community Shared Vision: "Activeville is the most physically active community in the United States"

6. Create a comprehensive action plan

7. Implement action plan

8. Monitor and manage the plan

9. Evaluate progress/modify action plan

10. Celebrate success and recycle the process each year! This is how, together and year after year of "planning their work and working their plan" ACTIVEVILLE USA achieved their shared Vision of being the most physically active community in the USA! Visit www.CreatingHealthy

Communities.org to learn more about how the ACTIVEVILLE story can be replicated in your community!!

ACKNOWLEDGEMENTS

Thank You to Judith and Sunil for the opportunity, To Lynn and Mary for your partnership and To Drs. R. Keelor and T. Hancock for your mentorship and Inspiration.

CONFLICT OF INTEREST

The authors confirm that this chapter contents have no conflict of interest.

REFERENCES

[1] Bize R, Johnson J, Plotnikoff R. Physical activity level and health-related quality of life in the general adult population: a systematic review. Prev Med. 2007;45(6):401-15.

[2] Rejeski WJ, Mihalko S. Physical activity and quality of life in older adults. J Gerontol A Biol Sci Med Sci. 2001 [cited 2013 Feb 23]; 56 (suppl 2): 23-35. Available from: Oxford Journals.

[3] Fries J. The theory and practice of active aging. Current Gerontology and Geriatrics Research, vol. 2012, Article ID 420637, 7 pages, 2012. doi:10.1155/2012/420637

[4] Finkelstein E, Ruhm C, Kosal, K. Economic caused and consequences of obesity. Ann Rev Public Health 2005 [cited 2013 Feb 23]; 26: 239-57. Available from: http://www.annualreviews.org/doi/full/10.1146/annurev.publhealth.26.021304.144628.

[5] Katzmarzyk P, Gledhill N, Shephard R. The economic burden of physical activity in Canada. CMAJ. 2000;163(11):1435-1440.

[6] Katzmarzyk P. The economic costs associated with physical inactivity and obesity in Ontario. Health and Fitness J. of Canada [online]. 2011 [cited 2013 May 18]; 4(4):31-40. Available from: http://www.healthandfitnessjournalofcanada.com/index.php/html/article/view/112/78.

[7] Colditz G. Economic costs of obesity and inactivity. Med Sci Sports Exerc. 1999; 31(11 Suppl):S663-7.

[8] Chenoweth D, Leutzunger J. The economic cost of physical inactivity and excess weight in American adults. J of Phys Act and Hlth. 2006; 3: 148-163.

[9] Haskell WL, Lee I, Pate RR, *et al.* Physical activity and public health: updated recommendation for adults from the American College of Sports Medicine and the American Heart Association. Med Sci Sports Exerc. 2007;39(8):1423.

[10] Warburton D, Nicol C, Bredin S. Health benefits of physical activity: the evidence. CMAJ. 2006;174(6):801- 809.

[11] Mathers C, Stevens G, Mascarenhas M. Global health risks: mortality and burden of disease attributable to selected major risks: World Health Organization; 2009.

[12] Hallal PC, Andersen LB, Bull FC, Guthold R, Haskell W, Ekelund U. Global physical activity levels: surveillance progress, pitfalls, and prospects. The Lancet. 2012.

[13] Caspersen CJ, Powell KE, Christenson GM. Physical activity, exercise, and physical fitness: definitions and distinctions for health-related research. *Public health rep.* 1985;100(2):126.

[14] U.S. Department of Health and Human Services, Centers for Disease Control and Prevention, National Center for Chronic Disease Prevention and Health Promotion, The President's Council on Physical Fitness and Sports. Physical activity and health: a report of the Surgeon General. Sudbury: Jones & Bartlett Learning; 1996.

[15] Sturgeon J, Meer J. The first fifty years 1956-2006: The President's Council on Physical Fitness and Sports revisits its roots and charts its future. In: The President's Council on Physical Fitness & Sports the first 50 years: 1956-2006. Tampa: Fairount, 2006; p. 40-66.

[16] Berryman JW. Celebrate 50 Years of science and medicine: 1954-2004: 50 Years of Progress and Service. Med Sci Sports Exerc. 2004;36(1):A17.

[17] Cooper KH. Aerobics. New York: M. Evans and Company; 1968.

[18] Pate RR, Pratt M, Blair SN *et al*. Physical activity and public health. JAMA. 1995;273(5):402-407.

[19] Day K. Active living and social justice: planning for physical activity in low-income, black, and Latino communities. J Am Plann Assoc. 2006;72(1):88-99.

[20] Heath GW, Parra DC, Sarmiento OL, Andersen LB, Owen N, Goenka S, *et al*. Evidence-based intervention in physical activity: lessons from around the world. The Lancet. 2012.

[21] Chan C, Ryan D, Tudor-Locke C. Health benefits of a pedometer-based physical activity intervention in sedentary workers. Prev Med. 2004;39(6):1215-22.

[22] Janssen I, LeBlanc A. Systematic review of the health benefits of physical activity and fitness in school-aged children and youth. Int J Behav Nutr Phys Act. 2010 [cited 2013 May 22];7:40. Available from: Biomed Central.

[23] Biddle SJH, Fox KR, Boutcher SH, editors. Physical activity and psychological well-being. London: Routledge; 2000.

[24] Faulkner G, Taylor A, editors. Exercise, health and mental health: Emerging relationships. London: Routledge; 2005.

[25] Trudeau F, Shephard RJ. Physical education, school physical activity, school sports and academic performance. Int J Behav Nutr Phys Act. 2008 [cited 2013 May 2];5:10 doi: 10.1186/1479. Available from: http://www.ijbnpa.org/content/5/1/10.

[26] Dwyer T, Sallis JF, Blizzard L, Lazarus R, Dean K. Relationship of academic performance to physical activity and fitness in children. Pediatr Exerc Sci 2001; 13: 225-238.

[27] Cox M, Shephard RJ, Corey P. Influence of an employee fitness programme upon fitness, productivity and absenteeism. Ergonomics. 1981; 24(10): 795-806.

[28] Levy E, Levy P, Le Pen C, *et al*. Economic cost of obesity: the French situation. Int J Obes Relat Metab Disord. 1995;19(11):788-792.

[29] Seidell J. The impact of obesity on health status: some implications for health care costs. Int J Obes Relat Metab Disord. 1995;19(6 Suppl):S13-16.

[30] Segal L, Carter R, Zimmet P. The cost of obesity: the Australian perspective. Pharmacoeconomics. 1994;5(1 Suppl):45-52.

[31] World Health Organization. 2008-2013 action plan for the global strategy for the prevention and control of noncommunicable diseases [homepage on the Internet]. c2008 [cited 2013 Feb 23]. Available from: http://www.who.int/nmh/publications/9789241597418/en/index.html

[32] World Health Organization. Global strategy on diet, physical activity and health [homepage on the Internet]. c2004 [cited 2013 Mar15]. Available from: http://www.who.int/dietphysicalactivity/strategy/eb11344/strategy_english_web.pdf

[33] Chaddock L, Erickson KI, Prakash RS, *et al*. A neuroimaging investigation of the association between aerobic fitness, hippocampal volume and memory performance in preadolescent children. Brain Res. 2010;1358:172-83.

[34] Davis CL, Tomporowski PD, Boyle CA, *et al*. Effects of aerobic exercise on overweight children's cognitive functioning: a randomized controlled trial. Research Quarterly Exerc and Sport. 2007; 78(5): 510-19.

[35] Hillman C, Pontiflex L, Raine D, Hall EE, Kramer, A. The effect of acute treadmill olled trial. Research Quarterly Exerc and Sport. 2007; 78(5): 510-19. walking on cognitive control and academic achievement in preadolescent children. Neuroscience 2009; 159: 1044-1054.

[36] Hallal P, Victora C, Azevedo M, Wells J. Adolescent physical activity: a systematic review. Sport Med. 2006; 36(12): 1019-1030.

[37] Handy S, Boarnet M, Ewing R, Killingsworth R. How the built environment affects physical activity: views from urban planning. Am J Prev Med 2002; 23(2s): 64-73.

[38] Anderson L, Quinn T, Glanz K, *et al*. The effectiveness of worksite nutrition and physical activity inteventions for controlling employee overweight and obesity: a systmeatic review. Am J Prev Med 2009: 37(4): 340-357.

[39] Falls among older adults: an overview. CDC Website [cited 2013 May20] Available from: http://www.cdc.gov/homeandrecreationalsafety/Falls/adultfalls.html.

[40] Clemson L, *et al.* Integration of balance and strength training into daily life activity to reduce rate of falls in older people (the LiFE study): randomised parallel trial. *BMJ.* 2012;345:e4547.

[41] Sherrington C, Whitney JC, Lord SR, Herbert RD, Cumming RG, Close JCT. Effective exercise for the prevention of falls: a systematic review and meta-analysis. J Am Geriatric Soc. 2008; 56:2234-43.

[42] Langlois F, Minh Vu T, Chasse K, Dupuis G, Kergoat MJ, Bherer L. Benefits of training on cognition and quality of life in frail older adults. J Geront Series B: Psych Sci and Soc Sci [online] 2012 [cited 2013 May 15]; 68(3) 400-404. Available from: Oxford Journals

CHAPTER 11

Prevention of Cardiovascular Disease: Behavioral Modification

Lekshmi Dharmarajan[*,1,2]

[1]*Chief, Division of Cardiology, Lincoln Medical and Mental Health Center, Bronx, New York, USA; and* [2]*Professor of Clinical Medicine, Weill Medical College of Cornell Univerity, New York. USA*

Abstract: Cardiovascular disease is the leading cause of death in the United States, overtaking communicable diseases, a trend that is likely to get worse. American Heart Association impact goals for cardiovascular health recommends behavioral modification pertinent to life style measures such as physical activity, diet, smoking, and alcohol consumption. Global burden of cardiovascular disease stresses the importance of public and private sectors and governmental involvement in addressing the problem. A heart healthy diet is of value in primary prevention of cardiovascular disease, based on the Mediterranean diet or Dietary Approaches to Stop Hypertension eating pattern. Dietary measures must be taken in conjunction with physical activity, with some physical activity always better than none. Smoking cessation is never too late to implement; physicians need to spend adequate time in effective counseling. Alcohol consumption is not to be encouraged; excessive drinking is harmful, while benefits may be apparent with alcohol consumption in moderate amounts.

Keywords: Addressing lifestyle, AHA goals, alcohol use, behavior, cardiovascular disease prevention, DASH diet, diet, global health, healthy lifestyle, mediterranean diet, nutrition, physical activity, primary prevention, risk, sodium intake, tobacco use, wellness.

INTRODUCTION

Cardiovascular disease is overtaking communicable diseases as a leading cause of death globally. However, the American Heart Association has targeted key behaviors to reverse this trend in the USA and more globally. Specific behavioral targets include lifestyle measures such as physical activity, diet, smoking, and alcohol consumption. This chapter addresses the global burden of cardiovascular disease and stresses the importance of public and private sectors and governmental involvement in addressing the problem. Specific topics include a

***Corresponding author Lekshmi Dharmarajan:** 31 Pheasant Run, Scarsdale, NY 10583, USA; Tel: (718) 579-4876; Fax: (914) 723-4297; E-mail: dharmarajanl@yahoo.com

Judith Wylie-Rosett & Sunil S. Jhangiani (Eds)

heart healthy diet, physical activity, smoking cessation, and limiting alcohol intake focusing on what physicians can do to provide effective counseling.

GLOBAL AND UNITED STATES OF AMERICA PERSPECTIVES

Aging trends demonstrate an increase in life expectancy worldwide. Yet, the United States of America (USA) which has a life expectancy at birth of about 80 years for females and 75 years for males lags behind the European countries and Japan in this regard. Several factors contribute to the difference. It is likely that an interplay of factors including globalization, differing disease patterns and importantly, adopted life style and obesity may play roles [1]. Across the world, there has been a shift in the cause of death with cardiovascular disease (CVD) becoming the leading cause of death overtaking communicable diseases, a trend that is likely to get worse [1].

In the past three decades there have been major shifts in cardiovascular science and medicine, with better risk stratification and pharmacogenomics to tailor choice [2]. Collaboration between cardiologists and other disciplines has increased. The U.S. faces an epidemic of obesity with approximately 30% of obese adults [2]. Risk factors are inadequately addressed, indicating the need for support from governmental agencies, patient advocates and professional societies to tackle the issues. As CVD is a leading cause of mortality worldwide, with more than 80% of CVD deaths occurring in low and middle income countries (LMICs), this is clearly a global burden. However, there has been insufficient investment and implementation of CVD prevention efforts in the LMICs [3]. Suggested domains to be addressed include policy approaches, health communication programs and healthcare delivery interventions [3]. Global control is possible but requires both public and private sector involvement.

As such there are proposals for a 2025 Global Non-Communicable Disease (NCD) mortality target initiative; the project has four proposed targets and has received immense support. The targets include addressing physical inactivity, control raised blood pressure, encouraging reduction in salt intake and cessation of tobacco smoking [1]. Additional targets that received some support include: a reduction in total energy intake from saturated fat, halting the rise in prevalence of obesity, 10% reduction in overall alcohol consumption and 20% reduction in the prevalence of raised total cholesterol. Targets also include provision of drug therapy and counseling to prevent heart attacks and stroke in 50% of eligible people (see CHAPTER 1 Lifestyle Diseases in the Modern Era: A Major Threat to Global Health!), and the provision of essential medications to treat major NCDs [1].

Cardiovascular disease is the number one cause of death among the top ten causes of death worldwide by broad income group, based on World Health Organization data [4]. Among the 58 million people who died in 2005 worldwide, cardiovascular disease accounted for 29.34% of deaths [5]. The top causes of death vary between underdeveloped and developed countries. Tobacco use is a major contributor to many causes of death, including CVD. Life expectancy is clearly higher in the high income countries, compared to middle income and low income groups (Table **1**).

Table 1. WHO data on top six causes of death worldwide, based on income and in descending order [4, 5].

Worldwide	Low Income Countries	Middle Income Countries	High Income Countries
Ischemic heart disease	Lower respiratory infections	Ischemic heart disease	Ischemic heart disease
Cerebrovascular disease	Diarrheal diseases	Cerebrovascular disease	Cerebrovascular disease
Lower respiratory infections	HIV / AIDS	Chronic obstructive pulmonary disease	Lung cancer
Chronic obstructive pulmonary disease	Ischemic heart disease	Lower respiratory infections	Alzheimer's and other dementias
Diarrheal diseases	Malaria	Diarrheal diseases	Lower respiratory infections
HIV / AIDS	Cerebrovascular disease	HIV / AIDS	Chronic obstructive pulmonary disease

Interventions for the primary prevention of CVD differ worldwide. Examples include: primary risk factor screening and improving life style in Canada [6]; tobacco, exercise and diet related messages sent as text-based interventions to prevent CVD [7] and individual assessment of risk and modulation of frequency and intensity of interventions [8] in Australia; screening for cardiovascular risk followed by polypill prescriptions, with demonstrated health gain in the Netherlands [9]; implementing cardiovascular prevention through an integrated hospital-field model in Italy [10]; and emphasizing the doctor-patient relationship through spending more time with patients utilizing a focus on education in France [11].

In the U.S. cardiovascular disease (CVD) remains a leading cause of death. Based on the Centers for Disease Control and Prevention (CDC) and prevention data, in adults aged 25 -44 years, heart disease is the third most common cause of death, a trend that has remained the same from 1980 to 2008. Heart disease was the leading cause of death in the 45-64 years old age group in 1980 and has since become the second cause of mortality for that age range in 2008. However, in over 65 years old age group, diseases of the heart have remained the number one cause of death both in 1980 and in 2008 [12]. Based on the data, one can understand the rationale and priority to take global steps for the prevention of CVD.

This chapter will focus on the AHA impact goals for cardiovascular health and recommendations for behavioral modification pertinent to physical activity, diet, smoking, and alcohol. See also CHAPTER 12 (Cardiovascular Disease: Addressing Risk Factors) which addresses in depth the risk factors for cardiovascular disease, focusing on obesity, hypertension, diabetes and hypercholesterolemia in addition to issues pertinent to women.

RISK FOR CARDIOVASCULAR DISEASE

Table **2** provides information on life expectancy at birth in select countries worldwide; the data confirm the longer life expectancy in females compared to males across the globe and also that at birth, life expectancy in the listed countries is much longer in 2009 *versus* 1980. Table **3** provides data on life expectancy at ages 65 and 75 years by sex and race in the United States; the data demonstrate the same gender patterns (with females outliving males) for all races, though race by itself also results in differences. Table **4** provides information on the causes of death and the numbers of death for three age groups in the U.S.: 25-44 years, 45-64 years and 65 years and over. Table **4** confirms that heart disease is the third leading cause of death even in the age group 25-44 years; it is the second most common cause of death in the age group 45-64 years and the leading cause of death in the 65 and over age group, well ahead of the second cause, cancer. The information supports the need to implement preventive health measures to address the increasing prevalence of heart disease and related mortality with aging. These efforts, if properly targeted, stand to significantly benefit a large segment of the increasingly vulnerable older population.

The absolute risk of coronary artery disease (CAD) has been validated in many cohorts and estimated by index age (45, 55, 65, and 75 years), based on an analysis of 905,115 person years data over a 44 year period (1964-2008) [13]. At an index age of 45 years the lifetime risk for CVD was 60.3% and 55.6% for men and women; at age 55, despite an optimal risk factor profile (normal blood pressure and cholesterol, non-smoker, no diabetes), there was a life time risk greater than 40% and 30% in men and women respectively [13]. The lifetime risk for CVD is hence high for all persons, even for those with optimal risk factor profiles; however, optimal profiles were associated with longer morbidity free survival [13].

Table 2. Life expectancy in years at birth, in 1980 and 2009 for select countries [12].

Country	Male in 1980	Male in 2009	Female in 1980	Female in 2009
United States of America	70.0	76.0	77.4	80.9
Australia	71.0	79.3	78.1	83.9
Canada	71.7	76.3 (2000)	78.9	81.7 (2000)
France	70.2	77.7	78.4	84.4
Greece	73.0	77.8	77.5	82.7
Italy	70.6	79.1 (2008)	77.4	84.5 (2008)
Japan	73.3	79.6	78.6	86.4
Mexico	64.1	72.9	70.2	77.6
Sweden	72.8	79.4	78.8	83.4
United Kingdom	70.2	78.3	76.2	82.5

Table 3. Additional years of life expectancy at age 65 years and 75 years by sex and race in the United States of America in the year 2009 [12].

Race and Age in Years	Both Sexes	Male	Female
White, not Hispanic, at 65 years	19.1	17.6	20.3
White, not Hispanic, at 75 years	12.1	11.0	12.9
Black, not Hispanic, at 65 years	17.7	15.7	19.1
Black, not Hispanic, at 75 years	11.7	10.2	12.5
Hispanic, at 65 years	20.9	19.4	22.0
Hispanic, at 75 years	13.6	12.4	14.3

Table 4. Leading causes of death and number of deaths by age in the USA in 2008.

Age 25-44 Years, Cause of Death		Number of Deaths
All causes		118,645
1.	Unintentional injuries	30,653
2.	Malignancy	16,220
3.	**Heart disease**	**14,590**
4.	Suicide	12,003
5.	Homicide	7,516
Age 45-64 Years, Cause of Death		**Number of Deaths**
All causes		482,724
1.	Malignancy	154,494
2.	**Heart disease**	**104,603**
3.	Unintentional injuries	33,136
4.	Chronic lower respiratory disease	18,434
5.	Diabetes mellitus	16,992
Age 65 years and over, Cause of Death		**Number of Deaths**
All causes		1,799,830
1.	**Heart Disease**	**495,730**
2.	Malignant disease	391,729
3.	Chronic lower respiratory diseases	121,223
4.	Cerebrovascular disease	114,508
5.	Alzheimer's disease	81,573
6.	Diabetes mellitus	50,883

PHYSICIAN AWARENESS AND ADHERENCE TO PREVENTION GUIDELINES

Although CVD is common and the leading cause of death in both men and women, in practice, uniform care may not be provided by physicians to all patients. Unfortunately many patients who are at risk are not screened, risk stratified or counseled; surely there are both patient and physician related factors that account for this finding [14]. Physicians need to be aware of current guidelines and incorporate the information in routine practice. The provider must ensure that gender disparities in care do not exist; sex disparities in CVD outcomes are apparent, for reasons that are not clear [15-17]. Barriers in adopting guidelines appear to exist among primary care physicians and specialty based physicians such as cardiologists [18]. A study of 500 physicians revealed that physicians did not rate themselves as very effective in implementing preventive measures for CVD, and less than a fifth of physicians were aware that more women than men died of CVD annually. The study concluded that educational interventions are indicated to lower morbidity and mortality in both men and women [18].

Many risk factors are easy to identify and can be assessed through routine examination at low cost: gender, smoking status, blood pressure, blood sugar and lipid status [19]. If the patient does have cardiovascular disease, the person is clearly at high risk and requires management; here a risk calculation is not needed; the same approach is required should the patient have diabetes or hyperlipidemia [19]. For those at intermediate risk, the patient should be reassessed periodically and may be helped further through the use of novel risk markers such as coronary artery calcium, hs-CRP and ankle-brachial index [20]. In a study of 11,049 men, the life time risk for CVD was estimated for fitness levels at ages 45, 55 and 65 years; a single measure of low fitness in middle life was associated with a higher life time risk for CVD death, especially if there were also associated CVD risk factors [21].

American Heart Association (AHA) Goals for "Health Promotion and Disease Reduction" have listed seven metrics for ideal cardiovascular health [22]. The presence of adverse risk factors in young and middle aged patients suggests substantial elevation in lifetime risk of CVD and stroke. Addressing risk factors is the best approach toward avoiding clinical events, improving longevity and quality of life. Preventive practice strategies to deal with CVD risk factors must be implemented in childhood and adolescence. A large number of men and women with ideal health do survive to old age [22]. To attain ideal cardiovascular health, we are required to address seven broad components, listed in Table **5**. Primary and secondary measures are to be identified and monitored both in children and adults. Apparently if healthy men and women get to 50 years with optimal health, the life expectancy is likely to be at least another 40 years, largely free of heart disease [22].

Table 5. The seven metrics for ideal cardiovascular health [22].

1.	Abstinence or cessation of cigarette smoking
2.	Weight for adults >20 years: normal BMI of 18.5 to 24.9 kg/m^2
3.	Physical activity: >150 mins/wk moderate intensity or >75 mins /wk of vigorous intensity
4.	Diet, consistent with National and AHA guidelines, 4-5 components
5.	Total Cholesterol < 200 mg/dl
6.	Blood pressure < 120/80 mm Hg
7.	No diabetes; ideal fasting blood glucose below 100 mg %

The AHA 2010 and 2020 Impact Goals

The AHA 2010 Impact Goal was developed in 1999; the final version in 2004 had the intent to reduce the death rate due to CVD and stroke by 25% by the year 2010; reduce the prevalence of smoking, hyperlipidemia, uncontrolled hypertension and physical inactivity by 25%; and eliminate the growth of obesity and diabetes [22]. In fact, the targets for several components were met before 2010. However, the goals set for smoking, physical inactivity, obesity and diabetes have represented major challenges [22]. In 2010, the AHA defined the Strategic Impact Goals for the following decade: "By 2020, to improve the cardiovascular health of all Americans by 20% while reducing deaths from cardiovascular diseases and stroke by 20%" [23]. The goals included addressing health behavior, public policy, primary prevention, and chronic disease management, in addition to measuring progress and outcomes [23]. Interventions were to focus on high risk individuals, including children and adolescents. As an example, the goal was not just to normalize the blood pressure in hypertensive individuals, known to be at the highest risk, but also to target the many people with just over the mean blood pressure [24-26]. Based on the 2010 Dietary guidelines, the goals are to restrict sodium intake to less than 1.5 grams in 24 hours [25]. The efforts also included measures to deal with the food industry to regulate sodium content of foods rather than solely focus on sodium intake by individuals.

The ideal cardiovascular health (in terms of goals) involving health behaviors [22] for adults over age 20 years, are listed below:

- Body mass index < 25 kg/m^2
- Physical activity $\geq$ 150 minutes/week of moderate intensity or $\geq$ 75 minutes/week of vigorous intensity or a combination

- Healthy diet score meeting 4-5 components of selected 5 aspects of diet to define a healthy dietary score
- Smoking: never smoked or quit > 12 months ago
- Total cholesterol <200 mg/dl
- Blood pressure <120/< 80 mm Hg
- Plasma glucose (fasting) < 100 mg/dl

In a large study of nurses that provided evidence for a healthy life style, better health behavior was achieved through adoption of a combination of five factors. They included nonsmoking status, BMI <25 kg/m^2, participation in 30 minutes or more of moderate to vigorous physical activity daily, consumption of half a glass of wine daily and a healthy diet (low glycemic index, high fiber, high folate, low trans fats); the behavior tended to correlate with a lower risk for incident coronary heart disease [27]. The benefits were not altered by medications used for hypertension or hyperlipidemia, suggesting that drug treatment did not alter the importance of life style [28]. The benefits of healthy behavior to lower cardiovascular risk also appear applicable to the old, supported by a study where the average age of men and women was 73 years [29].

Physical Activity

Encouraging physical activity is an integral part of behavioral therapy. A little activity is always better than none and more activity is better than less. Exercise refers to a purposeful, repetitive planned or structured activity, designed to improve body function and is generally not inclusive of daily routines. Based on Center for Disease Control and Prevention (CDC) data, the prevalence of inactivity did not change from 2000 to 2001 (27.4% to 26.0%), suggesting that the increases in recommended activity (from 26% in 2000 to 45% in 2001) were due to the expanded definition of physical activity to include yard work and housework [30]. Previous guidelines recommended appropriate physical activity to be ≥20 minutes per day, ≥3 days a week. Based on the CDC data, the majority of U.S adults are not physically active at levels that help promote health. The CDC data for the period 1997-2006 showed that 26% of people aged 65 to 74 engaged in regular physical activity (defined in this case as light to moderate activity for 30 minutes at least 5 times a week); people older than 75 were less active, while 30% of those between 45 and 64 years of age met the requirements [30].

Ideally, physical activity has a threshold for energy intake that must be optimal and balanced with energy expenditure. Below a given threshold for physical activity level, excess energy intake leads to obesity (the unregulated zone). Above the threshold (or the regulated zone), energy intake and body weight are sensitive to each other. Optimally, a healthy body is maintained by a high level of physical activity and a high energy intake [31]. Food restriction alone is not an answer; while this approach produces weight loss, and a decrease in energy expenditure, an increase in hunger may follow [31]. An increase in physical activity is key to getting people into the regulated zone of energy balance.

The AHA Impact goals have emphasized the importance of "Physical Activity Guidelines" to complement "Dietary Guidelines". As the amount of physical activity increases through an increase in intensity or frequency, the benefit increases for cardiac health. However, the greatest benefits are seen with an increase in activity at the lower levels [32]. This has been demonstrated in a recently published study where individuals engaged in the equivalent of 150 mins/wk of moderate intensity leisure time physical activity had a 14% lower CAD risk compared to those reporting no leisure time physical activity [32]. At higher levels of physical activity the risks were modestly lower, emphasizing that much gain is obtained with even modest activity. The conclusion was that "some activity was better than none and additional benefits occur with more activity". The accompanying clinical perspective commented that the "biggest bang for the buck for coronary heart disease risk reduction occurs at the lower end of the activity spectrum: at very modest achievable levels of physical activity" [32]. A brief overview of physical activity is provided in Table **6**.

Exercise is an activity that benefits almost every body part and function, if properly incorporated into life style, in conjunction with addressing other CVD risk factors. Sadly, even after elective percutaneous coronary interventions, patients do not participate in supervised home-based exercise training programs. Remaining inactive appears as harmful as cigarette smoking, in contrast to studies demonstrating a low level of cardiac events in the rehabilitation setting. As health care costs are escalating, physicians are encouraged to incorporate into mainstream the promotion of physical activity as a life style intervention, a measure that is also cost-effective medicine in terms of health outcomes [33].

A higher level of physical activity in a study of nearly 900 people, mean age 82 years, was associated with a reduced risk of death [34]. The findings did not vary with gender, education or dementia status [34]. Thus, healthy outcomes and longevity may be linked to increased physical activity. Society is looking forward to opportunities available to increase physical activity on the job; "activity breaks" are becoming increasingly popular in the form of 10 minute structured group exercise breaks, with the suggestion for the medical profession to lead the way in adopting such practices [35].

Table 6. Physical activity [22, 30, 32, 36, 37].

Defining Key Terms
• Physical activity: defined by the WHO as any body movement deployed by skeletal muscle that requires energy expenditure
• Exercise: Is physical activity that is planned, structured, repetitive and purposeful to condition any part of the body.
• Intensity: refers to the rate of energy expenditure during exercise and expressed as metabolic equivalents (METs)
• MET (Metabolic Equivalent of Task) or metabolic equivalent is the physiological measure of energy cost of physical activity, or its energy consumption. The reference metabolic rate is 3.5 ml O_2 /kg/min.
Intensity of exercise
• Moderate intensity exercise is performed at an intensity of 4 to 6 METs
• Vigorous intensity exercise is performed at an intensity of over 6 METs
Examples of Activities and Energy Requirements;
• Mild (<3 METs) ; Walking at <2 mph, playing a musical instrument, sitting, walking within the house, vacuuming, watching television
• Moderate (3-5 METs): brisk walking (3-4 mph), slow swimming, slow cycling, gardening, *etc.*
• Vigorous (over 5 METs): doubles tennis, jogging, swimming, climbing a hill
Recommendations
• Moderate Intensity: 150 minutes per week; one can talk, but is unable to sing during the activity
• Vigorous intensity: 75 minutes per week of activity; one cannot say more than a few words without pausing for breath
Type of Activity
• Ensure that the exercise is easy to perform and enjoyable
• Individualize: encourage patient's preferred activity
• Walking is the safest and initial preferred mode of exercise
• Other choices; cycling, rowing, swimming, jogging.
• Advance the exercise prescription as the patient becomes better conditioned
• Options for forms of exercise: endurance, strength, balance, flexibility
• Use short periods of down time when available to perform an exercise
• Stick with what is easy and what works
The activity requires ongoing monitoring

The National Institute of Aging and the National Institutes of Health have put forth a simple, easy to follow manual on physical activity [36]; some of the suggestions along with the 2008 Physical Activity guidelines [37] are incorporated into Table **6**. Exercise falls largely into 4 types: *Strength*, to increase muscle strength, *e.g.,* by lifting weights; *Balance*, to prevent falls, *e.g.,* Tai Chi or standing on one foot; *Flexibility*, *e.g.,* stretch of shoulder or arm, and yoga; *Endurance or aerobic*, to improve cardiopulmonary function, *e.g.,* walking, dancing, jogging. As a general rule, the exercise prescription must be made an enjoyable one for the patient, an activity that is easy and safe to perform regularly [36]. Encourage the patient to engage in a preferred form of activity, one that is tailored to the individual, safe and easy to perform. Changing the form of exercise is encouraged if a chosen activity does not work; the patient should be monitored for progress.

Diet in Conjunction with Physical Activity

Diet goes hand in hand with physical activity; the approach to behavioral modification must always include both components, utilizing an individualized approach, rather than depend solely on one or the other means. Diet adds significant relevance to several factors linked to cardiovascular health, including body weight, serum lipids, blood sugar, and blood pressure. Less well defined are the benefits of anti-oxidants. Dietary guidelines have been updated in late 2010 [25]. The United States Preventive Services Task Force (USPSTF) has issued a clinical guideline to promote behavior to adhere to a healthful diet to prevent CVD in adults [28]. Dietary recommendations must also address relevant comorbid states.

Medium to high intensity dietary counseling, with or without physical activity, has resulted in small but statistically significant improvements in adiposity, blood pressure, blood glucose and serum cholesterol levels, with the evidence better for high intensity interventions [38]. The positive news is that none of the healthful dietary intervention trials reported adverse events. The optimal eating strategy to lose weight continues to be debated and may not be easily resolved. The total caloric intake appears more relevant than the intake of specific components. Although the exact mechanisms between dietary composition and weight maintenance are not clear, caloric restriction is more important than weight loss regimens [39].

The 2010 Dietary Guidelines mention that Americans in general consume on average less than the optimum amount of vegetables, fruits, whole grains, fiber, low fat milk or milk products and sea food. On the other hand, the intake is excessive for solid fats, sugars, refined grains and sodium [25]. The dietary plan recommended must be flexible rather than rigid, and suit the individual's preferences. The goals are to reduce overweight states and obesity in the U.S. population by reducing overall caloric intake. The guidelines call for a shift to more plant based diets including whole grains, vegetables, fruits, nuts and seeds, in addition to intake of lean meats, poultry and eggs. Suggestions also include methods for the safe handling of food as well as the provision of educational programs in schools to educate children (and their families) [25].

The fact that modest reductions in dietary salt could substantially reduce cardiovascular events and health care costs, has led to suggestions for the recommendation to be made a public health target [40, 41]. Most of the high salt intake in the U.S. diet comes from processed foods and reducing this amount may result in improved public health [40]. The matter is not without controversy. An editorial states that there are two possible paths forward: a rash route through universal sodium restriction, through implementing change in the diet of all residents (in the U.S.); the alternate more cautious approach is through large population based randomized clinical trials [41]. The editorial calls for a prudent course of action.

In particular, the Dietary Approaches to Stop Hypertension (DASH) plan [42] has shown good results in several studies. The AHA Impact Goals state that the overall dietary pattern may be consistent with a DASH eating plan as expressed below [22]:

- Fruits and vegetables: at least 4.5 cups per day
- Fish: ≥ two 3.5 oz. servings per week (preferably oily fish)
- Fiber rich whole grains (≥ 1.1 g fiber per 10 g carbohydrate): ≥ three 1 oz servings/day
- Sodium: < 1500 mg/day for blacks, middle age and older people and for those with hypertension.
- Sodium: < 2300 mg per day for general adult population, with amounts to decline over time for this population [29].

- Sugar sweetened beverages: ≤450 kcal (36 oz) per week

Additional components of a heart healthy diet suggested by the AHA include: avoidance of trans fat (partially hydrogenated fat) and reduction in saturated fat to < 7% of total energy intake; reduction in the intake of processed meats and processed foods in general; increasing the intake of unsalted nuts and legumes (to ≥ 4 servings a week); increasing the intake of food rich in fiber such as fruits, vegetables and whole grains; and use of non-fat dairy products to improve intake of calcium [22].

The value of a Mediterranean diet supplemented with extra-virgin olive oil or nuts in the primary prevention of cardiovascular disease was demonstrated in a study of nearly 7500 persons, age range 55 to 80 years, with 57% women [43]. The diet reduced the incidence of major cardiovascular events, with no diet related adverse effects [43].

The National Cholesterol Education Program (2002) has also suggested the importance of diet as part of the Therapeutic Life Style Changes. The recommendations are that less than 25-35% of calories come from fat, with < 7% from saturated fat, and cholesterol intake to be <200 mg/day.

The Influence of Alcohol

More than a quarter of the U.S. population misuses alcohol, based on a USPSTF meta-analysis, with several men consuming more than 4 drinks per day and many women in excess of 2 drinks per day [44]. Among the 10% who exceed the daily and weekly limits for drinking, the prevalence of alcohol abuse and dependence is almost one in two [45]. Physicians are expected to question patients regarding alcohol consumption routinely and methodically as part of their examination, in a non-judgmental manner, similar to any other aspect of the history. The National Institute on Alcohol Abuse and Alcoholism recommends fewer than seven drinks per week for women (and not to exceed 3 drinks any day) and fewer than 14 drinks per week for men (and not to exceed 4 drinks any day). The AHA recommends no more than a drink a day for women and one to two for men. A standard drink is defined as 12 oz of beer, 5 oz of red or white wine and 1.5 oz of 80% proof alcohol. Older individuals are recommended a lower alcohol intake than younger adults; women are recommended lesser amounts than men. The water compartment declines with age, and alcohol levels attain a higher level in the older adult than in the young for a given amount consumed [46]. This decline in body water with aging is even more pronounced in women compared to men.

The concept of wine being beneficial for the heart has long been discussed. The recommendation for wine consumption is similar for red as for white wine. While there is no doubt that excessive drinking is harmful to cardiovascular health and increases the likelihood of cardiac disease and mortality, it is possible that light drinking may be cardio-protective to some [47-49]. Alcohol related benefits have been attributed to an increase in high density lipoprotein (HDL), a decrease in the plaque build-up in blood vessels and an inhibition of platelet aggregation and clotting mechanisms [47-49]. Although alcohol consumption in excess can increase the plasma triglycerides and very low density lipoprotein (VLDL), it also increases the HDL.

Is alcohol cardio-protective and is it wine specifically that results in benefit, and if so, is it red wine? These are questions often asked by patients to providers. Several studies have looked at the relationship, as well described in a science advisory [49]. The belief is that alcohol in small amounts may be cardio-protective, while heavy intake increases mortality. However the net results are confounded by life style, including exercise, diet and several other factors. The benefit for red wine over other alcoholic beverages is not clear. The benefits of wine may be mediated through antioxidants; the presence of polyphenols such as flavanoids may be antioxidant in effect, but the same substances are also found in grape juice [49].

A systematic review and meta-analysis discuss pooled data from 4235 studies on the risk of alcohol on cardiovascular outcomes. The lowest risk of coronary heart disease mortality occurred with 1-2 drinks a day and for stroke mortality it occurred with $\leq$ 1 drink per day [50]. The well-established relationship between regular alcohol consumption and decreased risk for CVD is not evident until middle age or older in men; women may benefit at a much younger age [41]. These benefits from alcohol are negated when alcohol is consumed in a heavy episodic drinking pattern especially in the middle aged and older men [51]. Thus the ultimate influence of alcohol on cardiovascular outcomes is largely dependent on the amounts consumed over time, and additional factors such as age, gender and existing comorbidity. The linkage to benefits reported in some studies may be the influence of lifestyle factors rather than alcohol, including increased physical activity, and a diet high in fruits and vegetables but lower in saturated fats.

Besides cardiomyopathy, excessive alcohol consumption over time can cause hypertension and ultimately, its consequences to the heart and brain such as stroke, cardiac arrhythmia and sudden death [45, 49, 52]. Well controlled comparison trials are required to compare the specific effects of wine *versus* other forms of alcohol and risk of heart disease. Given these facts and additional risks incurred from alcohol consumption, the AHA cautions people not to start drinking, if they do not already drink alcohol. A discussion may be held with the physician on the benefits and risks of consuming alcohol in moderation (Table 7).

Table 7. Alcohol: standard drinks, consumption and related hospital discharges [45, 49, 52].

	Standard Drinks
•	Beer: 12 oz (~5% alcohol) (22 oz = 2 drinks)
•	Wine: 5 oz (~7% alcohol) (750 ml bottle = 5 drinks)
•	80 proof spirits 1.5 oz (~40% alcohol) (A pint (16 oz) = 11 drinks)
	Per capita gallons of ethanol consumption, United States, age 14 and older
•	Year 2010: Beer 1.13 Wine 0.39 All beverages 2.26
•	Year 2005: Beer 1.19 Wine 0.36 All beverages 2.24
•	Year 2000: Beer 1.22 Wine 0.31 All beverages 2.18
	Alcohol related hospital discharges
•	In 2010, 390,000 hospital discharge episodes had principal alcohol related diagnosis
•	Alcohol related psychosis and cirrhosis of the liver were the prime diagnosis, followed by alcohol dependence syndrome

Smoking Cessation

Cigarette smoking is the number one preventable cause of death, largely from cardiovascular disease [53]. The main ingredient in cigarette smoke is nicotine, although there are several additional toxic ingredients. Smoking causes harm through several mechanisms. These include an increase in endogenous catecholamines with resultant increase in blood pressure and cardiac rate, activation of platelets, impaired fibrinolysis, cardiac arrhythmias, alteration in lipoproteins (raised triglycerides and lower HDL) and an overall proneness to endothelial changes and atherosclerosis [53]. Smoking is a strong risk factor for premature mortality even in old age; cessation of smoking is beneficial at any age [54]. Most smokers underestimate the associated risks and feel they are too old to quit! It is worth noting that it is not just the smoker who suffers consequences, but exposure to passive smoke affects many others around; educating nondaily smokers on the dangers of secondhand smoke to others is a more powerful message than traditional smoking cessation counseling [55]. It is ideal to get smokers and non-smokers in the household to understand the consequences of nicotine use and accept behavioral intervention.

"It is never too late to quit smoking", is a statement that can be safely made to any patient who smokes. Smokers who quit smoking reduce their risk of coronary events by half in a year or two and match the risk of non-smokers after 5-15 years; in addition, cessation of smoking is associated with a marked reduction in risk of mortality compared to those still smoking [53, 56]. The AHA Get With The Guidelines CAD (GWTG-CAD) program has significantly improved compliance with smoking cessation counseling (SCC) in patients with CAD and stroke [57]. Challenges to successfully implement measures involve patient and health provider. Patients lack motivation even when they recognize the risks of quitting. Physicians see little success in SCC and tend to not intervene, although advice does lead to at least a few quitting [58]. SCC initiated while the patient is hospitalized is said to be more effective.

Following acute myocardial infarction (AMI) the most important behavioral modification for a smoker is to quit smoking [59]. Persistent smoking post AMI increases risk of recurrent MI; the issue of safety of smoking cessation treatments is thus relevant in discussing this intervention [59, 60]. Nicotine replacement therapies are commonly used but their safety is not supported by adequate data. Bupropion, an anti-depressant was tried in a recent trial based on its other properties. Bupropion suppresses nicotine withdrawal symptoms, is an anti-depressant (relevant as depression is common following an AMI), and it has little effect on heart rate and blood pressure [60]. The 2008 U.S. Department of Health and Human Services guidelines supports the use of bupropion for the post AMI patient to help quit smoking [61]. In a recent trial, bupropion was well tolerated and found safe for use following an AMI, however, two thirds of patients returned to smoking at 12 months [60]. The guidelines also call for hospitals to be smoke-free and to initiate smoking cessation measures for patients while still in the hospital.

Elective surgery offers a great opportunity for physicians and surgeons to help smokers quit smoking. Perioperative smoking is linked to surgical complications such as wound infection, besides pulmonary and cardiac complications [62]. Studies suggest that smoking cessation 4 to 8 weeks prior to surgery reduces post-operative complications; hence the pre-operative period is an opportunity to convince patients to quit smoking; the opportunity should not be missed by health care providers [62]. However, the cessation should be taken in context of any withdrawal manifestations that could occur during the peri-operative period.

A Cochrane review of 50 tobacco treatment trials did not find benefit for counseling to quit smoking in the hospital when it was less intensive, while addition of nicotine replacement therapy to intensive counseling increased rate of quitting [63]. However, nicotine medications can increase heart rate and blood pressure, and cause vasoconstriction [59].

Table 8. Smoking cessation options [53, 54, 55, 59, 64, 65, 66].

Interaction with the Patient who Smokes	
o	"It is never too late to quit": the first rule!
o	Obtain a focused history on present and past history of smoking
o	Physicians must emphasize to smokers the importance of quitting, including around the time of surgery [64]
o	Provide simple direct evidence based warning on risks of morbidity and death
o	Provide education: through both verbal communication and written or other forms of material
o	Smoking cessation may be followed by withdrawal symptoms in the immediate post cessation period, and by weight gain in the long term
Follow Joint Commission Recommendations for Hospitals (in the U.S.)	
o	Must identify and document smoking behavior on patients
o	Effective counseling is a must for all smokers
o	Arrange for transition to outpatient status, including follow up
o	Address other relevant comorbid states: *e.g.,* depression
o	Anticipate recurrence of the smoking behavior and address appropriately
o	Document smoking status a month after discharge
Medications for nicotine replacement therapy and adverse profiles	
•	Medication prescription needs to be individualized
•	Nicotine patch: several strengths; adverse effects: local skin reactions
•	Nicotine gum and lozenge: associated with oral sores and dyspepsia
•	Nicotine inhaler or spray: associated with nasal and oral irritation
•	Bupropion: adverse effects include insomnia, dreams and extra-pyramidal movements. Avoid if patient has a seizure disorder.
•	Varenicline: may increase cardiovascular events in adults with CVD
•	Combination varenicline and bupropion may offer another option [65]

Buproprion is not free of sympathomimetic activity in higher doses; varenicline, a selective nicotinic receptor antagonist, while an effective option, is not totally without adverse cardiac effects either [59]. Combination varenicline and bupropion may increase prolonged abstinence, but with little difference at 52 weeks [65]. Data from 12 Cochrane reviews of 26 different treatments suggested that combination therapy was most effective in achieving cessation; further, none of the therapies was associated with serious adverse events (Table **8**) [66].

CONCLUSION

The presence of risk factors and burden for CVD remains high although the rate of deaths has declined; the control of traditional risk factors has remained an issue for Americans [67]. Heart disease is the number one killer in the U.S. as one ages, and a major cause globally. While CVD causes one of every 6 deaths in the U.S., stroke accounts for one of every eighteen deaths [67]. The AHA 2020 Impact goals target is to improve the cardiovascular health of all Americans by 20% while reducing deaths from cardiovascular diseases and stroke by 20% [12].

Addressing life style and modifying behavior is a major component in the primary prevention of cardiovascular disease. A heart healthy diet is of value in primary prevention of cardiovascular disease, based on the Mediterranean diet or DASH diet eating pattern. Dietary measures must always be taken in conjunction with physical activity. A little physical activity is better than none, while more is better. The most benefit, relatively stated, is obtained at the lower end of the spectrum with some activity as opposed to none. More than choosing the dietary components, the total caloric intake is what matters. Smoking cessation is never too late to implement; physicians need to spend time in effective counseling. Tobacco control is associated with a reduction in premature deaths and an extension of life span [68].Alcohol consumption in restricted amounts may have some benefits; however it is never a recommendation to begin drinking, and taken in excess is always harmful.

ACKNOWLEDGEMENTS

Declared none.

CONFLICT OF INTEREST

The authors confirm that this chapter contents have no conflict of interest.

REFERENCES

[1] Smith SC, Collins A, Ferrari R, *et al*. Our time: A call to save preventable death from cardiovascular disease (heart disease and stroke). Circulation.2012; 126: 2769-75.
[2] Zoghbi WA, Homes DR, Jr. Improving cardiovascular health: a balance between discovery and delivery. JAMA 2013; 309: 1117-8.
[3] Fuster V, Kelly BB, Vedanthan R. Gobal cardiovascular health: Urgent need for an intersectoral approach. J Am Coll Card 2011; 58: 1208-10.
[4] World Health Organization: The top 10 causes of death. [Cited April 8, 2013]. Available from: http://www.who.int/mediacentre/factsheets/fs310/en/.
[5] List of causes of death by rate, from Wikipedia. [Cited April 8, 2013]. Available from http://en.wikipedia.org/wiki/List_of_causes_of_death_by_rate.
[6] Cox JL, Carr B, Vallis TM, Szpilfogel C, O'Neill BJ. A novel approach to cardiovascular health by optimizing risk management (ANCHOR): a primary initiative examining the impact of health risk factor assessment and management on cardiac wellness. Can J Cardiol 2011; 27(6): 809-17.
[7] Chow CK, Redfern J, Thiagalingam A, *et al*. Design and rationale of the tobacco, exercise and diet messages (TEXT ME) trial of a text messge-based intervention for ongoing prevention of cardiovascular diseae in people with coronary disease: a randomized controlled trial protocol. BMJ Open 2012; 2 (1): e000606.
[8] Carrington MJ, Kok S, Jansen K, Stewart S. The Green, Amber, Red Delineation of Risk and Need (GARDIAN) management system: a pragmatic approach to optimizing heart health from primary prevention to chronic disease management. Eur J Crdiovasc Nurs 2012. Jun 29 (ahead of print).
[9] Van Gils PF, Over EA, Hamberg-van Reenen H, *et al*. The polypill in the primary prevention of cardiovascular disease: cost-effectiveness in the Dutch population. BMJ Open 2011; 1(2): e000363.
[10] Griffo R, Biondett M, Stellini F, Camerini A, Picciotto R. Implementing cardiovascular prevention in the real world: presentation of an integrated hospital-field model. Monaldi Arch Chest Dis 2003; 60(2): 155-60.
[11] Cheryy CO, Steichen O, Mathew A, Duhot D, Hebbrecht G, Schuster RJ. A culture of care: the French approach to cardiovascular risk factor management. J Am Board Fam Med 2012; 25(4): 477-86.
[12] Health, United States 2013. [Cited Feb 10, 2013]. Available from: http://www.cdc.gov/nchs/data/hus/hus13.pdf.
[13] Wilkins JT, Ning H, Berr J, Zhao L, Dyer AR, Lloyd-Jones DM. Lifetime risk and years lived free of total cardiovascular disease. JAMA 2012; 308: 1795-1801.
[14] Cabana MD, Rand CS, Powe NR, *et al*. Why don't physicians follow clinical practice guidelines? A framework for improvement. JAMA 1999; 282: 1458-65.
[15] Kim C, Hofer TP, Kerr EA. Review of evidence and explanations for suboptimal screening and treatment of dyslipidemia in women: a conceptual model. J Gen Intern Med 2003; 18: 854-63.
[16] Jha A, Varosy PD, Kanaya AM, *et al*. Differences in medical care and disease outcomes among black and white women with heart disease. Circulation 2003; 108: 1089-94.
[17] Mosca L, Appel LJ, Benjamin EJ, *et al*. Evidence-based guidelines for cardiovascular disease prevention in women. Circulation.2004; 109: 672-93.
[18] Mosca L, Linfante AH, Benjamin EJ, *et al*. National study of physician awareness and adherence to cardiovascular disease prevention guidelines. Circulation 2005; 111: 499-510.

[19] Gaziano JM, Wilson PWF. Cardiovascular risk assessment in the 21st century. JAMA 2012; 308: 816-7.
[20] Yesboah J, McClelland RL, Polonsky TS, *et al.* Comparison of novel risk markers for improvement in cardiovascular risk assessment in intermediate-risk individuals. JAMA 2010; 308: 788-95.
[21] Berry JD, Willis B, Gupta S, *et al.* Lifetime risks for cardiovascular disease mortality by cardiorespiratory fitness levels measured at ages 45, 55 and 65 years in men. The Cooper Center Longitudinal Study. J Amer Coll of Cardiol 2011; 57: 1604-10.
[22] Lloyd-Jones DM, Hong Y, Labarthe D, *et al.* On behalf of the American Heart Association Strategic Planning Task Force and Statistics Committee. Defining and setting national goals for cardiovascular health promotion and disease reduction: the American Heart Association's Strategic Impact Goal through 2020 and beyond. Circulation 2010: 121: 586-213.
[23] Roger VL, O'Donnell CJ. Population health, outcomes research and prevention. Example of the American Heart Association 2020 Goals. Cir Cardiovascular Qual Outcomes 2012; 5: 6-8.
[24] Centers for Disease Control and Prevention (CDC) application of lower sodium intake recommendations to adults-United States 1999-2006; MMWR Morb Mortal Wkly Rep.2009; 58: 281-3.
[25] Report of the Dietary Guidelines Advisory Committee on the Dietary Guidelines for Americans, 2010. [Cited February 24, 2013]. Available from: http://www.cnpp.usda.gov/Publications/DietaryGuidelines/2010/PolicyDoc/ExecSumm.pdf.
[26] Appel LF, Brands MW, Daniel SR, *et al.* Dietary approaches to prevent and treat hypertension: a scientific statement from the American Heart Association. Hypertension 2006; 47: 296-308.
[27] Stampfer MJ, Hu FB, Manson JE, Rimm EB, Willett WC. Primary prevention of coronary heart disease in women through diet and lifestyle. N Eng J Med 2000; 343: 16-22.
[28] Chiuve SE, McCullough ML, Sacks FM, Rimm EB. Healthy life style factors in the primary prevention of coronary heart disease among men: benefits among users and nonusers of lipid lowering and antihypertensive medications. Circulation 2006; 114: 160-67.
[29] Mozaffarian D, Kamineni A, Carnethron M, Diousse L, Mukamal KJ, Siscovick D. Lifestyle risk factors and new-onset diabetes mellitus in older adults: the Cardiovascular Health Study. Arch Intern Med 2009; 169: 798-807.
[30] Prevalence of physical activity, including lifestyle activities among adults-United States, 2000-2001. MMWR Weekly 2003; 52(32): 764-9.
[31] Hill JO, Wyatt HR, Peters JC. Energy balance and obesity. Circulation 2012; 126: 126-32.
[32] Sattelmair J, Pertman J, Ding E, Kohl HW 3rd, Haskell W, Lee IM. Dose response between physical activity and risk of coronary heart disease. Circulation 2011; 124: 789-95.
[33] Boden WE, Franklin BA, Wenger NK. Physical activity and structured exercise for patients with stable ischemic heart disease. JAMA 2012; 309: 143-4.
[34] Buchman AS, YU L, Boyle PA, Shah RC, Bennett DA. Total daily physical activity and longevity in old age. Arch Intern Med 2012; 172: 444-6.
[35] Yancey AK, Sallis RE, Bastani R. Changing physical activity participation for the medical profession. JAMA 2012; 309: 141-2.
[36] Exercise and physical activity. National Institute on Aging. National Institute of Health. Publication No. 09-4258, Jan 2009, reprinted September 2010.
[37] U.S. Department of Health and Human Service 2008 Physical Activity Guidelines for Americans. [Cited January 18, 2011]. Available from: http://www.health.gov/paguidelines/guidelines/chapter5.aspx.
[38] Lin JS, O'Connor E, Whitlock EP, Beil TL. Behavioral counseling to promote physical activity and a healthful diet to prevent cardiovascular disease in adults: A systematic review for the U. S. Preventive Services Task Force. Ann Intern Med 2010; 153: 736-50.
[39] Bray GA. Diet and exercise for weight loss. JAMA 2012; 307: 2641-2.
[40] Bibbins-Domingo K, Chertow GM, Coxson PG, *et al.* Projected effect of dietary salt reductions on future cardiovascular disease. N Eng J Med 2010; 363: 590-9.

[41] Alderman MH. Reducing dietary sodium. The case for caution. JAMA 2010; 303: 448-9.
[42] Your guide to lowering your blood pressure with DASH. U.S. Department of Health and Human Services. National Institutes of Health, National Heart Lung and Blood Institute. NIH publication No. 06-4082, revised 2006. [Cited February 24, 2013]. http://www.nhlbi.nih.gov/health/public/heart/hbp/dash/new_dash.pdf.
[43] Estruch R, Ros E, Salas-Salvado J *et al.* Primary prevention of cardiovascular disease with a Mediterranean diet. New Eng J Med 2013; 368 (14): 1279-90.
[44] Jonas DE, Garbutt JC, Amick HR, *et al.* Behavioral counseling after screening for alcohol misuse in preventive care: A systematic review and meta-analysis for the U.S. Preventive Services Task Force. Ann Intern Med 2012. 157: 645-54.
[45] National Institute on Alcohol Abuse and Alcoholism. Surveillance Report #94. Trends in alcohol-related morbidity among short stay community hospital discharges, United States, 1979-2010. [Cited February 23, 2013]. http://pubs.niaaa.nih.gov/publications/Surveillance94/HDS10.htm.
[46] Dharmarajan TS. The physiology of aging. In Pitchumoni CS, Dharmarajan TS eds. Geriatric Gastroenterology. New York, Springer 2012; 17-31.
[47] Klatsky AL. Alcohol and cardiovascular mortality: common sense and scientific truth. J Am Coll Card 2010; 55: 1336-8.
[48] Klatsky AL. Alcohol and cardiovascular health. Physiol Behav 2010; 100: 76-81.
[49] Goldberg IJ, Mosca L, Piano MR, Fisher EA. Wine and your heart. A scientific advisory for healthcare professionals from the Nutrition Committee, Council on Epidemiology and Prevention and Council on Cardiovascular Nursing of the American Heart Association. Circulation 2001; 103: 472-5.
[50] Ronksley PE, Brien SE, Turner BJ, Mukamal KJ, Ghali WA. Association of alcohol consumption with selected cardiovascular outcomes: a systematic review and meta-analysis. BMJ 2011; 342d671.
[51] Snow WM, Murray R, Ekuma O, Tyas SL, Barnes GE. Alcohol use and cardiovascular health outcomes: a comparison across age and gender in the Winnipeg Health and Drinking Survey Cohort. Age Ageing 2009; 38(2): 206-12.
[52] National Institute on Alcohol Abuse and Alcoholism. Surveillance Report #95. Understanding the impact of alcohol on human health and well-being. [Cited February 23, 2013]. http://pubs.niaaa.nih.gov/publications/Surveillance95/tab1_10.htm.
[53] Pasternak RC. Comprehensive rehabilitation of patients with cardiovascular disease. In Zipes DP, Libby P, Bonow RO, Braunwald E eds. Braunwald's Heart Disease. 7th ed. Philadelphia, Saunders 2003; 1085-1102.
[54] Gellert C, Schottker B, Brenner H. Smoking and all-cause mortality in older people. Arch Intern Med 2012; 172: 837-44.
[55] Schane RE, Prochaska JJ, Giantz SA. Counseling nondaily smokers about secondhand smoke as a cessation message: a pilot randomized trial. Nicotine Tob Res 2013; 15(2): 334-42.
[56] Critchley JA, Capewell S. Mortality risk reduction associated with smoking cessation in patients with coronary heart disease. A systematic review. JAMA 2003; 290: 86.
[57] Huang PH, Kim CX, Lerman A, *et al.* Trends in smoking cessation counseling: experience from American Heart Association-Get With The Guidelines. Clin Cardiol 2012; 35: 396-403.
[58] Lancaster T, Stead L. Physician advice for smoking cessation. Cochrane Database Syst Rev 2004; CD000165.
[59] Benowits NL, Prochaska JJ. Smoking cessation after acute myocardial infarction. JACC 2013; 61: 533-5.
[60] Eisenberg MJ, Grandi SM, Gervais A, *et al.* Bupropion for smoking cessation in patients hospitalized with acute myocardial infarction. JACC 2012; 61: 524-32.
[61] Fiore MC, Jaen CR, Baker TB *et al.* Treating Tobacco Use and Dependence 2008 Update. Clinical Practice Guideline. Rockville, MD: U.S. Department of Health and Human Services. Public Health Service, May 2008.
[62] Joseph AM, Fu SS, Lindgren B, *et al.* Chronic disease management for tobacco dependence: a randomized, controlled trail. Arch Intern Med 2011; 171: 1894-900.

[63] Lam TH. Absolute risk of tobacco deaths. Arch Intern Med 2012; 172: 845-6.
[64] Khullar D, Schroeder SA, Maa J. Helping smokers quite around the time of surgery. JAMA 2013; 10: 993-4.
[65] Ebbert JD, Hatsukami DK, Croghan IT, *et al.* Combination varenicline and Bupropion SR for tobacco-dependence treatment in cigarette smokers. A randomized trial. JAMA 2014; 311(2): 155-63.
[66] Cahill K, Stevens S, Lancaster T. Pharmacological treatments for smoking cessation. JAMA 2014; 311 (2): 193-4.
[67] Roger VL, Go AS, Lloyd-Jones DM, *et al.* Executive summary: Heart disease and stroke statistics - 2012 update: A report from the American Heart Association. Circulation; 2012: 125: 188-97.
[68] Holford TR, Meza R, Warner KE, *et al.* Tobacco control and the reduction in smoking-related premature deaths in the United States, 1964-2012. JAMA.2014; 311(2): 164-171.

CHAPTER 12

Cardiovascular Disease: Addressing Risk Factors

Lekshmi Dharmarajan*,[1,2] and T.S. Dharmarajan[3]

[1]Chief, Division of Cardiology, Lincoln Medical and Mental Health Center, Bronx, New York, USA; [2]Professor of Clinical Medicine, Weill Medical College of Cornell Univerity, New York, USA; [3]Vice Chairman, Department of Medicine, Clinical Director, Geriatrics, Montefiore Medical Center (Wakefield Campus), Bronx, New York, USA; Professor of Clinical Medicine, Albert Einstein College of Medicine, Bronx, New York, USA

Abstract: Cardiovascular disease is the leading cause of death in the United States. The American Heart Association has an influence on goals for cardiovascular health, recommending behavioral modification as the foundation to heart health and medications as a supplement to prevent cardiovascular disease. Diet, in conjunction with physical activity is a vital component both for primary and secondary prevention and at any stage of the disease. Several new ACC/ AHA guidelines have been released in 2013 pertinent to assessment of cardiovascular risk, management of high cholesterol, addressing overweight and obesity status, and emphasizing the use of life style for these disorders. The 2013 European Society of Hypertension /European Society of Cardiology and Joint National Committee 8 guidelines for hypertension are also discussed in the chapter. Information is provided on women's cardiovascular health, aspirin and omega-3 fatty acids.

Keywords: Aspirin, body mass index, cardiovascular disease prevention, cardiovascular disease, cardiovascular risk assessment, diabetes, guidelines for cardiovascular risk assessment, guidelines for hyperlipidemia, healthy life style, hyperlipidemia management, hyperlipidemia screening, obesity management, obesity, screening for hypertension, statins and omega-3 fatty acids, women's cardiovascular health.

INTRODUCTION

The World Heart Federation (WHF) sponsors programs which are intended to increase public awareness and bring knowledge across governments to help develop programs and policies [1, 2]. The WHF goal is to reduce by 25% the premature mortality from cardiovascular disease by 2025 [3]. The need for quality improvement [4] and redesigning health care services are discussed taking into

***Corresponding author Lekshmi Dharmarajan:** 31 Pheasant Run, Scarsdale, NY 10583, USA; Tel: (718) 579-4876; Fax: (914) 723-4297; E-mail: dharmarajanl@yahoo.com consideration all stakeholders, economics and locality [5, 6]. This chapter focuses on risk assessment and addresses the selected interventions. It is noteworthy that guidelines from different sources on a topic are not necessarily consistent. Several guidelines released in 2013 offer detailed information [7-14].

GLOBAL PERSPECTIVES

Successful implementation of programs as a targeted population approach for the prevention of heart disease is not a novel idea and is a complex task. World Heart Day, celebrated every September, is aimed at actually increasing public awareness and bringing this knowledge across governments to help develop programs and policies [1, 2]. To this effect, the World Heart Federation (WHF) has been developed as a non-governmental organization, with headquarters in Geneva, Switzerland, and a membership of over 100 countries. The organization is largely dedicated to lowering mortality from non-communicable diseases; half this mortality is attributable to cardiovascular disease (CVD). To be successful, the government alone cannot be held accountable; initiatives must be supported by non-governmental organizations and also endorsed by the public.

Moving from political declaration to action for reducing the global burden of cardiovascular diseases is an intent of the Global Cardiovascular Diseases Taskforce, working in collaboration with the World Health Organization (WHO). The intent is to assess and define specific metrics for CVD to achieve the global target of “25 by 25”, referring to the global target of 25% reduction in overall mortality from cardiovascular disease, diabetes, cancer and chronic respiratory disease by 2025; and a WHF goal to reduce by 25% the premature mortality from cardiovascular disease by 2025 [3].

A national registry of over 150,000 coronary artery disease (CAD) patients in an outpatient cardiology setting, revealed that over a third failed to receive optimal secondary prevention, suggesting the need for quality improvement [4]. Hence, health care services need to be redesigned to include all stakeholders, economics and locality [5, 6].

Secondary prevention is utilized after the disease has had its onset; the intent in secondary prevention is to prevent complications and morbidity. As the disorder may not be clinically apparent, the approach is addressed during early case findings of asymptomatic disease. The approaches focus on screening or detecting disease at an asymptomatic stage; without treatment these patients have potential for significant cardiovascular disease and poor outcomes. Screening tests are used in several areas in health care. Examples include screening for cardiovascular disease, peripheral arterial disease, obesity, diabetes, diabetes, hypertension, hyperlipidemia, infections such as tuberculosis, cancer of the breast or cervix, osteoporosis and others. Secondary prevention is particularly helpful when the disorder has a long latency period as with diabetes and hyperlipidemia, and is clearly relevant to cardiovascular disease (CVD).

The American College of Cardiology (ACC), the American Heart Association (AHA) and the National Heart, Lung and Blood Institute (NHLBI) have recently released guidelines for obesity, lifestyle for CVD prevention and cholesterol management [7-10]. Several extensive and comprehensive reviews on secondary prevention and risk reduction therapy in CVD provide relevant information [11-14].

PRACTICE GUIDELINES

Assessment of Cardiovascular Risk

A practice guideline on the assessment of cardiovascular risk has just been released by the ACC/AHA Task force [10]. In this report, the focus on atherosclerotic risk extends beyond the heart to add stroke to coronary events. The focus now is to recognize a 10-year risk of atherosclerosis related events and a secondary focus on assessing the life time risk for adults 59 years old and younger who are not at high, short term risk, utilizing formulas for assessing risk by race and gender as well as the use of markers such as coronary artery calcium in selected cases [10]. A downloadable tool enables estimation of the 10-year risk for atherosclerotic CVD, which is the risk of developing a first atherosclerotic CVD event, defined as a nonfatal myocardial infarction, CAD death or fatal / non-fatal stroke over ten years, in those who are free of the disease at the beginning of the period.

The predictors of 10-year risk in this report include age, gender, race, total cholesterol high density lipoprotein cholesterol (HDL-C), blood pressure, diabetes and current smoking status. In addition, when the risk based treatment decision is uncertain, one may resort to use four additional markers: family history, high sensitivity C-reactive protein (Hs-CRP), ankle-brachial index (ABI) and coronary artery calcium (CAC) score, to enable informed decision making (10). The risk for CVD may be assessed every 4 to 6 years in adults aged 20 to 79 years and free from atherosclerotic CVD.

The report also mentions about the use of statins when the 10-year risk of atherosclerotic CVD exceeds ≥7.5%. Even if an individual has acceptable cholesterol levels, but other factors such as age, smoking status and blood pressure increased the cardiovascular risk to over 7.5%, guidelines now recommend the use of a statin [10]. Statins are a class of cholesterol lowering drugs that work through inhibiting the HMG-CoA reductase enzyme in the liver, the site where most of the cholesterol production takes place in the body.

Importance of Lifestyle

Lifestyle guidelines are addressed in CHAPTER 11 emphasizing behavioral modification and primary prevention of cardiovascular disease. They include aerobic physical activity of moderate to vigorous intensity, and consumption of a diet that is consistent with a Mediterranean or Dietary Approaches to Stop Hypertension (DASH) type diet. The Mediterranean style of diet has taken precedence over low fat diets; rather than reducing fat intake, the recommendation is to reduce the calories consumed from saturated and trans fats [8].

The strength of recommendations based on evidence are A (strong), B (moderate), C (weak), D (against), E (insufficient) and N (no recommendation).

A detailed guideline on the management of lifestyle to prevent CVD was released in 2013 by the ACC/AHA Task Force [8]. For lowering LDL cholesterol, the diet includes whole grains, fruits and vegetables, vegetable oils, legumes and nuts plus low fat, low sugar and limited meat; 5-6% of calories from saturated fat, and avoidance of trans fat [8]. The U.S. National Health and Nutrition Examination Survey (1999-2010) revealed association between higher dietary fiber intake and a lower prevalence of cardio-metabolic risks, suggesting a need to develop strategies to increase dietary fiber intake. For patients with hypertension the sodium intake must be no more than 2400 mg/d, with a further reduction to 1500 mg/d desirable. The average sodium intake in the US is around 3.5 g/day [8]. Physical activity is recommended to include aerobic physical activity for hypertension, and the lowering of LDL-C and non-HDL-C. All these recommendations have a strength of evidence A; while lowering sodium intake is an A recommendation, the amount of sodium intake per day carries a B recommendation. This guideline recommends aerobic physical activity 40 minutes per session 3-4 times a week [8].

Obesity

New guidelines from the National, Heart, Lung and Blood Institute (NHLBI) in collaboration with the ACC/AHA have been released in 2013, on the management of overweight and obesity disorders, designed to help health care providers to better help their overweight or obese patients [7]. The ACC/AHA Task Force issued the recommendations in conjunction with the Obesity Society (TOS). Americans consume more calories and perhaps far more salt than required; the consequence over the years has been the development of several preventable health disorders such as overweight to morbid obesity states, hypertension, diabetes, hyperlipidemia, osteoarthritis, gall bladder disease, sleep apnea and some cancers, in addition to premature mortality [7, 15]. Obesity increases the risk of all cause and CVD mortality [7]. Based on the report of the United States Dietary Guidelines Advisory Committee, over the past 40 years, the calorie consumption has gradually increased by 200 to 600 calories per individual per day.

The obesity epidemic entails huge health care costs, leave alone the resultant morbidity and mortality; further, the challenges posed are a result of the trends in daily routines involving diet and exercise [16]. The prevalence of obesity is on the increase worldwide, more in urban settings, with women more likely to be obese than men. Much research is required to collect required to collect data on the Do's and Don'ts in preventive strategies targeting the disorder, and additionally for methods to tackle obesity once it is established [16]. Obesity research needs to focus on changing the environment and lifestyle early in life; it is now a established knowledge that once children are obese, the likelihood of developing diabetes later in life is high [17]. Community programs, in collaboration with government policy changes and support for research are most relevant here [17]. Exercise and diet induced weight loss can prevent or delay the development of diabetes [18].

The obesity guideline recommendations may be summarized as follows: identify those who need to lose weight; counsel those who need to lose weight regarding the benefits of weight loss; prescribe a diet to achieve reduced calorie intake; enroll in comprehensive lifestyle intervention programs; and finally recognize the use of bariatric surgery in some when appropriate [18].

The body mass index (BMI) derived from height and weight has been retained to define "overweight" (BMI 25-29.9) and "obese" (≥30) states. Waist circumference is an indicator of risk for type 2 diabetes, cardiovascular disease and all-cause mortality [7]. Height, weight and BMI must be calculated annually in adults and more often when indicated [7]. While the upper limits for waist circumference for males is 40 inches and for women 35 inches in the U.S., different values may be applicable to other ethnic groups such as Asian Indians. The guidelines state that weight reducing diets must be individualized to patient preferences and their health status [7]. Diet prescriptions must be specific such as stating the kcals/day, adjusted for body weight and energy deficit, or could be an evidence based diet that restricts certain food types [7]. In addition to informing patients of the need to lose weight, they must be additionally counseled on the means to achieve their targets through utilization of physical activity and reduction in caloric intake as part of programs on a group or individual basis. Overweight and obese adults must be told that they are at elevated risk of CVD and also informed about the cut off points for the differing severities of the disorder (overweight to morbid obesity) [7].

The best approach by the government may be to regulate the intake of food products that are considered harmful to health, an approach already been taken in New York City [15]. There are currently regulations in relation to use of sodium, trans fats and portion sizes of high caloric sugary beverages [15]. In the Look AHEAD Trial, life style induced weight loss by itself in type 2 diabetics was modest (6% weight loss *vs* 3.5% in controls), resulting in no reduction in cardiovascular morbidity and mortality [19]. However, when life style does not prove effective, there remains the option of drugs for weight loss, an area where research is on the increase, including obtaining FDA approval for anti-obesity drugs [20].

As many anti-obesity drugs work on the principle of stimulation of sympathetic activity, the agents have the potential to increase heart rate and blood pressure, and contribute to enhancing cardiovascular disease [21]. The Food and Drug Administration recommends that anti-obesity drugs may be tried for 12 weeks, at which time, if deemed ineffective, they should be discontinued [7, 22, 23]. Medications used as an adjunct to long-term life style measures lead to greater mean weight loss relative to placebo [23]. Based on the FDA, pharmacotherapeutic agents for obesity are broadly categorized into short-term (weeks) and long-term use groups [23]. Whether a reduction in weight through the use of obesity drugs will offset the increase in cardiovascular risk from these agents is a matter of debate; for example, an increase in major adverse cardiac events led to withdrawal of sibutramine from the market [21].

Unfortunately, life style measures have limitations and often fail to produce the desired results [24]. When lifestyle and anti-obesity drugs have failed to produce the desired effect, the value of gastric by-pass surgery becomes a consideration to offset the health and cardiovascular disease risks. Compared to non-surgical approaches, a Roux-en-Y gastric bypass (RYGB) approach was associated with higher rates of diabetes remission and lower risk of adverse cardiovascular and other health outcomes over 6 years [25]. In the Diabetes Surgery Study, a multicenter, Randomized Controlled Trial (RCT), life style combined with RYGB achieved far greater weight loss at one year compared with life style alone; in nearly half of the bariatric surgery groups, the outcome achieved for weight loss was in addition to meeting the American Diabetes Association (ADA) guideline end points for diabetes treatment (essentially HbA1c <7%), LDL cholesterol <100 mg % and a systolic blood pressure target below 130 mm Hg [26]. In another study published around the same time, 1738 of 2438 patients aged 18 to 78 years underwent RYGB; at 3 years there was evidence of substantial weight loss, with the majority experiencing maximum weight change at the end of year one; but there was variability in the amount and trajectory of weight loss, diabetes, blood pressure and lipid outcomes [27]. At this time, the short and medium term outcomes following bariatric surgery are encouraging [24].

Nevertheless, although the results following bariatric surgery are generally impressive, it is equally important to ensure adequate long-term follow up of the patient in the post-surgical period, as there are variations in response as well as possible adverse outcomes, besides recurrence of obesity. Table **1** provides information on the epidemiology of obesity.

Hypertension

Hypertension has long been recognized as a modifiable risk factor for CVD. The prevalence of hypertension increases with age and affects half the adults over the age of 65 years. Systolic hypertension, referring to the systolic blood pressure being over 140 mm Hg with a diastolic blood pressure less than 90 mm Hg is a phenomenon observed exclusively in the older population. In these adults, there is an increase in pulse pressure; a widened pulse pressure, over 60 mm Hg is considered to be a poor prognostic risk factor for heart disease, and is typically present in systolic hypertension [30].

The Joint National Committee Seventh (JNC 7) report on hypertension was released in 2003. An updated and delayed report, the JNC 8, was ultimately

Table 1. Obesity: Global facts [28, 29].

• Obesity is recognized as a global epidemic by the World Health Organization
• Worldwide, over 1.5 billion adults are overweight or obese (WHO)
• The prevalence has doubled across the world between 1980 and 2008
• Women are mostly likely to be obese, compared to men
• Obesity rates have a higher prevalence in urban settings in most countries
• Obesity is highest in the regions of the Americas and lowest in south-east Asia
• China: a dilemma of over-nutrition from lifestyle changes involving diet and physical activity; however overall obesity rates are below 5%
• In Sub-Saharan Africa, obesity is not common
• In India, urbanization and modern settings are contributory, obesity rates are lower in rural areas and more in women, especially in higher socioeconomic class
• Japan has a low rate of obesity
• In United Kingdom, nearly a quarter are obese, a dramatic increase of four-fold has been observed in 30 years
• In Canada, nearly a quarter of adults are obese
• In Australia, three of five people are overweight, and a quarter obese
• United States has the second highest obesity rates in the developed world; over a third of men and women are obese, highest in African American women

released 10 years later, in 2013 [31, 32]. Around the same time, guidelines were released from the American Society of Hypertension (ASH) and International Society of Hypertension (ISH) [33]. Earlier, the European Society of Hypertension (ESH) and the European Society of Cardiology (ESC) released the 2013 ESH/ESC guidelines for the management of arterial hypertension [30]. The terminology for blood pressure staging or grading and values for systolic and diastolic hypertension differ between the JNC 7 and the 2013 ESH/ESC guidelines (outlined in Table **2**) [30, 34]. JNC 8 has retained the same nomenclature for staging of hypertension as with JNC 7.

Medication prescribing practices have changed since the publications of the Antihypertensive and Lipid-Lowering Treatment to Prevent Heart Attack Trial (ALLHAT) and JNC7 guidelines, which reflected better hypertension control rates over time [35]. Over the years, antihypertensive treatment appears to be initiated at lower blood pressure levels with improvement in hypertension control rates.

The new ESH/ESC guidelines outline the need to estimate total cardiovascular risk along with a diagnosis of hypertension. These include cardiovascular risk factors, symptomatic target organ damage, presence of diabetes, symptomatic CVD or chronic kidney disease (CKD). Accordingly, CVD risk is classified as low, moderate, high or very high, referring to the 10-year CV mortality. Treatment must always address lifestyle factors; and additionally ensure prompt initiation of drug therapy for hypertension grades 2 and 3, and with any level of CV risk.

There is no more controversy regarding treatment of hypertension in the geriatric population [36, 37], with many trials substantiating the benefits. There is good evidence for recommending drug therapy in all adults, irrespective of age, with a goal to bringing the systolic blood pressure down to between 150 and 140 mm Hg, and below 140 in the fit elderly. For those over 80 years, prudence is used to reduce the systolic pressure below 150 mm Hg. There is little evidence for benefit in lowering the systolic blood pressure below 130 mm Hg in patients with diabetes and chronic kidney disease; the goal currently, is a target of below 140 mm Hg [30].

A Consensus Statement has also been put forth on Hypertension in the Elderly by the American College of Cardiology Foundation (ACCF) Task Force and the American Heart Association (AHA) in 2011 [36]. The statement emphasizes (similar to the ESH/ESC guidelines) the importance of the entities white coat hypertension (elevated readings in the office or clinic), pseudo hypertension (false readings from sclerotic arteries) and resistant hypertension (hard to control blood pressure). The importance of ambulatory blood pressure recordings is emphasized [36]. The target goals are similar to the ESH/ESC guidelines with the same goals in the below 80 year age group. Diuretics have been suggested as the second drug, if not used as the initial therapy. Secondary causes of hypertension must be considered in the elderly, especially if the blood pressure is hard to control; examples include renal artery stenosis, primary aldosteronism, obstructive sleep apnea and hyperthyroidism [36]. Finally, a strategy to target populations who are more likely to benefit from therapy may be more rewarding in improving outcomes [38].

The JNC 8 Report released the 2014 Evidence- based guideline for the Management of High Blood Pressure; the recommendations are based on RCT quality evidence [31] but differ from JNC 7 in several aspects. JNC 8 does not redefine values for different stages of hypertension, but rather states the threshold for pharmacological treatment for categories of patients, including age below and above 60 years, and race and disease (diabetes and CKD). Life style management remains the same. Choices of drugs include 4 classes: angiotensin converting enzyme inhibitors (ACEI), angiotensin receptor blockers (ARBs), calcium channel blockers and diuretics; this is based on evidence and is tailored to the categories of patients. The target blood pressure is 150/90 mm Hg for those above age 60 years and below 140/90 mm Hg for those ages below 60, and patients with CKD or diabetes. The approach is simple and practical.

The guidelines for management of hypertension from the ASH/ISH also offer a straight forward practical approach and have set targets of <140/90 mm Hg as the treatment goal. As opposed to age group of ≥60 for a threshold blood pressure of ≥150/90 mm Hg to start treatment in JNC 8, the ASH/ISH report recommends a systolic blood pressure of <150/90 mm Hg for those 80 or older [33]. The guideline emphasizes the importance of systolic blood pressure as the basis for diagnosis; in the age >80 years the threshold for starting treatment is at levels ≥ 150/90 mm Hg. The ASH/ISH guideline does not redefine stages of hypertension outlined by JNC.

Tables **2**, **3** and **4** provide summarized material from the three guidelines.

Table 2. **Definitions of hypertension: a comparison of two guidelines [30, 34].**

2003 Joint National Committee 7 Report on High Blood Pressure	2013 European Society of Hypertension/European Society of Cardiology Guidelines
Normal blood pressure: <120 and <80 mm Hg	Optimal: <120 and <80 mm Hg
Pre hypertension: 120-139 or 80-89 mmHg	Normal: 12 0-129 and/or 80-84 mm Hg
	High normal: 130-139 &/or 85-89 mm Hg
Stage 1 hypertension: 140-159 or 90 -99 mm Hg	Grade 1 hypertension: 140-159 &/or 90-99 mm Hg
Stage 2 hypertension: ≥160 or ≥100 mm Hg	Grade 2 hypertension: 160-179 &/or 100-109 mm Hg
	Grade 3 hypertension: >180 and >110 mm Hg
	Isolated systolic hypertension: >140 and <90 mm Hg

Blood Cholesterol and Cardiovascular Risk

The ACC/AHA guidelines on the treatment of blood cholesterol to reduce atherosclerotic cardiovascular risk in adults were released in 2013 [9]. The guidelines which focus on CVD risk reduction, identified four statin benefit groups on the basis of evidence, and additionally the statement categorizes those needing statins as high, moderate, and low intensity groups based on the required reduction in LDL-C levels from the use of daily statin therapy for secondary and primary prevention. There is no support for further use of specific LDL-C and non-HDL-C treatment targets [9]. The guidelines claim that non-statin therapy does not provide acceptable risk reduction compared to the potential benefits *versus* adverse effects from the use of statins [9].

Table 3. Management of hypertension based on 2013 ESH/ESC guidelines [30].

	Life Style Therapy: Indicated for All Hypertensive Patients
•	Salt restriction: 5-6 grams of salt based on ESH/ESC guidelines; sodium less than 1.5 g/day based on the report of the Dietary Guidelines for Americans, 2010
•	Avoid added salt to food and high salt containing items (*e.g.* processed foods)
•	Moderation of alcohol intake: no more than 20 to 30 g/d in men, 10-20 g/d in women
•	Alcohol consumption should not exceed 140 g for men and 80 g for women per week
•	Consumption of vegetables and fruits, plus a low fat diet. The Mediterranean diet is encouraged. Soy milk appears beneficial.
•	No firm recommendations for or against coffee consumption (in hypertension)
•	Weight reduction recommended, as excess body weight correlates with hypertension, best achieved through regular exercises of low to moderate intensity 5-7 days a week
•	Smoking cessation is recommended, as smoking is a major risk factor for CVD
	Pharmacological Therapy: A Supplement to Life style Measures
•	Any class of drug may be used for the initiation and maintenance of treatment
•	Medications may be used as mono therapy or a combination
•	Differences between classes are similar or differ by only a small degree
•	Choices include diuretics, beta blockers, calcium antagonists, angiotensin converting enzyme inhibitors and angiotensin receptor blockers
•	Compelling choices may be made for certain conditions such as diabetes, chronic kidney disease and heart failure.
•	Contraindications to certain medications exist with certain disorders

A discussion between provider and patient is recommended before initiating statins, including elaboration of safety recommendations. Statins have consistently shown reduction in CVD events in randomized controlled trials (RCTs), but there appears little evidence for titrating cholesterol lowering drug therapy to achieve target LDL-C or HDL-C levels, as formerly stated in the Adult Treatment Panel III report. Healthy diet and life style measures will always remain essential background therapy nevertheless. The older approaches of treatment to target and that "lowest cholesterol is best" are no longer advocated, as adverse effects of therapy may pose problems.

Table 4. 2014 evidence-based guideline on management of high blood pressure (JNC8) and clinical practice guidelines for management of hypertension from ASH / ISH [31, 33].

Evidence Based Guideline on Management of High Blood Pressure, JNC8 (2014)
• Strong evidence to use drug therapy to lower blood pressure in those > 60 years at systolic BP >150 and diastolic BP >9 0 mm Hg
• If in the above group, drug therapy already lowered the BP <150 mm, no further therapy should be given, if therapy is tolerated without side effects
• In the age group <60 years, treatment should be initiated at diastolic BP ≥ 90 mm and systolic ≥140 mm
• In adults with CKD or diabetes, blood pressure goal is <140 / 90 mm
• In non-blacks, initial drug may be thiazide type diuretic, CCB, ACEI or ARB
• In blacks, including diabetics, a thiazide type diuretic or CCB is recommended to use as the first drug
• In presence of CKD, moderate evidence supports the use of ACEI or ARB as initial therapy
• Choice of diuretics: chlorthalidone, indapamide and hydrochlothiazide
Clinical Practice Guidelines for Management of Hypertension from ASH / ISH (2013)
• The guidelines do not redefine hypertension
• Main risk event is tied to systolic hypertension
• Treatment goal is <140 for systolic and <90 for diastolic hypertension
• For those over age 80, a target of < 150/90 mm Hg is recommended; the threshold for starting treatment is ≥ 150/90 mm Hg
• In the age group below 50, data is inadequate for threshold value to start treatment
• In CKD and diabetes, a value of < 140/90 mm Hg is the target
• In blacks, the choice of drug can be a CCB or a diuretic
• In whites below age 60, an ACEI or ARB is reasonable; over 60, a CCB or thiazide is the choice
• ACEI and ARB should not to be combined
• Diuretics recommended for hypertension are: chlorthalidone, indapamide and hydrochlothiazide

Four major statin benefit groups were identified in whom the benefit of statin therapy for CVD risk reduction outweighed the risk of adverse events. The four groups are (1) those with atherosclerotic CVD; (2) those with primary elevation of LDL-C ≥ 190 mg/dl; (3) diabetes aged 40 to 75 years with LDL-C 70 to 189 mg/dl and without clinical atherosclerotic CVD; and (4) those without clinical atherosclerotic CVD or diabetes, with LDL-C 70 to 189 mg/dl and an estimated 10 year atherosclerotic CVD risk ≥ 7.5% [9].

The guidelines further define high, moderate and low intensity therapy. High intensity refers to a daily dose that lowers LDL-C by approximately ≥ 50%; moderate intensity refers to a daily dose that lowers LDL-C by approximately 30% to < 50% and low intensity refers to a daily dose that lowers LDL-C by

< 30%. The guideline details several subcategories which are recommended for differing intensities of therapy. The doses of statins for different intensity therapies based on their use in RCTs, and as recommended in the guideline, are provided in Table **4**.

The discussion between patient and provider often involves the adverse effects from statin therapy, involving the liver or muscle. Ultimately, data suggests that the benefits of statin use far outweigh the risks; statins likely have pleotropic effects and their benefits expand beyond control of lipid levels. A study of 18 RCTs in over 50,000 men and women from several countries demonstrated a reduction in all cause mortality, CVD and stroke events, favoring the use of statins; the incidence of adverse events did not differ between the groups, suggesting that overall benefits of statin therapy outweighed the hazards [39].

In a 2013 Cochrane review of Asian Indians, a population with the highest risk of premature CAD and diabetes, statins lowered all-cause mortality, adverse CVD events and incidence of coronary artery revascularization procedures [40]. In a Netherlands study, age differences in drug use for prevention and treatment of CAD attenuated over time while gender differences persisted, suggesting opportunities for improved treatment, especially in young women and the elderly [41]. The benefits of statin use in women and men are comparable, both in areas of primary and secondary prevention of CAD [11]. Sex disparities in addressing cholesterol levels exist, with women less likely than men to have their LDL-C levels lowered to the desired ranges through use of statins [42]. Additionally, in nearly all patients after a myocardial infarction discharged on secondary prevention medications, dose increases are infrequent and are below proven efficacy requiring performance measures for improvement (Table **5**) [43]. Other lipid abnormalities involving triglycerides and HDL should also be addressed although the details are beyond the scope of discussion in this chapter.

Diabetes Mellitus

Targeted screening for diabetes mellitus Type 2, based on age and risk is a cost-effective measure compared to universal screening. The 2013 recommendations on screening for type 2 diabetes from the American Diabetes Association (ADA) have been outlined in Table **6**. Targeted screening in blacks 45 to 54 years of age has been the most cost-effective [12].

Table 5. Statin therapy recommendations based on 2013 ACC/ AHA guidelines [9].

• Action of statins: inhibition of 3-hydroxy-3methylglutaryl-coenzyme A reductase	
• Statins are only a supplement to life style measures, the foundation for CVD prevention	
• No recommendations for target levels of LDL-C or HDL-C	
• Intensity of therapy is directed to select categories	
High intensity statin therapy (daily dose lowers LDL-C by ≥ 50%)	
○ Atorvastatin	40 - 80 mg
○ Rosuvastatin	20 - 40 mg
Moderate intensity statin therapy (daily dose lowers LDL-C 30 to < 50%)	
○ Atorvastatin	10 - 20 mg
○ Rosuvastatin	5 - 10 mg
○ Simvastatin	20 - 40 mg
○ Pravastatin	40 - 80 mg
○ Lovastatin	40 mg
○ Fluvastatin XL	80 mg
○ Fluvastatin	40 mg bid
○ Pitavastatin	2 - 4 mg
Low intensity statin therapy (daily dose lowers LDL-C by < 30%)	
○ Simvastain	10 mg
○ Pravastatin	10 - 20 mg
○ Lovastatin	20 mg
○ Fluvastatin	20-40 mg
○ Pitavastatin	1 mg

All adult diabetics over 40 years of age are recommended low dose aspirin at 75-162 mg/day; the measure is also recommended in younger adults who are diabetic and smoke or have additional risk factors. All diabetics need to be counseled on life style measures. Diabetics must have aggressive modification of risk factors including weight reduction, control of hyperlipidemia and blood pressure maintained in the recommended ranges [12, 13].

The foundation of management includes addressing life style measures (diet, exercise, smoking cessation, alcohol restriction), supported by the use of medications including insulin and oral agents. Hemoglobin A1C (HbA1C) must be monitored at least twice a year with stable glycemic control and every quarter when control fails to meet goals [44]. The ADA recommends target goals for

HbA1C below or around 7% to reduce microvascular complications of diabetes and a more stringent goal of < 6.5% for select individuals [44].

In particular, diabetics and smokers must also be assessed for the presence of peripheral arterial disease, through a focused history and physical examination, followed by the assessment of ankle-brachial index (ABI) as a screen. An ABI of < 0.9 suggests peripheral artery disease with good sensitivity and specificity [14]. Only a small number of those with peripheral artery disease are symptomatic. Since the majority are asymptomatic, the disorder often remains undiagnosed until late in the course.

Table 6. American diabetes association criteria for diagnosis of diabetes (2013) [44].

• Hemoglobin A1C ≥ 6.5%
• Hemoglobin A1C 5.7 to 6.4 indicates pre-diabetes
• Fasting blood glucose ≥ 126 mg % (7.0 mmol/L)
• Two hour post prandial plasma glucose ≥200 mg % (11.1 mmol/L)
• Random plasma glucose ≥200 mg % (11.1 mmol/L) in the symptomatic
• Results should be confirmed by repeat testing
• Screening should begin at age 45 years and
• Screen overweight adults with BMI over 25, hypertension (over 140/90 mm Hg), first degree relatives of diabetics, high risk ethnic groups and a history of cardiovascular disease

Cardiovascular Disease in Women

In the past several years, awareness to address health issues has been increased, especially cardiovascular disease without an exception, particularly in women. CVD is the most common cause of death in women worldwide; In the United States more women than men are dying of CVD. CVD being a preventable disorder, translates to the fact that CVD is largely addressable in women [45].

The guidelines for prevention of CVD in women classify the risk for CVD as high risk, at risk and ideal cardiovascular health, based on the presence of comorbidity and calculation of the 10- year Framingham global risk [46]. There is an acknowledgement that all women are at risk for CVD, emphasizing the need for women to adopt a heart-healthy lifestyle [45]. The use of hormone therapy and aspirin has changed. The Women's Health Initiative (WHI) findings lead to a dramatic cut down of the use of hormones [47] and aspirin is now considered in women based on the risks and benefits [45].

The guideline has been updated in 2011, and emphasizes certain interventions that should not be used in women and may even be harmful: hormone therapy and selective estrogen receptor modulators should not be used for primary or secondary prevention of CVD; antioxidant vitamin supplement (vitamin E, C, beta carotene) and folic acid should not be used for primary or secondary prevention of CVD; aspirin should not be routinely used in healthy women below age 65 for prevention of MI [46].

Menopausal hormone therapy has a complex pattern of risks and benefits evidenced from the follow up of the WHI hormone therapy trials; the findings do not support the use of estrogen plus medroxy progesterone acetate for chronic disease prevention, although it is appropriate for symptom management in some women [48]. This large study once again confirms the initial findings from estrogen *versus* estrogen plus progestin; most risks and benefits were reduced but persisted in the estrogen plus progestin group, whereas risks and benefits were balanced in the estrogen group only [48]. The study also validates the fact that human biology varies by sex, and that women and minorities must be included in trials [49].

An AHA National Survey published 15 year trends in awareness of heart disease in women. Although awareness in women has improved over the past 15 years, a significant racial/ethnic minority gap still persists, suggesting that efforts must be taken to address the gap through public health campaigns and evidenced based strategies to motivate women to take action [50].

ADDITIONAL CONSIDERATIONS

Aspirin

Aspirin use is associated with significant benefits in both primary and secondary prevention. While in primary prevention, the appropriate use of aspirin is individualized and based on clinical judgment of risks *versus* benefits, there is little disagreement that the use of aspirin is beneficial in secondary prevention, such as in patients who survive a prior occlusive event, whether it is an acute myocardial infarction or an acute thrombotic stroke. In these settings, use of aspirin results in a reduction of subsequent myocardial infarction, stroke and vascular death [51]. In spite of the effectiveness, the adherence to a proper aspirin regimen has been suboptimal, ranging from 72 to 92% rate, relating to a combination of patient and medication related factors [52].

Risk factors for non-adherence to aspirin include forgetfulness, cognitive impairment, presence of depression, poor understanding of the disease or benefits of medication, low education, inadequate support, side effects, polypharmacy, provider related aspects (relating to difficulty in addressing barriers and providing appropriate instructions) and others [52]. The dose of aspirin including efficacy and safety, based on data from trials, shows no difference between 75-150 mg/day and 160-325 mg/day, the most common doses used are 81 and 325 mg /day. In summary, patients who suffer a myocardial infarction or an occlusive stroke must be placed on aspirin, and continued long-term [51].

The mechanism of action for aspirin is by irreversibly acetylating cyclo-oxygenase, needed for production of thromboxane A2, a promoter of platelet aggregation. Aspirin irreversibly inhibits platelets. Additional mechanisms may explain the action of aspirin; for example, the production of nitric oxide which also inhibits platelet aggregation, besides playing a role in vascular homeostasis [51].

Omega-3 Fatty Acids

Effects of seafood consumption and long chain n-3 polyunsaturated fatty acids (PUFAs) on cardiovascular diseases have drawn attention [52, 53]. The precise physiological effects and mechanisms of action are not yet clear; in addition, results of trials have raised mixed findings, raising concerns [52]. Fish (including finfish and shell fish) is the food source of long chain n-3 PUFA, including eicosapentaenoic acid (EPA) and docosahexaenoic acid (DHA); fish also provides vitamin D and additional minerals and nutrients [53].

The U.S Dietary Guidelines (2010) recommend consumption of a minimum of two 4 oz servings or 8 oz of fish a week for the prevention of CVD; this would provide about 250 mg / day of EPA and DHA. Long chain omega 3 fatty acids EPA and DHA are recommended in the form of oily fish or as EPA and DHA supplements [52-54]. The governmental regulations of supplements for standards of purity and safety are not as tightly implemented as for prescription medications, a factor that should be kept in mind with the use of omega-supplements. A variety of benefits have been attributed to omega-3 fatty acids, including: anti-inflammatory activity, reduction in triglyceride levels, reduction in non-HDL levels, increase in HDL level, attenuation of atherosclerotic plaques, lowering of blood pressure, decline in cardiac arrhythmias and antithrombotic properties [53, 54]. The reduction in triglyceride levels that is necessary is usually not possible only through the consumption of fish, therefore a fish oil supplement is also recommended. A modestly higher incidence of diabetes has been associated with n-3 PUFA consumption [53].

Omega-3 fatty acids are available as both dietary supplements in numerous forms, and as prescription formulations. Unlike with supplements, the prescription formulations contain consistent active compounds, to be usually taken with meals. It is essential for providers to be aware of the differences between the two forms. It is also necessary to differentiate between the consumption of fish oil and fish; as fish contains additional nutrients but may not be suitable for all, supplements are reasonable for those who do not consume fish [53].

In some cases, the combination of EPA and DHA results in an increase in LDL-C levels, although they did lower triglyceride levels. In a meta-analysis of trials published till March 2013, involving over 15,000 patients, no statistically significant association was noted for all-cause mortality and stroke, but protective effects were observed for cardiac death, sudden death and myocardial infarction [54]. In another meta-analysis of comparative trials including 20,000 patients with CVD, omega-3 fatty acid supplements did not reduce the risk of a subsequent cardiovascular event [55].

Immunizations

The importance of appropriate vaccinations in those at risk for CVD should be emphasized. In a large meta-analysis involving older adults, the use of influenza vaccinations was associated with a lower risk of major adverse cardiovascular events. The greatest benefit was noted for those patients with the highest cardiovascular risk, and patients with more active coronary artery disease [56]. Patients with cardiovascular disease should receive annual influenza vaccination [11]. Pneumococcal vaccination is indicated in all adults over age 65 years; it is also indicated for those below age 65 years in the presence of risk factors such as diabetes mellitus, heart and lung disease, heart failure, smokers, kidney disease, and in the immune suppressed [57].

Psychosocial Factors

Psychosocial issues are often ignored, and deserve to be addressed in secondary prevention. These include personality factors such as type A behavior patterns, including hostility; depression has emerged as a risk factor for cardiac events,

Table 7. Addressing risk factors for cardiovascular disease [11, 44, 57, 58].

	Anti-Platelet Agents (ACC/AHA)
•	Aspirin 75-162 mg daily in all patients with CAD, unless contraindicated
•	Clopidogrel 75 mg daily is an alternative in those intolerant or allergic to aspirin
	Diabetes Mellitus (American Diabetes Association)
•	Testing to detect type 2 diabetes and pre-diabetes in asymptomatic adults at any age, when overweight or obese (BMI $\geq$ 25/kg m^2) and in those who have 1 or more additional risk factors for diabetes.
•	In those without risk factors, testing begins at 45 years; repeated at 3 year intervals
•	Target goals for HbA1C around or <7% to reduce microvascular complications
•	Target may be a more stringent goal of <6.5% for selected individuals
	Diabetes Mellitus (USPSTF)
•	Screen for diabetes in asymptomatic adults with sustained blood pressure greater than 135/80 mm Hg
	Lipid Disorders: Screening (USPSTF)
•	Screen men aged 35 years and older and women aged 45 years and older at increased risk for CAD (grade A)
•	Screen men aged 20-35 years who are at increased risk for CAD and women aged 20-45 years at increased risk for CAD (Grade B)
•	Men aged 20-35 years and women aged ≥20 years, not at risk for CAD: no recommendation
	Lipid Disorders: Management (ACC/AHA)
•	A lipid profile should be established in all patients with CAD; for hospitalized patients lipid lowering therapy must be initiated before discharge
•	Counseling on life style measures is an essential recommendation along with drug therapy (see Table 5)
•	Statin therapy intensity is variable and relates to the CVD risk reduction required
	Hypertension (USPSTF)
•	Screen for high blood pressure in adults 18 years and older (Grade A)
•	Screen every 2 years if BP < 120/80 mm hg
•	Screen every year with blood pressure 120-139 / 80-89 mm Hg
	Hypertension (AHA/ACCF)
•	All patients should be counseled on life style modification
•	Patients with blood pressure >140/90 mm Hg should be treated with medication
	Smoking Cessation (AHA/ACCF)
•	Patients should be asked about tobacco smoking at every office visit
•	Every tobacco user should be advised to quit at every visit
•	Patients should be assisted and follow up is recommended
•	Tobacco control reduces premature deaths and extends life span [58]
	Immunizations: (AHA/ACCF, USPSTF)
•	Influenza vaccination must be offered annually
•	Pneumococcal vaccine should be offered once to all adults 65 years and older; it should also be provided for those adults with diabetes, heart, lung, liver and kidney disease and those immune suppressed at any age, and in these patients it should be repeated at the age of 65.

commonly following myocardial infarction; stress and anxiety are common in today's life style and can trigger fatal cardiovascular events; poor socioeconomic support, which may also contribute to depression and stress; impaired cognition can impair cooperation from the patient and adherence to treatment recommendations [14].

A summary on recommendations to address risk factors for CVD are outlined in Table **7**.

CONCLUSION

Cardiovascular disease is a global problem and a leading cause of mortality worldwide, increasing with age. New guidelines have been released by the ACC/AHA in 2013; these guidelines address key areas in cardiovascular health, risk assessment and management. Overweight and obesity are risk factors for myocardial infarction and ischemic heart disease, regardless of the presence of the metabolic syndrome, emphasizing the value of addressing the BMI status [59]. Life style measures are the foundation when addressing cardiovascular health; measures include counseling for a healthy diet for heart [60, 61], adequate exercise and smoking cessation. The importance of higher dietary fiber intake with lower cardiometabolic risks has been substantiated from data in U.S. adults [60]. Alcohol consumption, if a must, must be limited to the recommended amounts. Three new guidelines have been released in 2013, pertinent to the management of hypertension; the recommendations do not concur in all aspects of management. The approach to overweight and obese individuals includes recognition of the disorder, evaluation and assessment, with an individualized approach that includes counseling on lifestyle measures, medications and where indicated, a surgical approach. New guidelines address the approach to high cholesterol levels by placing individuals in four statin groups, with no attempt at target levels. Statin therapy is associated with a reduction of CVD events; based on the desired reduction of LDL-C, therapy may be of high, moderate or low intensity. The benefits from use of omega-3 fatty acids as compared to fish consumption is not clear. An increased awareness is necessary for the occurrence of cardiovascular disease in women, including the need to address screening. Women are at high risk for cardiovascular disease and mortality; management measures must meet at least the same intensity utilized for men.

ACKNOWLEDGEMENTS

Declared none.

CONFLICT OF INTEREST

The authors confirm that this chapter contents have no conflict of interest.

REFERENCES

[1] Maranhao M, Tse T, Poole-Wilson P. Global cardiovascular disease prevention. Lancet 2001; 358: 1642

[2] Bonow RO, Smaha LA, Smith SC, Mensah GA, Lenfant C. World Heart Day 2002. The International Burden of Cardiovascular Disease: Responding to the Emerging Global Epidemic. Circulation.2002; 106: 1602-5

[3] Smith SC, Chen D, Collins A, *et al*. Moving from political declaration to action on reducing the global burden of cardiovascular diseases. A statement from the global Cardiovascular disease Taskforce. Circulation 2013; 128: 2546-8

[4] Maddox TM, Chan PS, Spertus JA, *et al*. Variations in CAD secondary prevention prescription among outpatient cardiology practices: Insights from the NCDR. J Am Coll Card 2014; 63(6): 539-46.

[5] Puspitaari HP, Aslani P, Krass I. Austalian community pharmacists' awareness and practice in supporting secondary prevention of cardiovascular disease. Int J Clin Pharm 2013; 35(6): 1218-28.

[6] Briffa T, Chow CK, Clark AM, Redfern J. Improving outcomes after acute coronary syndrome with rehabilitation and secondary prevention. Clin Ther.2013; 35(8): 1076-81

[7] Jensen MD, Ryan DH, Apovian CM, *et al* 2013 AHA/ACC/TOS guideline for the Management of Overweight and Obesity in Adults: A Report of the American College of Cardiology/American Heart Association Task Force on Practice Guidelines and The Obesity Society. Circulation, published on line Nov 12, 2013; http://circ.ahajournals.org/content/129/25_suppl_2/S102.full.pdf

[8] Eckel RH, Jakicic JM, Ard JD, *et al* 2013 AHA/ACC guideline on lifestyle management to reduce cardiovascular risk: a report of the American College of Cardiology/American Heart Association Task Force on Practice Guidelines.. J Am Coll Cardiol 2013; available at http://content.online jacc.org/journal.aspx; Circulation2013; available at: http//circ.ahajournals.org

[9] Stone NJ, Robinson J, Lichtenstein AH, *et al* 2013 ACC/AHA guideline on the treatment of blood cholesterol to reduce atherosclerotic cardiovascular risk in adults: A report of the American College of Cardiology/American Heart Association. J Am Coll Cardiol 2013; Available at: http://circ.ahajournals.org/content/early/2013/11/11/01.cir.0000437738.63853.7a.full.pdf

[10] Goff DC Jr, Lloyd-Jones DM, Bennet G, *et al* 2013 ACC/AHA guideline on the assessment of cardiovascular risk: a report of the American College of Cardiology/American Heart Association Task Force on Practice Guidelines.. J Am Coll Cardiol 2013; Available at: http://circ.ahajournals.org/content/129/25_suppl_2/S49.full.pdf

[11] Smith SC, Benjamin EJ, Bonow RO, *et al*. AHA/ACCF Secondary Prevention and Risk Reduction Therapy for patients with coronary and other atherosclerotic vascular disease: 2011 Update: A Guideline from the American Heart Association and American College of Cardiology Foundation. Circulation 2011; 124: 2458-73

[12] Weintraub WS, Daniels SR, Burke LE, *et al*. Value of primordial and secondary prevention for cardiovascular disease: A policy Statement from the American Heart Association 2011; 124: 967-900

[13] Gaziano JM, Ridker PM, Libby P. Primary and secondary prevention of cardiovascular disease. In Bonow RO, Mann DL, Zipes DP *et al*. eds. Braunwald's Heart Disease. 9th edition. Philadephia, Elsevier 2012; 1010-1035

[14] Fleg JL, Forman DE, Berra K, *et al*. Secondary prevention of atherosclerotic cardiovascular disease in older adults. A scientific statement from the American Heart Association. Circulation 2013; 128: 2422-46

[15] Farley T. The role of government in preventing excess calorie consumption. The example of New York City. JAMA 2012; 308(11): 1093-4

[16] Rodgers GP, Collins FS. The next generation of obesity research. JAMA 2012; 308(11): 1095-6

[17] Zeitler P, Hirst K, Pyle L, *et al*. (TODAY Study Group).A clinical trial to maintain glycemic control in youth with type 2 diabetes. N Eng J Med 2012; 366(24): 2247-56

[18] Knowler WC, Barrett-Connor E, Fowler SE, *et al*. Diabetes Prevention Program Research Group. Reduction in the incidence of type 2 diabetes with lifestyle intervention or metformin. N Eng J Med 2002; 346(6): 393-403

[19] Wing PR, Bolin P, Brancati FL, *et al*. Look AHEAD Research Group. Cardiovascular effects of intensive lifestyle intervention in type 2 diabetes. New Eng J Med 2013; 369(2): 145-54

[20] Morrato EH, Allison DR. FDA approval of obesity drugs. A difference in risk-benefit perceptions. JAMA 2012; 308(11): 1097-8

[21] Hiatt WR, Goldfine AB, Kaul S. Cardiovascular risk assessment in the development of new drugs for obesity. JAMA 2012; 308(11): 1099-1100

[22] Jensen MD, Ryan DH. New obesity guidelines: Promise and potential. JAMA 2014; 311(1): 23-24

[23] Yanovski SZ, Yanovski JA. Long term drug treatment for obesity. A systematic and clinical review. JAMA 2014; 311(1): 74-86

[24] Ikramuddin S, Livingston EH. New insights on bariatric surgery outcomes. JAMA 2013; 310(22): 2401-2.

[25] Adams TD, Davidson LE, Litwin SE, *et al*. Health benefits of gastric bypass surgery after 6 years. JAMA 2012; 308(11): 122-31.

[26] Ikramuddin S, Lorner J, LeeWJ, *et al*. Roux-en-Y gastric bypass *versus* intensive medical management for the control of type 2 diabetes, hypertension and hyperlipidemia: the Diabetes Surgery Study randomized controlled trial. JAMA 2013; 309 (21): 2240-9

[27] Courcoulas AP, Christian NJ, Belle HS, *et al*. Weight change and health outcome at 3 years after bariatric surgery among individuals with severe obesity. JAMA 2013; 310(22): 2416-25

[28] Epidemiology of obesity. [Cited 2013, November10]. Available from: http://en.wikipedia.org/wiki/Epidemiology_of_obesity

[29] Global Health Observatory: Obesity. [Cited 2013, November 10]. Available from: http://www.who.int/gho/ncd/risk_factors/obesity_text/en/

[30] Mancia G, Fagard R, Narkiewicz K, *et al* 2013 ESH/ESC guidelines for the management of arterial hypertension. The Task Force for the management of arterial hypertension of the European Society of Hypertension (ESH) and of the European Society of Cardiology (ESC). J Hypertens 2013; 31(7): 1281-357.

[31] James PA, Oparil S, Carter BL, *et al* 2014 Evidence-based guideline for the management of high blood pressure in adults. Report from the panel members appointed to the Eight Joint National Committee (JNC8). JAMA 2014; 311(5): 507-20

[32] Sox HC. Assessing the trustworthiness of the guideline for management of high blood pressure in adults. JAMA 2013. Dec 18, E1-E3

[33] Weber MA, Schiffrin EL, White WB, *et al*. Clinical Practice Guidelines for the Management of Hypertension in the Community. A Statement by the American Society of Hypertension and the International Society of Hypertension. J Clin Hypertension 2013; DOI: 10.1111/jch.12237

[34] Chobanian AV, Bakris GL, Black HR, *et al*. The seventh report of the Joint National Committee on Prevention, Detection, Evaluation and Treatment of high blood pressure: The JNC7 report. Hypertension 2003; 42: 1206-52

[35] Krousel-Wood M, Muntner P, Carson A, *et al*. Hypertension control among newly treated patients before and after publication of the main ALLHAT results and JNC7 guidelines. J Clin Hypertension 2012; 14(5): 277-83

[36] Aronow WS, Fleg JL, Pepine CJ, *et al.* ACCF/AHA 2011 Expert consensus Document on Hypertension in the Elderly. J Am Coll Card 2011; 57: 2037-2114

[37] Dharmarajan TS, Dharmarajan L. Geriatric hypertension. In Dharmarajan TS, Norman RA eds, Clinical Geriatrics. Boca Raton, Parthenon Publishing 2003; 545-60

[38] Rahimi K, MacMahon S. Blood pressure management in the 21st century. Maximizing gains and minimizing waste. Circulation 2013; 128: 2283-5

[39] Taylor FC, Huffman M, Ebrahim S. Statin therapy for primary prevention of cardiovascular disease. JAMA 2013; 310: 2451-2

[40] Enas EA, Kuruvila A, Khanna P, Pitchumoni CS, Mohan V. Benefits and risks of statin therapy for primary prevention of cardiovascular disease in Asian Indians-A population with the highest risk of prematurely coronary artery disease and diabetes. Indian J Med Res 2013; 138: 461-91

[41] Koopman C, Vaarties I, Heinties EM, *et al.* Persisting gender differences and attenuating age differences in cardiovascular drug use for prevention and treatment of coronary heart disease, 1988-2010. Eur Heart J 2013. 34 (41): 3198-205

[42] Virani SS. Statins in primary and secondary prevention of cardiovascular disease in women. Facts and myths. Texas Heart J 2013; 40(3): 288-9

[43] Arnold SV, Spertus JA, Masoudi FA, *et al.* Beyond medication prescription as performance measures. Optimal secondary prevention medication dosing after acute myocardial infarction. J Am Coll Cardiol 2013; 62: 1791-801

[44] Executive summary: Standards of Medical Care in Diabetes-2013. Diabetes Care.2013; 36: S4-S10

[45] Mosca L, Banka CL, Benjamin EJ *et al.* Evidence based guidelines for Cardiovascular Disease Prevention in Women: 2007 update. J Am Coll Card 2007; 49: 1230-60

[46] Mosca L, Banka CL, Benjamin EJ, *et al.* Effectiveness based guidelines for Cardiovascular Disease Prevention in Women: 2011 update. A Guideline from the American Heart Association. Circulation 2011; 123: 1243-1262

[47] Rossow JE, Anderson GL, Prentice RL, *et al.* For the Writing Group for the Women's health Initiative Investigators. Risks and benefits of estrogen plus progestin in healthy postmenopausal women: principal results from the Women's Health Initiative randomized controlled trial. JAMA 2002; 288-321-33

[48] Manson JE, Chlebowski RT, Stefanick ML, *et al.* Menopausal hormone therapy and health outcomes during the intervention and extended post-stopping phases of the Women's Health Initiative Randomized Trials. JAMA 2013; 210: 1353-68

[49] Nabel E. the Women's Health Initiative-A victory for women and their health. JAMA 2013; 310: 1349-50

[50] Mosca L, Hammond G, Mochari-Greenberger H, *et al.* Fifteen year trends in awareness of heart disease in women: Results of a 2012 American Heart Association National Survey. Circulation 2013; 127: 1254-63

[51] Hennekens CH, Dalen JE. Aspirin in the treatment and prevention of cardiovascular disease: past and current perspectives and future directions. American J Med 2013; 126: 373-8

[52] Duffy D, Kelly E, Trang A, Mills G. Aspirin for cardioprotection and strategies to improve patient adherence. Postgraduate Medicine 2014; 126(1): 18-28.

[53] Mozaffarian D. Omega-3 fatty acids and cardiovascular disease. Effects on risk factors, molecular pathways and clinical events. J Am Coll Cardiol 2011; 58: 2047-67

[54] Casula M, Sorrana D. Catapano AL, Corrao G. Long-term effect of high dose omega-3 fatty acid supplementation for secondary prevention of cardiovascular outcomes: A meta-analysis of randomized, double blind, placebo controlled trials. Atheroscler Suppl 2013; 14 (2): 243-51

[55] Secondary cardiovascular prevention: omega-3 fatty acids ineffective. Prescrire Int 2013; 22(14): 218 (no authors listed)

[56] Udell JA, Zawi R, Bhatt DL, *et al.* Association between influenza vaccination and cardiovascular outcomes in high-risk patients. A meta-analysis. JAMA 2013; 310: 1711-20

[57] Moyer VA, LeFevre ML, Siu AL. The Guide to Clinical Preventive Services 2012. Recommendations of the U.S. Preventive Services Task Force. Agency for Healthcare Research and Quality 2012

[58] Holford TR, Meza R, Warner KE, *et al*. Tobacco control and the reduction in smoking-related premature deaths in the United States, 1964-2012. JAMA.2014; 311(2): 164-171

[59] Thomsen M, Nordestgaard BG. Myocardial infarction and ischemic heart disease in overweight and obesity with and without metabolic syndrome. JAMA Intern Med 2014; 174(1): 15-22

[60] Grooms KN, Ommerborn MJ, Pham DQ, Clark CR. Dietary fiber intake and cardio-metabolic risks among US adults, NHANES 1999-2010. Am J Med 2013; 126: 1059-67

[61] Report of the Dietary Guidelines Advisory Committee on the Dietary Guidelines for Americans, 2010. [Cited 2013, February 4]. Available from http://www.cnpp.usda.gov/Publications/DietaryGuidelines/2010/PolicyDoc/ExecSumm.pdf.

CHAPTER 13

Obesity and Health: A Primer on Sleep

Yasmin Mossavar-Rahmani*,1 and Kathryn J. Reid[2]

[1]Division of Health Promotion & Nutrition Research, Department of Epidemiology & Population Health, Albert Einstein College of Medicine, Bronx, NY 10461, USA; [2]Department of Neurology, Northwestern University, Feinberg School of Medicine, Chicago, IL 60611, USA

Abstract: Sleep is one of three pillars of health along with diet and physical activity. Lack of sleep and sleep disturbances are associated with a host of negative health outcomes such as diabetes, stroke, heart disease, obesity, cognitive decline, and accelerated aging of the brain. Given the shortening of sleep duration in the US and globally, associated adverse health outcomes are of concern. The focus of this chapter is on the impact of sleep on health, how much sleep is adequate, how sleep contexts affect the quality of sleep, the circadian clock system, strategies for keeping body clocks in tune through sleep timing, food, and sleep environment, and resources for assessing sleep. These resources include self-report tools such as short questionnaires as well as objective methods such as actigraphy. Major advances include understanding the impact of diet, environment, and the circadian system on developing optimal sleep patterns. Further research is warranted on assessment of sleep patterns globally as well as understanding the impact of diet, environment, and the body clock on improving the quality of sleep.

Keywords: Actigraphy, body clock, caffeine, circadian system, diet, global health, nutrition, obesity, overweight, risk, sleep assessment questionnaires, sleep duration, sleep environment, sleep quality, wellness.

INTRODUCTION

Sleep is an important pillar of health on par with nutrition and physical activity, its importance to health has only recently been characterized. Sleep is associated with hormones relating to growth, weight regulation, and overall longevity [1, 2]. In addition, short sleep duration as well as poor sleep quality may be associated with stroke, heart disease, diabetes, insulin resistance, obesity, adverse pregnancy outcomes, sleep apnea, sleep-disordered breathing in children, behavioral issues in youth, cognitive decline, and accelerated aging of the brain [3-7]. When sleep

***Corresponding author Yasmin Mossavar-Rahmani:** Albert Einstein College of Medicine, Block Bldg. #339, 1300 Morris Park Avenue, Bronx, NY 10461; Tel: (718) 430-2136; Fax: (718) 430-8780; E-mail: yasmin.mossavar-rahmani@einstein.yu.edu

Judith Wylie-Rosett & Sunil S. Jhangiani (Eds)

is restricted the ability of fat cells to respond to insulin efficiently is impaired resulting in insulin resistance [8]. Long sleep durations, on the other hand, are associated with significant morbidity and mortality [9].

In this chapter we discuss the impact of sleep on health, how much sleep is adequate, how sleep contexts affect the quality of sleep, the circadian clock system, strategies for keeping your clocks in tune through sleep timing, food and sleep environment, and resources for assessing sleep. Resources include items such as short self-report questionnaires, sleep logs, wrist actigraphy, and assessment of circadian timing using melatonin.

HOW MUCH SLEEP IS ADEQUATE?

"Sleep is considered adequate when there is no daytime sleepiness or dysfunction [10]. While the amount of sleep varies individually, and is also related to a variety of factors such as age and physical activity, the overall recommendation is that healthy adults sleep 7-9 hours per day" [11]. According to the National Health Interview Survey (NHIS), "30% of adult civilians employed in US or approximately 40.6 million workers report an average sleep duration of ≤ 6 hr/day" [12] which is considered short sleep duration. Short sleep durations are typically defined as ≤ 6 or 7 hours, average as 7-8 hours, and long as ≥ 9 hours. However, the determination is best done based on the distribution of sleep duration in the specific population under study. Short sleep duration is associated with sub-optimal dietary patterns high in snacks and calories, increased exposure to light at night, sleep apnea, noisy and unsafe neighborhoods, alcohol consumption at night and early morning, and shift or rotating shift work [13-15].

"Based on the NHIS survey among all workers at the those who usually worked the night shift 44% (representing approximately 2.2 million night shift workers), have a much higher prevalence of short sleep duration than those who work the day shift (28.8%). This number was especially alarming for individuals in the transportation, warehousing (69.7%) and health-care and social assistance (52.3%) industries" [12]. Among ethnic groups, non-Hispanic Blacks reported the highest prevalence (38.9%) while non-Hispanic whites (28.6%) and Hispanics (28.8%) reported the lowest prevalence of short sleep durations. Furthermore, because the assessment was done based on questionnaires, it is likely that sleep duration times are over-reported because *sleep latency* or the time it takes to transition into sleep is typically not accounted for. That would mean that even more civilian workers may be considered to have short sleep durations.

When objectively assessed using sleep monitors, sleep duration consists of the difference between wake and sleep times minus the time it takes to fall asleep and any awakenings during the sleep period. The time it takes to fall asleep is labeled as *sleep latency*. For example in noisy neighborhoods or unfamiliar environments it might take longer to fall asleep. In addition to difficulty falling asleep, these environmental factors and health status (sleep apnea, nocturia) may also result in fragmented sleep. The duration of these interruptions to sleep may be short (seconds) or long (minutes to hours) but both can have significant consequences on health. While reported sleep may seem to be normal (*e.g.,* 7.0 hrs) it may have taken the individual over an hour to fall asleep or he or she may have awoken several times during the night in which case this individual would be considered a short sleeper, although the self-report (time in bed) would characterize this person as a normal sleeper. That is why further assessment of sleep using objective methods is needed. We discuss self-report and more elaborate objective methods using sleep monitors to assess sleep in the section on resources.

There are several stages of sleep. In the first stage the body transitions from fast to slower brain waves and the body temperature decreases preparing the body for sleep. In the second stage the brain waves are faster (known as sleep spindles) while Delta or very slow brain waves occur in stage three. The third stage is associated with an increase in growth hormone [16]. Failure to get adequate sleep particularly during stage 3 may impact development. After this stage the body becomes more restful and the rapid eye movement (REM) or dreaming stage occurs. This stage helps consolidate memories and without this stage, the body does not feel fully rested.

Sleep changes over the lifetime, not only in duration but in structure. Infants and young adults need more sleep, whereas adults and older adults need less; however, the fragmentation of sleep as evidenced by a shorter sleep duration with age and sleep arousals is paralleled by an increase in napping during the daytime. A meta-analysis of over 3,500 healthy individuals indicated that while most sleep parameters deteriorate with age, only sleep efficiency continues to decrease after 60 years of age [17]. "Polysomnographic assessment confirms the subjective decline in sleep quality with age. Although elderly people spend more total time in bed, nocturnal sleep is both shallow and decreased in total amount, due to reductions in slow wave sleep and prolonged periods of wakefulness" [18, 19]. "In addition to age-related changes in sleep regulation, other factors have been implicated to produce sleep fragmentation in the elderly, including sleep disorders, compensation for lost sleep, increased total time in bed and lack of social and physical activity" [20-22]. Many common sleep disorders, including insomnia, sleep-disordered breathing, and restless legs increase in prevalence with age [23-28]. Furthermore, evidence suggests that medical conditions such as diabetes, cardiovascular disease, respiratory disorders, and chronic pain contribute to poor sleep in the elderly [21, 29, 30].

While the sleep patterns older of adults have been studied for many years, sleep behaviours in adolescent and of young adults have become a particular concern as 46% of 13-18 year olds and 51% of 19 to 29 yr olds (*vs* 38% of 46-64 yr olds) report that they rarely/never get a good night's sleep on weekdays [11]. This is thought to be the result of a combination of factors including the interaction between basic physiological differences in adolescents (sleep architecture and later circadian timing) and social, behavioral, and environmental factors such as early school start times, homework, extracurricular activities, and use of social networking or other computer based technologies.

HOW SLEEP CONTEXTS AFFECT THE QUALITY OF SLEEP

Sleep occurs in a variety of contexts throughout the world; individually, with a partner, extended family, and in groups. The presence of another person or persons can impact the quality of sleep by different sleep cycles with one waking up as the other falls asleep. Whether it is important to sleep continuously or in segments or have short naps is a matter of evolution, age, and health status. For example, it was (and is) not uncommon in agricultural societies for the elder of a family sleeping together to be up in the middle of the night to protect the group from predators; sleeping continuously for 8 or 9 hours in these contexts may not be possible or even desirable if there is any outside threat. Poets and artists in the 15th and 16th centuries wrote that their creativity increased in the middle of the night between the "first" and "second" sleep [31].

Patients with neurodegenerative disease such as Alzheimer's disease may have particularly discontinuous sleep with awakenings at night. These awakenings occur because the suprachiasmatic nucleus in the brain that regulates circadian rhythms is affected by the development of plaques and tangles of Alzheimer's disease.

Work factors and school schedules remain important to sleep. "For shift-workers attempts to sleep during daylight hours, when melatonin levels decline and body temperature rises, usually results in shorter sleep episodes and more wakefulness" [32, 33]. For adolescents trying to go to a 6:30 am band rehearsal or swim meet, waking up is a challenge as the production of melatonin starts later in the evening for adolescents and lasts longer into the morning. As a result, some schools have changed school start times to later hours such as 8:30 am to allow adolescents more time to sleep. Stress also plays a key role in sleep disturbance and insomnia.

THE CIRCADIAN CLOCK SYSTEM AND HOW IT AFFECTS HEALTH

The circadian clock located in the suprachiasmatic nucleus (SCN) of the hypothalamus acts as a central pacemaker to control the regulation of many physiological processes including management of sleep-wake, blood pressure, core body temperature and secretion of melatonin, and cortisol *et cetera* [34]. Each of these physiological functions has a temporal relationship with each other that is controlled *via* the SCN and this is why circadian misalignment can result in symptoms ranging from insomnia, sleepiness, and gastrointestinal upset. "The basic molecular mechanism by which SCN neurons generate and maintain a self-sustaining circadian rhythm is *via* an autoregulatory feedback loop in which oscillating circadian gene products regulate their own expression through a complex system of transcription, translation, and post-translational processes" [35].

The sleep-wake cycle is regulated by a complex interaction of circadian and homeostatic processes [36]. A basic knowledge of how these processes normally interact is useful in understanding how the circadian system and sleep disruption can impact on health. The current model of sleep-wake regulation proposes that the SCN produces an alerting signal that promotes wakefulness during the day to oppose the homeostatic sleep load build up [36, 37]. Since the homeostatic drive for sleep also increases during the course of the day, the endogenous circadian clock provides an alerting signal to allow people to stay awake until the appropriate time (~16 hours after waking). However, sleep timing and duration are also influenced by behavioral (*e.g.,* work, family, social activities, *etc.*) and environmental factors (*e.g.,* ambient light, noise, *etc.*) Disruption of these processes either by altering sleep duration or timing perhaps contributes to the associations reported between sleep and cardio-metabolic health factors.

The central circadian clock is also thought to orchestrate or control the timing of clock genes in peripheral tissues such as the liver, heart, and adrenal glands [38]. This has important implications not only for the role of factors such as feeding, light exposure, and activity on the timing of the SCN, but also on the timing within peripheral tissues. Alterations in the timing of peripheral clocks are thought to play a role in the development of cardiovascular and metabolic disorders [38]. For example, short sleep duration is not the only consequence of shift/night work, but circadian misalignment is also considered to play a significant role in the increase of cancer, diabetes, and higher BMI in this population [39-41]. However, it is difficult to untangle the complicated relationship between circadian timing and poor sleep quality/duration. With greater understanding of the consequences of the desychrony of peripheral circadian clocks, the effects of these different factors may be better understood.

"Poor sleep quality in older adults may also be caused in part by a change in the circadian timing system and/or in the interaction between the circadian and homeostatic processes [42-44]. Habitual wake time, the rise of melatonin and cortisol secretion, and endogenous temperature nadir of older subjects occur at an earlier clock hour, suggesting that the earlier wake time may be due to an advance of the circadian clock" [45, 46]. There is also recent evidence that the interaction of a reduction in the homeostatic drive for sleep and a reduction in the strength of the circadian signal promoting sleep may be responsible for the impaired sleep of older adults in the early morning [42]. Therefore, at least in part, an alteration in circadian timing and/or amplitude may be responsible for the early insomnia symptoms in older adults.

GETTING IT RIGHT: MANAGING THE BODY CLOCK

Maintaining optimal circadian timing both internally and with the external environment is believed to be beneficial for health. Strategies to maintain or improve circadian timing therefore involve both to control the external environment (such as light exposure) and the internal synchrony of rhythms such (sleeping and eating at the right circadian time).

Sleep & Diet

While there is a genetic basis for some of the sleep disturbances, behavioral strategies may be helpful in enhancing the quality of sleep. Ideally sleep may be more restful if bed-time occurs 3-4 hours from a meal and preferably with no caffeine during that time. "Late eating has been shown to be associated with higher BMI [47-49]. The amount of protein and carbohydrates consumed within 4 hours of sleep and the amount and percentage of carbohydrate and fat consumed after 8:00 pm are associated with greater total calories. Thus, eating in the evening or before sleep may predispose individuals to weight gain through higher total calories" [50]. Ingestion of large meals close to time of sleep may also affect sleep latency. The composition of the diet also affects sleep quality. For example among adolescent girls a negative association between total fat intake and quantity of REM sleep has been reported [51]. "In adult women the percentage of nocturnal fat intake correlated with sleep efficiency, sleep latency, REM latency, stage 2 sleep, REM sleep, and wake after sleep onset (WASO) and food intake near the sleeping period (dinner and late night snack) was negatively associated with sleep quality variables" [52]. In addition, manipulation of sleep stages such as suppression of slow wave sleep without a reduction in sleep duration has been shown to alter insulin sensitivity and plays an important role in glucose homeostasis [53].

"Overall those who sleep less are more likely to consume fats and refined carbohydrates; they consume fewer portions of vegetables and have more irregular meal patterns" [54-56]. In an experimental paradigm in healthy young adults when sleep was restricted to 4 hours a night for two nights there was a 24% increase in hunger, and a 32% increase in carbohydrate rich foods compared to a 10-hour night sleep opportunity [57]. On the other hand, ingested food can affect sleep through sleep promoting foods such as milk and some herbal products [10]. The mechanism of action seems to occur through synthesis of melatonin and serotonin that help promote sleep.

Foods such as caffeine, glucose, amino acids, sodium, and ethanol can reset the body clock [58, 59]. For example, eating patterns associated with the morning *vs* evening or mid-range type may differ; late risers may have more caffeine later in the day than early risers. Dimming the lights and pulling down the shades help with the shutdown needed for melatonin production.

Foods promoting sleep include melatonin-rich nighttime milk (milk of cows that are milked in darkness at night-time), herbal products such as chamomile or Valerian tea, and certain fruits such as cherries and kiwifruits. Consuming two kiwi fruits an hour before bedtime improved both the total sleep time as well as sleep efficiency, or the amount of time one is asleep after going to bed and turning off the lights, during a 4-week open clinical trial with 24 healthy subjects wearing an actigraphy watch [60]. Limited clinical evidence indicates nutritional deficiencies of magnesium or B vitamins may impair sleep [10].

Sleep & Environment

The sleep environment can have a significant impact on sleep quality. It is recommended to have a quiet, cool, dark place to sleep. Attempts to control noise include: using earplugs or white noise makers, turning off the ringer on the phone or other electronic devices, asking others in the household to keep noise at a minimum, *etc*. Keeping the sleep environment at the right temperature can be a challenge depending on the resources available to heat and cool. Keeping the room dark may mean installing black out window coverings, placing aluminum foil, black plastic or a blanket over the window and/or avoiding light exposure from electronic devices such as smart phones and computer screens close to bed-time.

Meeting these recommendations may not always be possible or culturally appropriate. City or high density living may be associated with excessive noise that is difficult to control. In some cultures it may be the norm for parents and children to sleep in the same bed. Alternative work schedules may require a person to travel for work and sleep in an unfamiliar environment or in a different time zone (jet lag), night work requires sleeping during the daytime which is warmer, lighter, and usually noisier.

Sleep & Stress

Stress can adversely affect sleep. In animal studies, for example, acute and chronic stress alters stress hormones (catecholamine, cortisol, ACTH) and decreases slow wave and rapid eye movement (REM) sleep [61]. In humans, stress results in similar changes to stress hormones and can give rise to acute or chronic insomnia (difficulty falling asleep, staying asleep or waking too early). Reducing stress by relaxation and meditation techniques and simply having a wind down period prior to sleep can reduce the impact of stress on sleep. In addition, managing aspects of day-to-day living such as regular and balanced meals and regular moderate exercise for about 30 minutes 3-4 times a week (*e.g.*, stretching, jogging, biking or hiking) may help manage and reduce stress.

RESOURCES TO ASSESS SLEEP

There are numerous tools available to assess sleep and in this section we describe both self-reported and objective measures of sleep, sleep quality, and circadian timing. Sleep quality is not simply a function of duration but also the ability to fall asleep, stay asleep, and wake at the desired times. Recently, the timing of sleep and circadian timing have also been implicated in health outcomes such that later sleep times or evening chronotype are associated with a higher BMI [47]. Therefore, the assessment of many aspects of sleep can be beneficial.

Self-report: Sleep Questionnaires

Sleep Diary

There are many different types of sleep diaries available but generally they all assess the same key elements, even though the wording of the specific questions may differ. A comprehensive sleep diary should include at a minimum the following items during the week (work/school days) and on week-end (no-work/no school) days: time when sleep is attempted (bed time), time of sleep onset and offset, time out of bed, and minutes one is awake after falling asleep.

Sleepiness

As mentioned earlier the amount of sleep needed varies among individuals and is considered adequate when there is no excessive sleepiness when one is awake. A simple question such as "Do you feel excessively sleepy?" has been shown to be associated with poor physical and mental health related quality of life [62]. "Clinically, daytime sleep propensity and sleepiness is often assessed subjectively using the Epworth Sleepiness Scale (ESS). The ESS asks a measurement of a person's general level of daytime sleep propensity: it asks individuals to estimate the likelihood of dozing off or falling asleep in 8 different sedentary situations" [63, 64]. The ESS correlates to some extent with mean sleep latencies on the objective Multiple Sleep Latency Test (MSLT) and with the degree to which people complain of sleepiness [65, 66]. The ESS has been used extensively as a subjective measure of sleepiness.

Risk for Sleep Disordered Breathing

Medical conditions such as obstructive sleep apnea can negatively impact the quality of sleep and is associated with poor cardio-metabolic outcomes. Risk of sleep apnea can be assessed by questionnaires such as the Berlin or the STOP or STOP-Bang questionnaires [67, 68]. These questionnaires are designed to identify adult patients who are likely to have sleep apnea. They include questions about snoring behavior, wake time sleepiness or fatigue, and the presence of obesity or hypertension [69].

Sleep Quality

A questionnaire that is commonly used to assess sleep quality is the Pittsburgh Sleep Quality Index (PSQI). A score of 5 or greater on this questionnaire has been associated with poor sleep quality. "This self-rated 21 item questionnaire assesses individual sleep habits (bedtime, morning rising time, sleep-onset latency, and night sleep duration), insomnia, and hypnotic use over a 1-month time interval. The PSQI has been widely applied in a variety of clinical settings and epidemiological studies in many countries, because of its satisfactory psychometric properties" [70].

Chronotype

The timing of sleep can also impact on sleep quality. In general, there is a preferred timing of sleep that is thought to be associated with the timing of the internal circadian clock, but may also be influenced by social, occupational and environmental factors. Sleeping at the "wrong" time can result in disruptions in sleep and in extreme cases, circadian rhythm sleep disorders. There are two main tools that are used in research to assess chronotype: the Horne-Ostberg morning-evening questionnaire [71] and the Munich Chronotype questionnaire [72]. These questionnaires characterize individuals on whether they are likely to have an evening, morning, or intermediate preference to sleep and conduct daily activities. Chronotype is also associated with age, in that people tend to become more morning type, *i.e.,* they usually wake up early and go to bed early in the evening, as they become older [73].

Objective Data: Polysomnography, Actigraphy, and Salivary Melatonin

Sleep-wake cycles, sleepiness, and circadian timing can also be assessed objectively in various ways. These techniques are generally reserved for clinical or research purposes due to the technical expertise needed in the collection and interpretation, and the associated expense.

Polysomnography (PSG)

Polysomnography is the gold standard in determining sleep-wake. This technique includes measurements of electroencephalographic (EEG), electrooculographic

(EOG), and submental electromyographic (EMG) signals. However, due to the expense in recording and interpreting the findings and the inconvenience of the technique it is not always feasible to measure PSG for long periods of time over many days. PSG monitoring in the home is becoming more common but usually for a single night or a few days at most.

Actigraphy

Wrist actigraphy monitoring measures rest-activity cycles and is a surrogate marker of sleep-wake timing, and correlates well with PSG measures of sleep when sleep is normal [74, 75]. Several measures derived from the rest-activity cycle and commercially available algorithms used to determine sleep-wake timing become less reliable as sleep becomes more disturbed. However, it is an excellent tool in determining overall rest-activity patterns over extended periods. Actigraphy is used extensively in research and to some extent clinically to objectively assess patterns and timing of sleep-wake.

Multiple Sleep Latency Test (Sleep Propensity/Sleepiness)

For the Multiple Sleep Latency Test (MSLT), the person will lay in a quiet, temperature controlled, darkened room and be instructed to "lay still, close your eyes and try to go to sleep" during five, 20 minute nap opportunities every 2 hours beginning 2 hours after initial morning awakening [76]. Sleep onset latency is determined as the time from lights out to either 3 consecutive epochs of stage 1 or any one epoch of other sleep stages. In the absence of sleep, the nap opportunity is concluded after 20 minutes. There are published normal age-specific sleep onset latencies.

Melatonin as a Marker of Circadian Timing

Melatonin is a hormone produced by the pineal gland and its production is directly controlled *via* the suprachiasmatic nucleus or master circadian time keeper and is widely considered to be the best marker of circadian timing currently available in humans. Light exposure will directly suppress melatonin production so care is needed during sampling to keep light levels low (candle light) so as not to artificially alter the levels. Melatonin levels may be measured from blood, saliva, or *via* the primary metabolite 6-sulphatoxy-melatonin in urine. The timing of the melatonin rhythm is most commonly assessed by the dim light melatonin onset (DLMO) in either blood or saliva.

CONCLUSION

In summary, sleep is an important pillar of health. Further research on the impact of environment, genetics, diet (both quality and meal timing) and physical activity on sleep has the potential to provide important insights in the prevention of chronic disease and promotion of longevity.

ACKNOWLEDGEMENTS

Declared none.

CONFLICT OF INTEREST

The authors confirm that they do not have any conflicts of interest related to this chapter.

REFERENCES

[1] Ayas NT, White DP, Al-Delaimy WK, *et al.* A prospective study of self-reported sleep duration and incident diabetes in women. Diabetes Care 2003 Feb; 26(2): 380-4.

[2] Patel SR, Hu FB. Short sleep duration and weight gain: a systematic review. Obesity (Silver Spring) 2008 Mar; 16(3): 643-53.

[3] Ayas NT, White DP, Manson JE, *et al.* A prospective study of sleep duration and coronary heart disease in women. Arch Intern Med 2003 Jan 27; 163(2): 205-9.

[4] Chaput JP, Despres JP, Bouchard C, *et al.* Short sleep duration is associated with reduced leptin levels and increased adiposity: Results from the Quebec family study. Obesity (Silver Spring) 2007 Jan; 15(1): 253-61.

[5] Knutson KL, Spiegel K, Penev P, *et al.* The metabolic consequences of sleep deprivation. Sleep Med Rev 2007 Jun; 11(3): 163-78.

[6] Moore M, Bonuck K. Comorbid Symptoms of Sleep-Disordered Breathing and Behavioral Sleep Problems From 18-57 Months of Age: A Population-Based Study. Behav Sleep Med 2013; 11(3): 222-30.

[7] Stamatakis KA, Kaplan GA, Roberts RE. Short sleep duration across income, education, and race/ethnic groups: population prevalence and growing disparities during 34 years of follow-up. Ann Epidemiol 2007 Dec; 17(12): 948-55.

[8] Broussard JL, Ehrmann DA, Van Cauter E, *et al.* Impaired insulin signaling in human adipocytes after experimental sleep restriction: a randomized, crossover study. Ann Intern Med 2012 Oct 16; 157(8): 549-57.

[9] Patel SR, Malhotra A, Gottlieb DJ, *et al.* Correlates of long sleep duration. Sleep 2006 Jul; 29(7): 881-9.

[10] Peuhkuri K, Sihvola N, Korpela R. Diet promotes sleep duration and quality. Nutr Res 2012 May; 32(5): 309-19.

[11] Sleep Foundation. How much sleep do we really need? [updated 1/5/2014; cited 2/24/14]. Available from http://www.sleepfoundation.org/alert/how-sleep-works/how-much-sleep-do-we-really-need.

[12] Luckhaupt S. Short sleep duration among workers: United States 2010. Morbidity & Mortality Weekly Report 2012; 61(16): 281-5.

[13] Chaput JP, McNeil J, Despres JP, *et al.* Short sleep duration is associated with greater alcohol consumption in adults. Appetite 2012 Dec; 59(3): 650 5.

[14] Fonken LK, Workman JL, Walton JC, *et al.* Light at night increases body mass by shifting the time of food intake. Proc Natl Acad Sci U S A 2010 Oct 26; 107(43): 18664-9.
[15] Carnethon KK, Kim K, de Chavez PJ, *et al.* Racial/ethnic differences in sleep duration and quality in a population sample. Sleep 2012: 35.
[16] Van Cauter E, Plat L, Scharf MB, *et al.* Simultaneous stimulation of slow-wave sleep and growth hormone secretion by gamma-hydroxybutyrate in normal young Men. J Clin Invest 1997 Aug 1; 100(3): 745-53.
[17] Ohayon MM, Carskadon MA, Guilleminault C, *et al.* Meta-analysis of quantitative sleep parameters from childhood to old age in healthy individuals: developing normative sleep values across the human lifespan. Sleep 2004 Nov 1; 27(7): 1255-73.
[18] Allen SR, Seiler WO, Stahelin HB, *et al.* Seventy-two hour polygraphic and behavioral recordings of wakefulness and sleep in a hospital geriatric unit: comparison between demented and nondemented patients. Sleep 1987; 10(2): 143-59.
[19] Dement WC, Miles L, Carskadon M. "White Paper" on sleep and the elderly. J Am Geriatr Soc 1982; 30: 25-50.
[20] Ancoli-Israel S, Parker L, Sinaee R, *et al.* Sleep fragmentation in patients from a nursing home. J Gerontol 1989; 44(1): M18-21.
[21] Bliwise NG. Factors related to sleep quality in healthy elderly women. Psychol Aging 1992; 7(1): 83-8.
[22] Jacobs D, Ancoli-Israel S, Parker L, *et al.* Twenty-four-hour sleep-wake patterns in a nursing home population. Psychol Aging 1989; 4(3): 352-6.
[23] Ancoli-Israel S, Klauber MR, Butters N, *et al.* Dementia in institutionalized elderly: relation to sleep apnea. Journal of the American Geriatric Society 1991; 39(3): 258-63.
[24] Ancoli-Israel S, Kripke DF. Prevalent sleep problems in the aged. Biofeedback Self Regul 1991; 16(4): 349-59.
[25] Ancoli-Israel S, Kripke DF, Klauber MR, *et al.* Morbidity, mortality and sleep-disordered breathing in community dwelling elderly. Sleep 1996; 19(4): 277-82.
[26] Bliwise DL. Chronologic age, physiologic age and mortality in sleep apnea. Sleep 1996; 19(4): 275-6.
[27] Mant A, King M, Saunders NA, *et al.* Four-year follow-up of mortality and sleep-related respiratory disturbance in non-demented seniors. Sleep 1995; 18(6): 433-8.
[28] Youngstedt SD, Kripke DF, Klauber MR, *et al.* Periodic leg movements during sleep and sleep disturbances in elders. J Gerontol A Biol Sci Med Sci 1998; 53(5): M391-4.
[29] Foley DJ, Monjan AA, Brown SL, *et al.* Sleep complaints among elderly persons: an epidemiologic study of three communities. Sleep 1995; 18(6): 425-32.
[30] Maggi S, Langlois JA, Minicuci N *et al.* Sleep complaints in community-dwelling older persons: prevalence, associated factors, and reported causes. J Am Geriatr Soc 1998; 46(2): 161-8.
[31] Randall K. Decoding the science of sleep. Wall Street Journal 2012.
[32] Burgard S, Ailshire J. Putting work to bed: stressful experiences on the job and sleep quality. Population Studies Center research report 08-652. Ann Arbor, MI: : University of Michigan; 2008. Available from: http://www.psc.isr.umich.edu/pubs/pdf/rr08-652.pdf.
[33] Dijk DJ, Duffy JF, Riel E, *et al.* Ageing and the circadian and homeostatic regulation of human sleep during forced desynchrony of rest, melatonin and temperature rhythms. J Physiol 1999 Apr 15; 516 (Pt 2): 611-27.
[34] Klein DC, Moore RY, Reppert SM. Suprachiasmatic Nucleus - The Mind's Clock. New York: Oxford University Press, 1991.
[35] Dunlap JC. Molecular bases for circadian clocks. Cell 1999 Jan 22; 96(2): 271-90.
[36] Borbely AA. A two process model of sleep regulation. Hum Neurobiol 1982; 1(3): 195-204.
[37] Edgar DM, Dement WC, Fuller CA. Effect of SCN lesions on sleep in squirrel monkeys: evidence for opponent processes in sleep-wake regulation. J Neurosci 1993 Mar; 13(3): 1065-79.
[38] Albrecht U. Timing to perfection: the biology of central and peripheral circadian clocks. Neuron 2012 Apr 26; 74(2): 246-60.
[39] Esquirol Y, Perret B, Ruidavets JB, *et al.* Shift work and cardiovascular risk factors: new knowledge from the past decade. Arch Cardiovasc Dis 2011 Dec; 104(12): 636-68.

[40] Karlsson BH, Knutsson AK, Lindahl BO, *et al.* Metabolic disturbances in male workers with rotating three-shift work. Results of the WOLF study. Int Arch Occup Environ Health 2003 Jul; 76(6): 424-30.
[41] Van Amelsvoort LG, Schouten EG, Kok FJ. Duration of shiftwork related to body mass index and waist to hip ratio. Int J Obes Relat Metab Disord 1999 Sep; 23(9): 973-8.
[42] Dijk D-J, Edgar DM. Circadian and homeostatic control of wakefulness and sleep. In: Turek FW, Zee PC, editors. Regulation of Sleep and Circadian Rhythms. New York: Marcel Dekker, Inc.; 1999; p. 111-47.
[43] Miles LE, Dement WC. Sleep and aging. Sleep 1980; 3(2): 1-220.
[44] Weitzman ED, Moline ML, Czeisler CA, *et al.* Chronobiology of aging: Temperature, sleep-wake rhythms and entrainment. Neurobiol Aging 1982; 3: 299-309.
[45] Czeisler CA, Dumont M, Duffy JF, *et al.* Association of sleep-wake habits in older people with changes in output of circadian pacemaker. Lancet 1992; 340(8825): 933-6.
[46] Van Coevorden A, Mockel J, Laurent E, *et al.* Neuroendocrine rhythms and sleep in aging men. Am J Physiol 1991; 260: E651-E61.
[47] Baron KG, Reid KJ, Kern AS, *et al.* Role of sleep timing in caloric intake and BMI. Obesity (Silver Spring) 2011 Jul; 19(7): 1374-81.
[48] Corbalan-Tutau MD, Madrid JA, Garaulet M. Timing and duration of sleep and meals in obese and normal weight women. Association with increase blood pressure. Appetite 2012 Aug; 59(1): 9-16.
[49] Hsieh SD, Muto T, Murase T, *et al.* Association of short sleep duration with obesity, diabetes, fatty liver and behavioral factors in Japanese men. Intern Med 2011; 50(21): 2499-502.
[50] Baron KG, Reid KJ, Horn LV, *et al.* Contribution of evening macronutrient intake to total caloric intake and body mass index. Appetite 2013 Jan; 60(1): 246-51.
[51] Awad KM, Drescher AA, Malhotra A, *et al.* Effects of exercise and nutritional intake on sleep architecture in adolescents. Sleep Breath 2012 Jan 31.
[52] Crispim CA, Zimberg IZ, dos Reis BG, *et al.* Relationship between food intake and sleep pattern in healthy individuals. J Clin Sleep Med 2011 Dec 15; 7(6): 659-64.
[53] Tasali E, Leproult R, Ehrmann DA, *et al.* Slow-wave sleep and the risk of type 2 diabetes in humans. Proc Natl Acad Sci U S A 2008 Jan 22; 105(3): 1044-9.
[54] Grandner MA, Kripke DF, Naidoo N, *et al.* Relationships among dietary nutrients and subjective sleep, objective sleep, and napping in women. Sleep Med 2010 Feb; 11(2): 180-4.
[55] Shi Z, McEvoy M, Luu J, *et al.* Dietary fat and sleep duration in Chinese men and women. Int J Obes (Lond) 2008 Dec; 32(12): 1835-40.
[56] Weiss A, Xu F, Storfer-Isser A, *et al.* The association of sleep duration with adolescents' fat and carbohydrate consumption. Sleep 2010 Sep; 33(9): 1201-9.
[57] Spiegel K, Tasali E, Penev P, *et al.* Brief communication: Sleep curtailment in healthy young men is associated with decreased leptin levels, elevated ghrelin levels, and increased hunger and appetite. Ann Intern Med 2004 Dec 7; 141(11): 846-50.
[58] Sherman H, Gutman R, Chapnik N, *et al.* Caffeine alters circadian rhythms and expression of disease and metabolic markers. Int J Biochem Cell Biol 2011 May; 43(5): 829-38.
[59] Froy O. Metabolism and circadian rhythms--implications for obesity. Endocr Rev 2010 Feb; 31(1): 1-24.
[60] Lin HH, Tsai PS, Fang SC, *et al.* Effect of kiwifruit consumption on sleep quality in adults with sleep problems. Asia Pac J Clin Nutr 2011; 20(2): 169-74.
[61] Han KS, Kim L, Shim I. Stress and sleep disorder. Exp Neurobiol 2012 Dec; 21(4): 141-50.
[62] Reid KJ, Martinovich Z, Finkel S, *et al.* Sleep: a marker of physical and mental health in the elderly. Am J Geriatr Psychiatry 2006 Oct; 14(10): 860-6.
[63] Johns MW. A new method for measuring daytime sleepiness: the Epworth sleepiness scale. Sleep 1991 Dec; 14(6): 540-5.
[64] Johns MW. Reliability and factor analysis of the Epworth Sleepiness Scale. Sleep 1992; 15(4): 376-81.
[65] Chervin RD, Aldrich MS, Pickett R, *et al.* Comparison of the results of the Epworth Sleepiness Scale and the Multiple Sleep Latency Test. J Psychosom Res 1997 Feb; 42(2): 145-55.
[66] Fong SY, Ho CK, Wing YK. Comparing MSLT and ESS in the measurement of excessive daytime sleepiness in obstructive sleep apnoea syndrome. J Psychosom Res 2005 Jan; 58(1): 55-60.

[67] Chung F, Subramanyam R, Liao P, *et al.* High STOP-Bang score indicates a high probability of obstructive sleep apnoea. Br J Anaesth 2012 May; 108(5): 768-75.

[68] Vana KD, Silva GE, Goldberg R. Predictive abilities of the STOP-Bang and Epworth Sleepiness Scale in identifying sleep clinic patients at high risk for obstructive sleep apnea. Res Nurs Health 2013 Feb; 36(1): 84-94.

[69] Netzer NC, Stoohs RA, Netzer CM, *et al.* Using the Berlin Questionnaire to identify patients at risk for the sleep apnea syndrome. Ann Intern Med 1999 Oct 5; 131(7): 485-91.

[70] Buysse DJ, Reynolds CFd, Monk TH, *et al.* The Pittsburgh Sleep Quality Index: a new instrument for psychiatric practice and research. Psychiatry Res 1989; 28(2): 193-213.

[71] Horne JA, Ostberg O. A self-assessment questionnaire to determine morningness-eveningness in human circadian rhythms. Int J Chronobiol 1976; 4(2): 97-110.

[72] Zavada A, Gordijn MC, Beersma DG, *et al.* Comparison of the Munich Chronotype Questionnaire with the Horne-Ostberg's Morningness-Eveningness Score. Chronobiol Int 2005; 22(2): 267-78.

[73] Roenneberg T, Allebrandt KV, Merrow M, *et al.* Social jetlag and obesity. Curr Biol 2012 May 22; 22(10): 939-43.

[74] Practice parameters for the use of actigraphy in the clinical assessment of sleep disorders. American Sleep Disorders Association. Sleep 1995; 18(4): 285-7.

[75] Ancoli-Israel S, Cole R, Alessi C, *et al.* The role of actigraphy in the study of sleep and circadian rhythms. Sleep 2003 May 1; 26(3): 342-92.

[76] Arand D, Bonnet M, Hurwitz T, *et al.* The clinical use of the MSLT and MWT. Sleep 2005 Jan; 28(1): 123-44.

CHAPTER 14

Yoga and Meditation: Antidotes to Civilization

Sonia Suchday*[,1], Yvette Fruchter[2], Lauren Hagemann[2] and Anthony F. Santoro[2]

[1]Department of Psychology, PACE University, New York, NY 10007, USA; [2]Graduate Students, Department of Psychology Yeshiva University, Ferkauf Graduate School of Psychology, 1165 Morris Park Avenue, Bronx, NY, USA

Abstract: The rapid spread and chronic nature of diseases of civilization have created a scenario where local and traditional medicine is ill-equipped to deal with health and wellness. Low cost public health prevention and intervention efforts are key elements in stemming the tide of diseases arising from fast-paced globalization. Diseases travel across borders, so do modalities of health. The mingling of Eastern and Western methods of health and wellness has given rise to the practice of various mind-body techniques. Yoga and meditation, categorized as mind-body therapies, are examples of this cross-fertilization of treatments between the East and the West. Both yoga and meditation have been described as useful and effective health and stress management tools that can alleviate the negative physical effects of stress by improving neuroendocrine status, metabolic function, inflammation, HPA regulation and parasympathetic nervous system tone. Yoga and meditation benefit health *via* their effect on obesity and diseases such as coronary heart disease and diabetes mellitus. The inexpensive nature of yoga and meditation practice makes them attractive public health tools. With the increasing impact of globalization, the arsenal of public health tools should include traditional and modern medical approaches from both Eastern and Western traditions. This sharing of regional and culture-bound health practices offersthe opportunity to implement potentially effective public health programs within unexplored geographic locations and settings. Yoga and meditation are ancient wellness techniques that can be used in combination with traditional medicine to reduce the global escalation of obesity and related chronic illnesses.

Keywords: Yoga, meditation, obesity, relaxation, stress management, Eastern medicine, Western medicine, global health, overweight, wellness, risk, behavior, lifestyle-related diseases.

INTRODUCTION

Yoga and meditation are categorized as mind-body therapies, which are largely cross-fertilization of treatments between the East and the West. Both yoga and

***Corresponding author Sonia Suchday:** Dyson College of Arts and Sciences of Pace University 41 Park Row, Rm 1313, NY 10007, USA; Tel: (212) 346-1618; Fax: (212) 346-1618; E-mail: ssuchday@pace.edu

Judith Wylie-Rosett & Sunil S. Jhangiani (Eds)

meditation are used to alleviate the negative physical effects of stress by improving neuroendocrine status, metabolic function, inflammation, HPA regulation and parasympathetic nervous system tone. Yoga and meditation are also potentially beneficial in treating obesity and diseases such as coronary heart disease and diabetes mellitus. This chapter will examine how traditional Eastern wellness techniques and perspectives can be incorporated effectively into the contemporary, industrialized society. Specifically, the chapter will provide an overview of yoga and meditation as well as explore evidence of their efficacy for stress, obesity and metabolic syndrome. Additionally, the integration of yoga and meditation into a variety of unique settings and their usage as a public health technique will be discussed.

OBESITY AND CIVILIZATION

In recent decades, the prevalence of obesity and the metabolic syndrome has escalated in both the developed and developing countries [1, 2]. Researchers suggest that the growth of contemporary metropolitan societies has fueled the rise of obesity and describe the phenomenon as "the civilization syndrome" [3]. Rapid and drastic lifestyle changes in exercise, dietary habits, and various health behaviors were an outgrowth of the Industrial Revolution [4]. However, genetic adaptations that would allow humanity to flourish under these new conditions have lagged behind [5]. Obesogenic habits such as over-nutrition, inactive lifestyle, sleep deprivation and smoking are widespread worldwide [1, 3]. Chronic exposure to environmental stress is also hypothesized to be an important factor associated with such poor health habits as well as the increase in obesity rates throughout the world [1, 6]. Globalization, characterized by the spread of industrialization, urbanization, economic development, related consumer behaviors, unhealthy lifestyles (*e.g.*, high-density fast food) and a sedentary lifestyle as well as elevated stress, has led to the adoption of a "modern" lifestyle by the developing countries, particularly among individuals trying to reconcile beliefs/behaviors that are not native to the local culture with local, traditional beliefs and practices [2, 7, 8]. Thus, the "civilization syndrome" and "modern lifestyles" are worldwide phenomena, posing a growing threat to the health on a global scale [9].

Obesity is a prominent risk factor for various chronic diseases such as metabolic syndrome, heart disease and diabetes. Metabolic syndrome refers to a group of risk factors that increase the likelihood of chronic health conditions, including diabetes, heart disease and strokes [10]. Core features include insulin resistance, glucose intolerance, atherogenic dyslipidemia (*i.e.*, high triglycerides and low HDL cholesterol), visceral adiposity, and hypertension [11]. It is a complex condition that involves numerous interrelated factors such as hypercoagulation, chronic inflammation, endothelial dysfunction and oxidative stress [12]. Additionally, chronic stress and negative affective states such as depression and anxiety are associated with the symptoms of metabolic syndrome. Thus, it is essential to identify prevention and management strategies for this cluster of risk factors that effectively address the multilayered underlying components.

Mind-body therapies (MBT) may offer strategies that can be used in combination with diet, physical activity and medicine to improve symptoms associated with the metabolic syndrome and obesity. MBT, which originate from ancient, traditional Eastern medicine, include physical postures, mental exercises and breathing techniques to attain a balanced integration of mind, body and soul. Examples of mind-body medicine include meditation, yoga, relaxation, visual imagery, biofeedback, qi gong and tai chi [10]. Overweight and/or obese individuals and those with a sedentary lifestyle may be incapable of or uninterested in engaging in physical activity. Yoga and meditation are simple, inexpensive and noninvasive therapies that require minimal equipment and may provide added benefits of relaxation and serenity [10]. Research indicates that MBT, such as yoga and meditation, have beneficial effects in the treatment of cardiovascular disease, recurrent myocardial infarction, overweight/obesity, and impact on risky behaviors such as smoking and a sedentary lifestyle [13].

YOGA & MEDITATION: THE BASICS

The traditional Eastern practice of yoga and meditation does not clearly distinguish between them. Rather, both are viewed as part of a disciplined lifestyle towards achieving Nirvana or eternal bliss along with vegetarianism and breathing practices. Yoga and meditation are practiced early in the morning to accrue maximum benefits to health and well-being [14-22]. However, in the West, both yoga and meditation are regarded as techniques to achieve optimum health and well-being. Hence, yoga and meditation will be discussed as two distinct identities.

Yoga

Yoga is an approach to wellness that began during the Indus Valley Civilization around the year 3000 BC, although some research suggests a more ancient origin

[14]. The term yoga is derived from the Sanskrit word yoke, meaning to join or bring together, more specifically, joining nature (Prakriti), with spirit (Purusha) [15]. This “joining” rarely comes naturally and is in fact a very active process, requiring years of commitment and dedicated practice. Practitioners of yoga believe that through consistent practice of the physical postures, deep breathing, and meditative techniques, yoga can lead to an enduring life of happiness and health, with complete physical and mental peace and harmony [16-18].

A true yoga practice includes the compilation and implementation of eight “limbs”. This construct provides a holistic characterization of how the practice of yoga emphasizes the mind-body-spirit connection. These limbs include yama (universal ethics), niyama (individual ethics), asana (physical postures), pranayama (breath control), pratyahara (control of the senses), dharana (concentration), dhyana (meditation) and samadhi (bliss) [19].

As cultures and societies evolved and changed, yoga practice has been adapted, since for centuries in both the East and the West. This adaptation has resulted in the development of various forms of yoga to accommodate to cultural changes. For example, Eastern cultures view yoga and meditation as a way of life, whereas Western societies seek to implement these practices as a form of intervention, therapy, or an alternative or adjunct therapy along with conventional western medicine and exercise. The most commonly practiced styles of yoga in the Western world include Hatha, Iyengar, Sudarshan Kriya and Meditative yoga. Each of these styles stresses a different aspect of relaxation, ranging from a strict focus on postures (asanas), in order to bring about the physical and health benefits such as flexibility, muscle strengthening and fitness, to emphasizing one’s breath (pranayama) which has been shown to promote a state of awareness and mindfulness [20, 21]. Additionally, the aim of Raja yoga, also known as ashtanga yoga, is self-realization or liberation. It is considered as yoga of the mind because of its emphasis on the awareness of one’s state of mind [22].

Meditation

As mentioned earlier, the use of meditation in the Western cultures is another example of how the practice of yoga has transformed in recent decades. Meditation, which has already been identified as one limb of yoga, seems to have evolved into its own individualized skill and/or practice. The utility of meditation is designed to promote attention, focus and concentration, with the ultimate goal to achieve a heightened sense of well-being and the physiological responses related to relaxation such as lowering of blood pressure [21, 23].

Meditation has been well researched as being one of the most productive forms of stress reduction as well as being a useful tool to assist with the management of anxiety and depressive symptoms [24, 25]. Meditative techniques, such as mindfulness, or the focused attention on the present moment and acceptance, have also shown to aid in improving exercise habits, *i.e.*, increase in physical activity, leading to weight loss and other health benefits [26].

As with yoga, there are many variations of meditation. One of the most popular styles, Transcendental Meditation (TM), is mantra-based. A mantra is a sound, syllable, word, or a group of words. Transcendental meditation aims to promote focused attention and prevent distracting thoughts by active repetition of a word, sound or symbol [25]. Traditional Eastern perspectives indicate that this recitation is a key to spiritual transformation. According to Western therapies, specifically the cognitive-behavioral perspective, reciting a mantra on a regular basis trains the mind and serves multiple purposes, including the prevention of distressing cognitive activation such as worry and excessive thinking (often associated with anxiety/depression), achieving an enhanced sense of awareness and clarity, improved decision making, and enhancement of coping abilities [25]. Another popular form of meditation includes Mindfulness Meditation (MM) [27], which emphasizes on staying focused in the present moment, suspending judgment and accepting reality [28]. Mechanisms for achieving present-focused awareness include focusing on the experience of bodily sensations and states (*e.g.*, relaxation *versus* tension, breathing, *etc.*), and paying attention to ongoing thoughts and emotions. Specific techniques include guided imagery, body scans (focusing your attention on your body and how it feels, assessing tension/relaxation throughout your body) and deep breathing [29]. Tables **1** and **2** compare the characteristics and perspectives of yoga and meditation.

Prevalence of Yoga and Meditation

Healthcare is a global concern. There seems to be a constant race in the healthcare industry to develop new medications and interventions to help prevent, treat and cure disease. Barriers to accessing appropriate care, including financial, systemic or infrastructure deficits, inefficient education and training have led to evolving global interest in low cost prevention and intervention such as yoga and meditation.

Table 1. Characteristics of yoga and meditation.

	Yoga	Meditation
Definition	The joining of nature and spirit that leads to eternal peace and harmony	A conscious focus on a sound, object, or image that promotes awareness of the present moment
Benefits	Enhances the physical, mental, emotional, and spiritual dimensions of an individual	Promotes attention, focus and concentration Achieves a heightened sense of well being Attains physiological responses related to relaxation
Techniques/Styles	Hatha: Slow paced, gentle yoga practice which includes basic postures Iyengar: Emphasizes body alignment *via* holding poses for longer durations of time and use of props (blocks/straps) Sudarshan Kriya: Utilizes rhythmic breathing which better enhances the connection and flowing movement between postures and breath Meditative Yoga: Focuses on the mind, spirit, action and body and not just the body itself	Transcendental Meditation: Prevents distracting thoughts by active repetition of a mantra Mindfulness Meditation: Emphasizes staying present focused, suspension of judgment and promoting acceptance Guided imagery Body scans Deep breathing

Table 2. Perspectives of yoga and meditation.

	Yoga & Meditation
Eastern Perspectives	A way of life requiring daily practice and dedication A practice that creates a balanced state of mind and body to obtain spiritual union with a higher power
Western Perspectives	A leisure or recreational activity An intervention that achieves physical fitness, health benefits, emotional stability and peace of mind

In the West, alternative medicine (also referred to as complementary alternative medicine or CAM) has been defined as any medical intervention or approach that does not typically follow general medical philosophies. Although evidence is accumulating, these alternative methods to conventional medicine lack scientific explanation for effectiveness as compared to the traditional Western medicine approaches [30]. Research indicates a wide range of interest in the use of alternative methods of medicine in industrialized countries, such as the United States, Australia, Canada, United Kingdom and most of Europe. It has been noted that greater than 50% of the populations of these and other developed countries have endorsed engaging in some form of complimentary or alternative medicine, with yoga and meditation being popular choices [31, 32]. Prevalence of use in these countries is as follows: USA 42%, Australia 48%, France 49% and Canada 70% [32].

Alternative medicine is an expansive subject area ranging the gamut from herbal remedies and dietary supplements to acupuncture, massage therapy and chiropractic medicine [33]. Yoga and meditation are two examples of alternative therapies and contribute a significant fraction of the percentages outlined above. For example, of the population using alternative medicine in Australia, 17.5% utilized meditation and 12% practiced yoga [34]. Similar trends are evident in the United States, where roughly 8-10% of the population endorsing CAM use, report practicing yoga at least once in their lifetime [35]. Other CAM practices widely used in developed countries include herbal medicines and supplements, massage, relaxation and chiropractic medicine [30].

Research has identified certain social and demographic characteristics which appear to be associated with yoga and meditation use. A recent meta-analysis of studies conducted on non-clinical samples throughout the United States and United Kingdom indicated that across numerous studies, women far exceeded men in yoga use [36]. In fact, among women, there appears to be a two-fold increase in the use of such practices as yoga, meditation and guided imagery [36]. This gender disparity may be related to the notion that females tend to be more proactive about self-care and consequently seek medical and health care treatment, including alternative treatments, more readily as compared to men [37].

Although both education and income predict CAM use, however, in-depth analyses suggest that education may be more influential as compared to income in determining CAM use [31]. The picture regarding the utilization of yoga and meditation among individuals of different ages and ethnicities is complex. Their use has primarily been seen in young and middle-aged adults; however with the aging of the baby boom generation, this trend may shift; geriatric cohorts are becoming increasingly acceptable and are interested in exploring the benefits of yoga and meditation exercises. The variety of ethnicities drawn to yoga and meditation is also multi-faceted. A steady increase in interest is observed among Caucasians, African American, Hispanics and Asian populations [34].

Growing Popularity in Developing Countries

There has been a misconception that yoga/meditation and other alternative practices are primarily used by the "well-educated and wealthy" [31]. However, data indicating the widespread use of alternative therapies in the developing economies of South American and African population as compared to trends observed in more industrialized nations challenges the notion of it being primarily used among the affluent people of the world. For example, data indicate that 80% of the population in various South American and African countries reports engagement in some modality of alternative treatment including yoga and meditation as compared to 50% of the population of industrialized nations [32]. Additionally, it has been noted that most people in developing countries choose to remain loyal to local, traditional medicine instead of turning to more conventional Western pharmaceutical approaches to care popular in the industrialized countries [38].

Affordability may be an important factor contributing to the popularity of yoga and meditation in developing nations. Yoga is an inexpensive intervention that is easy to sustain, requiring little to no equipment or professional personnel [39]. When other forms of health care are not readily accessible, these countries can turn to yoga and meditation to enhance health and well-being.

The flexibility of yoga with its diverse forms and styles makes it easily adaptable to the needs of diverse medically vulnerable patients, including those struggling with obesity and other health risks. The availability of instructional DVDs, videos, books and other literature, as well as interactive video games, means that the practice of yoga is no longer confined to the walls of a yoga studio. The fact that such resources are available at a fraction of the cost of a typical treatment means that more of the world's population can access its various benefits.

Growing Popularity in the United States

Although yoga/meditation practices are rising in popularity in the Western world, specifically in the United States, it is important to acknowledge the vastly different ways in which they are utilized when compared to Eastern cultures. Since the early 1970's, yoga and meditation have become part of American society and trends show continued growth in popularity [15, 40]. The number of Americans who have used the techniques ranges from approximately 15 million to 30 million people [29, 41].

The appeal of yoga in Western culture is quite distinct from the traditional boundaries of practice. Unlike Eastern cultures, where yoga and meditation seem to be a way of life, requiring daily practice, the Western world has internalized the practice of yoga and meditation as interventions to attain health benefits, holistic self-awareness, emotional stability and peace of mind, and has developed a less regimented commitment [42].

According to the World Health Organization [43], more than 1.4 billion adults in the world are diagnosed as clinically obese, with the global population of obesity doubling within the past 30 years. There is an urgent need to develop universal and effective interventions that can be implemented on a global scale to combat this pandemic. The effectiveness and flexibility that yoga and meditation exhibit suggest that they are good global health strategies and should be paid special attention.

YOGA AND MEDITATION AS TREATMENT TOOLS

For Stress-Management

Globalization, with its accelerated pace of development, is an inherently stressful process which requires individuals and communities to adapt to rapidly changing realities. The overpowering influence of globalization and the related stress on human society in recent times make stress a particularly important by-product of civilization. Stress involves a threat to an organism's natural equilibrium or homeostasis [8]. Stressors may be external, such as relationship or employment problems, or internal, such as under-nutrition. The stress response comprises of behavioral and physiological reactions produced by animals to regain homeostasis, and entails a complex network of brain structures such as the hypothalamus, amygdala and prefrontal cortex. Although a short-term stress response is essential for individuals to cope with stress, over time this essential response can become maladaptive; especially if the stress is chronic and intense [44, 45]. Stress along with strain and worry, is at the root of many mental and physical disabilities [46]. As a result of chronic stress, bodily systems such as the hypothalamic pituitary adrenal (HPA) axis are overused and experience "wear and tear" [44]. Numerous studies suggest that stress can result in maladaptive neuroendocrine, metabolic, inflammatory and neuropsychological changes that are associated with an array of health problems, such as cardiovascular disease, atherosclerosis, poor immune system functioning and insulin resistance syndrome [12]. Individuals who face chronic stress are more likely to develop clinical depression, suffer from a flare up of an existing allergic or autoimmune condition, and exhibit accelerated progression of chronic diseases [47, 48]. Research also suggests that chronic exposure to environmental stress may contribute to obesity, potentially *via* HPA axis dysregulation [1].

With stress-related illnesses becoming more and more of a worldwide pandemic, it is important to identify useful and effective stress management techniques that can be easily and safely adopted by people with diverse medical problems and functional limitations. Yoga and meditation have been described as effective stress management tools that can be modified for use with diverse populations, across diverse settings, for assorted illnesses [49]. In fact, participation in any type of yoga or meditation is associated with improvements in various outcomes related to mood (*e.g.*, reducing anxiety, depression) and quality of life [50].

Mind-body therapies can reduce the impact of stress both directly by improvements in physiological functions and health and indirectly through reduction in distress (*e.g.*, depression and anxiety) and enhanced quality of life. Pathways responsible for the benefits of yoga and meditation include improved neuroendocrine status, metabolic function and decreased inflammation resulting from reduced activation of the HPA axis and increased parasympathetic nervous system tone [51, 52]. Data also indicates that yoga and meditation have a beneficial impact on perceptual and physiological responses to stress by decreasing hormone levels associated with stress (*e.g.*, cortisol) [44, 53]. Furthermore, researchers have found that yoga and meditation may enhance parasympathetic output and stimulate the vagus nerve [53-56]. The vagus nerve, the longest cranial nerve, deactivates the "fight or flight" response and calms the body. A systematic review noted that a majority of 42 studies provided some evidence that yoga reduces sympathetic function, enhances cardiovagal function, and shifts the autonomic nervous system balance to parasympathetic functioning [57]. Additionally, yoga and meditation may have indirect effects on health through reduced psychosocial stress and affective states such as anxiety and depression; such reductions in distress may lead to improved health outcomes through decreased autonomic reactivity to stress, engagement in self-care practices (*e.g.*, healthy diet, exercise, stress management) and quality of life [10].

The short and long term improvements in reaction to stress provocation following engagement in a yoga and meditation regimen are significant and remarkable [58]. Even brief yoga interventions, as short as one sixty-minute session, have been shown to reduce anxiety in a sample of dental students [59]. Other benefits to short term interventions include improvements in the areas of perceived stress, depression, sleep, memory, blood pressure and overall quality of life, in both diseased and healthy population samples (Table **3**) [60]. Longitudinal studies have shown the benefits of yoga for mental health functioning over time [61].

Table 3. Yoga, meditation, and stress management.

How Do Yoga and Meditation Impact Stress Management?	
Physiological Pathways	Improved neuroendocrine status Improved metabolic function Improved blood pressure Increased telomere lengths Greater vagal nerve stimulation Greater parasympathetic output Reduced inflammation Reduced HPA axis activation
Psychosocial Pathways	Reduced distress Reduced psychological symptoms (anxiety and depression) Improved self-care practices Improved quality of life Improved concentration Improved mindfulness/awareness

For Physical Health

Although not originally conceptualized as exercise, yoga is considered to be a popular form of physical activity and has been recognized as one of the most widely adopted methods of fitness worldwide. According to a recent survey, yoga has been identified as one of the top fifteen modalities of physical activity adopted by populations across the globe for the past several years [62]. Since the early twentieth century, yoga has been studied as a therapeutic and health care intervention, with a particular focus on the psychological and physiological benefits. Asanas, or physical postures can increase physical flexibility and strength, while the breathing practices help calm down, focus the mind, and can increase the quality of life [57].

A recent literature review examined studies comparing the effects of yoga and other forms of physical activity/exercise and noted that in both healthy and diseased populations, yoga may be equal or superior in its ability to improve health outcomes, including heart rate variability, blood glucose, blood lipids, salivary cortisol and oxidative stress [19]. Physical fitness is the only outcome measure that was associated with other forms of exercise to a greater extent as compared to its association with yoga [19]. However, potentially more strenuous forms of yoga could provide equivalent physical fitness benefits as compared to strenuous physical exercise and are worthy of additional investigation. Another critical review indicated moderate effect sizes for aspects of physical fitness within older adults including body strength, balance, body flexibility and weight loss [63]. Thus, integrating yoga into treatment for chronic illness may have a multifaceted, beneficial impact on patient health.

Meditation has also been studied in medical and rehabilitation settings as a complementary treatment for a variety of chronic illnesses and pain conditions—particularly for its ability to target affective states that are distressing like anxiety, depression and stress, which frequently accompany chronic illness and pain conditions [27]. A systematic review of meditation techniques for medical purposes concluded that when stress or mood disorders (*e.g.*, depression or anxiety-related disorders) contribute to the pathophysiology and morbidity of a medical illness, meditation can be a particularly effective treatment alternative [64]. It has been suggested that meditation, particularly mindfulness meditation, may counteract chronic states of stress arousal by increasing telomere lengths, the protective caps at the end of chromosomes [27]. Telomere length is linked to age, cardiovascular risk factors, atheroscerlosis and diabetes. Therefore, meditation's ability to increase telomere length may lead to protective effects on the body. Studies have also indicated that meditation is associated with changes in the heart rate, blood pressure, electroencephalographic (EEG) ratings, hormones and immunological functioning [65]. Thus, meditation may also be conceptualized as a potential supplement to traditional treatment of obesity and related chronic diseases.

YOGA, MEDITATION & OBESITY/OVERWEIGHT

Yoga and meditation may have direct and indirect effects on obesity-related health issues.

Yoga and Obesity

Yoga can be helpful for physically inactive people who are overweight and consider strenuous physical activity difficult. A variety of studies have demonstrated beneficial effects for obese participants who engaged in yoga practice. One study of 177 obese individuals found that a combination of yoga asanas or positions with an emphasis on breathing techniques significantly reduced body mass index (BMI) after a week [66]. A combined dietary and yoga program for 47 obese participants yielded short term benefits including a decrease in BMI, waist and hip circumferences, fat-free mass, total cholesterol, high density lipoprotein (HDL) cholesterol, and fasting serum leptin levels [67]. Additionally, 56 overweight or obese participants who engaged in a 21-day treatment involving the dietary use of natural plant-based products and yoga experienced a significant reduction in obesity parameters with the exception of fat percentage and HDL [68]. A retrospective, observational study of over 15,550 adults aged 53-57 found that regular yoga practice for at least four years was significantly associated with weight loss in overweight patients [69]. Similar results were observed in studies focused on individuals with coronary artery disease (CAD), where significant weight loss was achieved through yoga practice [70-72].

Potentially, yoga may assist those who are obese or overweight to adopt a lifestyle that encourages weight loss. Asian adolescent obese males, a population that may not necessarily appear as typical yoga users, have positive outcomes from yoga practice; one study found that an 8-week yoga training program significantly reduced body weight, BMI, total cholesterol, and percent body fat, and significantly increased fat-free mass and basal metabolic rate compared to baseline values [73]. Even short-term yoga programs have evidenced positive effects on individuals struggling with weight issues. For example, though a seven-day yoga program did not demonstrate significant differences in weight or BMI, there were significant reductions in waist-hip ratio and diastolic blood pressure in diabetic and hypertensive participants. Interestingly, these results contrast with several studies noted above, which did find BMI differences even after just a short period of yoga practice [66, 74]. Thus, health care professionals may consider integrating a short-term yoga program into a variety of individual's treatment plans.

Meditation and Obesity

Research indicates that changes in lifestyle, regardless of weight loss, appear to protect individuals from obesity-related diseases including cardiovascular disease and diabetes [75]. Research [76-78] that has examined the relationship between meditation and eating behaviors or weight loss has focused on mindfulness meditation. Engaging in mindfulness while eating may impact eating patterns by increasing awareness of physical sensations of hunger and fullness and breaking the association between automatic eating and emotional reactions [76].

Mindfulness meditation may replace or absolve the need for self-destructive methods of self-soothing as a response to stress, including binging or overeating [77, 78].

Overall, it appears that mindfulness meditation may facilitate weight loss and improvement in obesity-related areas. For example, 10 obese men experienced significant increase in mindfulness and cognitive restraint with eating through participation in 6 weekly 2 hour-group classes of mindfulness training [79]. Participants also demonstrated significant decreases in weight, eating too many unhealthy foods, perceived stress, physical symptoms, negative affect (*e.g.*, anxiety, depression) and C-reactive protein [79]. Additionally, a randomized controlled trial found that women who took part in a mindfulness-based weight loss intervention engaged in significantly more physical activity and had significantly greater BMI reductions as compared to a control condition (when non-participating intervention women were excluded) [80]. Furthermore, a 4-month mindfulness training program focused on stress eating for obese and overweight women found that mindfulness, anxiety, and based on environmental cues rather than hunger pangs eating improved compared to a waitlist group; no significant differences were found in weight or abdominal fat over time, but intervention participants maintained body weight while control participants gained weight [81]. Finally, one randomized controlled trial compared 25 individuals enrolled in a 3-month diabetes self-management education program with 27 individuals enrolled in 3-month mindful eating program [82]. Three months after the intervention, change in weight and glycemia were compared between the groups, indicating modest reductions in both variables. Thus, results indicated that mindful eating is comparable to diabetes self-management in its ability to improve dietary intake, weight loss and glycemia [82].

YOGA & MEDITATION: TREATING COMORBIDITIES

Heart Disease

Researchers have also examined yoga and meditation's effectiveness as a complementary treatment for heart disease when adopted in conjunction with traditional medical practices. A randomized controlled study demonstrated that yoga slowed down progression of atherosclerosis in patients with severe coronary artery disease [70]. Furthermore, post-myocardial infarction, patients who practiced yoga combined with conventional medicine showed greater clinical improvements as compared to patients who did not practice yoga [83]. Yoga may also be helpful during patient's recovery from myocardial infarction by contributing to sleep, appetite, general well-being, and decrease physiological arousal [84].

Similar to research on yoga, there is an extensive research that evaluates the effects of meditation on the prevention and treatment of cardiovascular disease. Studies have examined the impact of meditation on lifestyle behaviors or risk factors that increase the likelihood of cardiovascular disease, as well as cardiovascular morbidity and mortality [85]. One randomized controlled study revealed that use of TM for 16 weeks in coronary heart disease patients improved blood pressure and insulin resistance compared with a health education control group [86]. Another randomized controlled trial found that transcendental meditation practice significantly decreased carotid intima-media thickness (measure of atherosclerosis) in hypertensive African American participants compared to a heart disease education group [87]. Meditation has also demonstrated beneficial effects in heart failure patients: African American participants recently hospitalized for heart failure who practiced transcendental meditation had better functional capacity on a 6-minute walk test compared to health education control group [88]. A 9-year randomized controlled trial indicated that African Americans with heart disease, who practiced transcendental meditation, had lower rates of cardiovascular clinical events that included mortality, nonfatal myocardial infarction, and nonfatal stroke compared to a health education control group [89]. Researchers have also examined mindfulness meditation with heart disease patients: one study assessed an 8-week psycho-educational intervention which included the practice of mindfulness reduced anxiety and depression in congestive heart failure (CHF) patients and also led to significantly better CHF symptoms at 12 months compared to control CHF patients who did not have the intervention [90]. Thus, in order to further improve heart disease patients' well-being, health care workers should consider integrating yoga and meditation into cardiac rehabilitation programs.

Diabetes

Studies indicate that yoga and meditation can help people control symptoms and complications associated with type 2 diabetes mellitus [91]. Diabetes patients with pre-existing complications exhibited significant progress after participating in studies involving yoga practice [52]. Furthermore, 14 diabetic patients participating in a pilot mindfulness-based stress reduction intervention demonstrated reduced glycosylated hemoglobin, mean arterial blood pressure, depression, anxiety and general psychological distress [92]. A recent literature review that examined the effects of yoga on type 2 diabetes concluded that yoga has a significant impact on short-term parameters of diabetes, including fasting plasma glucose levels and lipid profiles, but further research is necessary regarding long-term parameters, such as body mass index and glycosylated hemoglobin levels [91]. Another review of complementary and alternative medicine for diabetes suggested that more rigorous study of mind-body interventions is necessary before firm conclusions can be made regarding its efficacy for diabetes [93].

Chronic Health Risk Factors

Hypertension, Heart-Rate Variability, and Baroreflex Sensitivity

Yoga

Beneficial effects of yoga on hypertension include direct effects and indirect effects through stress; stress has been implicated in the etiology, morbidity and the pathophysiology of hypertension [94, 95]. An abundance of empirical literature suggests that yoga reduces blood pressure; in fact, a recent literature review of studies published between 2006 and 2011 noted this finding in eight out of nine studies centered on hypertensive and pre-hypertensive individuals [94]. Another literature review reported that the majority of 37 studies examined, demonstrated a reduction of systolic and diastolic pressure, including 12 randomized controlled trials, 12 nonrandomized clinical trials, 11 uncontrolled studies, 1 cross-sectional study and 1 single yoga session examination [52]. However, some of the studies were limited by potential biases and confounding factors, making it unclear whether the outcomes were particular to yoga effects. Studies also found that baroreflex sensitivity, a major cause of hypertension, can be restored through the use of particular yoga postures, including the head-up or head-down tilt [96, 97]. Furthermore, slow breathing, as part of yoga practice, may re-synchronize cardiovascular rhythms, thereby enhancing heart rate variability and baroreflex sensitivity [97].

Meditation

Meditation has been used in numerous studies as an intervention to prevent or treat high blood pressure. Potentially, meditation can be viewed as an efficacious and cost-effective technique for combating hypertension. According to a recent literature review, transcendental and mindfulness meditation techniques, are associated with small but significant decreases in blood pressure when used alone or in conjunction with traditional pharmacotherapy [98]. Additional randomized control trials of meditation and blood pressure are needed as various reviewed studies showed potential biases due to lack of blinding, poor measurement or lack of baseline blood pressure, minimal follow-up and lack of direct comparisons of different meditation techniques [98]. Regardless, a meta-analysis of nine randomized controlled trials of Transcendental Meditation interventions found that Transcendental Meditation was associated with an approximate 5/3 mm Hg reduction in systolic and diastolic blood pressure, respectively [99]. Evidence also indicates that meditation may also increase heart rate variability, thereby further reducing cardiovascular and obesity-related risks [86, 56, 100, 101].

Lipid Levels

High lipid levels (serum cholesterol, triglycerides and low density lipoprotein-cholesterol), often a by-product of obesity, are a risk factor for cardiovascular disease and diabetes. Yoga has been identified as a method of improving blood lipid levels in multiple studies [12]. For example, individuals at high risk for coronary heart disease exhibited reduced total triglycerides, reduced low density lipoprotein cholesterol (LDL-C), and greater high density lipoprotein cholesterol (HDL-C) after an eight-day yoga intervention [102]. A longer term study followed asymptomatic individuals who were at increased risk for coronary artery disease as well as men with angina who underwent a four day yoga program and then engaged in a year of private home yoga practice. Participants exhibited decreased lipid levels (with the exception of HDL) after the fourth week of practice [103]. At least two studies that examined raja yoga practitioners found that serum cholesterol levels improved in long-term and short-term meditators compared to non-meditators [104, 105].

Blood Glucose Levels

Numerous studies have examined the effect of yoga and meditation on blood glucose levels, a risk factor for obesity, heart disease and diabetes; the majority found that yoga reduced blood glucose levels [106, 107]. After participating in a yoga-lifestyle intervention that included three to four hours of practice over eight days, healthy adults exhibited decreased levels of fasting plasma glucose [102]. In another study, fasting glucose levels dropped significantly in adults with type 2 diabetes who had engaged in four months of yoga practice [108]. With regards to meditation, type 2 diabetics who practiced a version of sitting breathing meditation experienced a beneficial post prandial hypoglycemic effect [109].

Randomized controlled trials have also found significant positive effects of yoga and meditation on blood glucose. Both yoga and physical exercise were associated with a significant decrease in fasting blood glucose levels in a group of 186 type 2 diabetics at three months and six months in a blinded randomized controlled trial that compared the effects of 6 months of weekly classes and home practice of yoga with aerobic exercise and stretching [110]. Another randomized control trial found heart disease participants in the Transcendental Meditation intervention who experienced improved fasting blood glucose and insulin levels compared with the control group [86]. These findings suggest that yoga and/or meditation can be used as a supplement to Western medicine when treating metabolic disorders.

YOGA & MEDITATION AS PUBLIC HEALTH TECHNIQUES

Currently, obesity represents as one of the most prominent and alarming public health issues across the globe. There is an urgent need to develop and implement effective, feasible interventions and programs in Eastern and Western civilizations. Due to the large and indiscriminating scope of health-related problems linked to obesity, multidisciplinary and innovative public health techniques with universal appeal are needed to combat this pandemic [111, 112]. With the increasing impact of globalization, the arsenal of public health tools has expanded to include traditional and modern medical approaches from both Eastern and Western traditions. This sharing of regional and culture-bound health practices affords the opportunity to implement potentially effective public health programs within diverse geographic locations and settings. Yoga and meditation may be potentially effectual and underutilized public health techniques to aid in the fight against obesity (Table **4**) [113].

Public health initiatives that address the health-related problems related to obesity need to be approached considering individual, community, and government engagement [113]. In evaluating the viability of translating an individual practice or intervention into an effective large-scale public health technique, there are a number of aspects that need to be taken into consideration. At face value, it appears that yoga and meditation techniques lend themselves well to the arena of public health. Interventions and health-promoting programs that incorporate these mind-body techniques are applicable and effective among ethically and culturally diverse groups and across the lifespan. These interventions are cost-effective and easily understood, taught and implemented. Moreover, these practices are flexible and can be individually tailored to meet the needs of diverse groups of individuals within a variety of settings. However, it is yoga and meditation's empirical robustness as a protective variable against stress-related illnesses that affords these practices in the essence of potentially useful tools for public health initiatives. In evaluating the appropriateness of endorsing yoga and meditation programs as a public health technique, specific attention should be given to the feasibility of implementing related intervention within non-clinical environments. It is those programs the efficacy of which extends beyond the confines of traditional treatment settings that show promise as an effective public health technique.

Table 4. Yoga and meditation as public health techniques for obesity.

Why are yoga and meditation appropriate public health techniques for obesity?
Research indicates obese individuals experience benefits from yoga and meditation
Yoga and meditation have positive impacts on both mental and physical health
Originated in Eastern countries and has spread to Western countries
Flexible practices that can be individually tailored to meet needs of diverse individuals (including school age children, office employees, and prison inmates)
No equipment necessary for use in a variety of settings
Can be used in combination with diet, exercise and medicine
Cost-effective, noninvasive and straightforward to implement

Integrating Yoga & Meditation into Schools

Mind-body techniques have been found to increase self-awareness, self-control and concentration abilities in children [114, 115]. Implementing programs that teach these techniques may be especially attractive to integrate into classroom settings [116]. Assessing the feasibility of implementing a mind-body intervention in an elementary school setting, researchers assessed the effects of an in-school yoga intervention in children with emotional and behavioral disorders [116]. In this study, children received two one-hour yoga sessions each week for three and a half months. The protocol included relaxation training, yoga exercises and postures, group exercising or partnering up, imagery techniques and meditation. The study shows support for the feasibility of facilitating a yoga-based intervention in an urban school setting. Moreover, teachers reported improvements in children's attention and adaptive skills, as well as a decrease in depressive and behavioral symptoms post-intervention. Given that this intervention was well received by teachers, parents and students, and was shown to bring about positive changes, there appears to be merit in further exploring the use of mind-body based interventions in a school setting.

Integrating Yoga & Meditation into the Workplace

It is a common knowledge that the workplace stress is widespread. Work-related stress poses a threat to health and well-being, and is linked to mental and physical health challenges [117]. In a recent study of 1,700 workers, data indicated that 20% of participants were characterized as experiencing either very high or extremely high degrees of stress. Moreover, this work-stress was associated with negative physiological outcomes, poor mental performance and greater risk of having an accident on the job [118]. Stress reactions at work are probably compounded by prolonged exposure to the environment where the stress manifests since most individuals spend a large portion of their day at work; thus the workplace may be an appropriate and crucial setting to address health issues [117, 119]. A recent study showed the effectiveness of mind-body interventions in the workplace in a sample of 239 employees [120]. One of these interventions was the Viniyoga Stress Reduction Program, which includes teaching yoga postures, guided relaxation and breathing techniques. The other intervention consisted of the mindfulness at work stress management program. Within the mindfulness program, each participant learned the basic tenets of mindfulness-based meditation with a particular focus on combating workplace-specific stress. Each intervention was implemented once a week for a total of 12 weeks. Compared to a control group, participants in both the mind-body intervention groups showed health benefits post-intervention. Both the yoga-based intervention and the mindfulness-based intervention appeared to be effective in reducing perceived stress, as well as sleep disturbances. This study supports the feasibility of implementing effective health-promoting yoga-based and mindfulness-based interventions in the workplace.

Although more research on yoga and meditation within the workplace is warranted, preliminary evidence indicates that these interventions are starting to find their way into the workforce [121, 122]. Since stress can hamper productivity, it would appear to be in the best interest of the corporation or organization to make implementing programs that combat the negative effects of stress, a corporate priority [123]. Meditation within the corporate setting is becoming especially popular, and various major companies are starting to set up these on-site programs. Meditation appears especially applicable to the workplace because of its face validity as a mechanism to combat stress and shows extremely robust, positive effects in combating current stress, as well as in serving as a protective agent against future stress. Yoga and meditation techniques can be practiced independently; these interventions may easily be implemented during lunchtime or after-work workshop. Likewise, a yoga or meditation intervention could be added into an employee-training day.

Integrating Yoga & Meditation into Juvenile Detention and Correctional Facilities

As yoga and meditation practices are making their way into our schools and workplaces, recent studies have investigated how these interventions fare when employed in more restrictive settings, such as juvenile detention and correctional facilities. A recent study evaluated the applicability of a mindfulness-based 10-week intervention within a sample of incarcerated adolescents in a juvenile detention facility setting and demonstrated increased self-regulation and lower levels of perceived stress [124]. The results of this study suggest that mind-body interventions may even promote health within youth with behavioral considerations or restrictions.

Expanding the application of mind-body interventions to adults in correctional facilities, Sumter, Monk-Turner, and Turner evaluated the utility of a meditation intervention program within a sample of incarcerated females [125]. Each meditation group was held once a week and lasted two and a half hours. After seven weeks, when compared to the control group, women who participated in the meditation group reported a reduction in sleep-related disturbances, feelings of guilt and less of an inclination to physically harm others. Likewise, women who completed the meditation program reported feeling more hopeful about their future. These women also showed less medical and emotional symptomology indicating the potential in these mind-body interventions and programs to meaningfully promote health benefits in settings in which other health promoting public health techniques are inappropriate or ineffective.

CONCLUSION

In general, meditation and yoga present low cost public health interventions that have found widespread appeal. Although the evidence base for their use and mechanisms by which they exert their influence is still being accumulated, preliminary data indicate their efficacy and appeal among a wide variety of populations, settings and disorders. Their adoption as techniques in the West compared to their being viewed as a lifestyle in the east, does not appear to decrease their efficacy in aiding mental and physical health and well-being. The effects of yoga and meditation along with other practices associated with a "yoga lifestyle" are synergistic, including practice of breathing exercises in the morning, and vegetarianism. Hence, adoption of any one of these practices may have a beneficial effect on health.

ACKNOWLEDGEMENTS

Declared none.

CONFLICT OF INTEREST

The authors confirm that this chapter contents have no conflict of interest.

REFERENCES

[1] Bose M, Olivan B, Lafarrere, B. Stress and obesity: The role of the hypothalamic pituitary-adrenal axis in metabolic disease. Curr Opin Endocrinol Diabetes Obes 2009; 16(5): 340-346.
[2] Misra A, Khurana L. Obesity and the metabolic syndrome in developing countries. J Clin Endocrinol Met 2008; 93(11): s9-s30.
[3] Bjorntorp P. Visceral obesity: a 'civilization syndrome'. Obes Res 1993; 1: 206-222.
[4] Cordain L, Eaton SB, Sebastian A., *et al.* Origins and evolution of the Western diet: Health implications for the 21st century. Am J Clin Nutr 2005; 81(2): 341-354.
[5] Carrera-Bastos P, Fontes-Villalba M, O'Keefe JH, Lindeberg S, Cordain L. The western diet and lifestyle and disease of civilization. Res Rep Clin Cardiol 2011; 2:15-35.
[6] Johnson, SS, Kushner RF. Mind/body medicine: An introduction for the generalist physician and nutritionist. Nutr Clin Care 2001; 4(5): 256-264.
[7] Kawachi I, Wamala S. Globalization and Health. New York, NY: Oxford University Press; 2007.
[8] McEwen BS. Allostasis & allostatic load: Implications for Neuropsychopharmacology. Neuropsychopharmacol 2000; 22(2): 108-122.
[9] World Health Organization. Obesity: preventing and managing the global epidemic. World Health Organ Tech Rep Ser 2000; 894.
[10] Anderson AS, Taylor AG. The metabolic syndrome and mind-body therapies: A systematic review. J Nutr Metab 2011; 1-8.
[11] Reilly M, Rader D. The metabolic syndrome: More than the sum of its parts? Circ 2003; 108: 1546-1551.
[12] Innes KE, Vincent HK. The influence of yoga-based programs on risk profiles in adults with type 2 diabetes mellitus: A systematic review. Evid Based Complement Alternate Med 2006; 4(4): 469-486.
[13] Koithan, M. Mind-body solutions for obesity. J Nurse Pract 2009; 5(7): 536-537.
[14] Cheema BS, Marshall PW, Chang D, Colagiuri B, Machliss B. Effect of an office worksite-based yoga program on heart rate variability: A randomized controlled trial. BMC Public Health 2011; 11: 578-583.
[15] De Michelis E. A History of Modern Yoga: Patanjali and Western Esotericism. London & New York. Continuum; 2004.
[16] Bryant EF. The Yoga sūtras of Patañjali: a new edition, translation, and commentary with insights from the traditional commentators. North Point Press; 2009.
[17] Eggleston B. Psychosocial determinants of attending yoga classes: An application of the theory of planned behavior [unpublished dissertation]. Indiana University; 2009.
[18] Ross A, Friedmann E, Bevans M, Thomas S. Frequency of yoga practice predicts health: Results of a national survey of yoga practitioners. Evid Based Complement Alternat Med; 2012.
[19] Ross A, Thomas S. The health benefits of yoga and exercise: A review of comparison studies. J Altern Complement Med 2010; 16(1): 3-12.

[20] Reder A. Reconcilable differences: Yoga and religion. Yog J 2001; 78-85.
[21] Cabral P, Meyer HB, Ames D. Effectiveness of yoga therapy as a complementary treatment for major psychiatric disorders: A meta-analysis. Primary Care Companion CNS Disord 2011; 13(4).
[22] Nazarith M, Herbert M. What is raja yoga [homepage on the internet]. No date [cited June 3, 2013]. Available from http://www.rajayogis.net/content/raja-yoga
[23] Slagter HA, Davidson RJ Lutz, A. Mental training as a tool in the neuroscientific study of brain and cognitive plasticity. Front Hum Neurosci 2011; 5(17).
[24] Carlson LE, Garland S. Mindfulness-based stress reduction (MBSR) on sleep quality in cancer patients. Int J Behav Med 2005; 12(4): 278-285.
[25] Manocha R. Why meditation? Aust Fam Phys 2000; 29(12): 1135-1138.
[26] Sharpe PA, Blanck HM, Williams JE, Ainsworth BE, Conway JM. Use of complementary and alternative medicine for weight control in the United States. J Altern Complement Med 2007; 13(2): 217-222.
[27] Horowitz S. Health benefits of meditation: What the newest research shows. Altern Complement Ther 2010; 16(4): 223-228.
[28] Baer R. Mindfulness training as a clinical intervention: A conceptual and empirical review. Clin Psychol: Sci Pr 2003; 10(2), 125-143.
[29] Ospina MB, Bond K, Karkhaneh M, *et al.* Clinical trials of meditation practices in healthcare: Characteristics and quality. J Complement Altern Med 2008; 14(10): 1199-1213.
[30] Eisenberg DM, Kessler RC, Foster C, Norlock FE, Calkins DR, Delbanco TL. Unconventional medicine in the United States—prevalence, costs, and patterns of use. New Engl J Med 1993; 328(4): 246-252.
[31] Bishop FL, Lewith GT. Who uses CAM? A narrative review of demographic characteristics and health factors associated with CAM use. Evid Based Complement Alternat Med 2010; 7(1): 11-28.
[32] Bodeker G, Kronenberg F. A public health agenda for traditional, complementary and alternative medicine. Am J Public Health 2002; 92(10): 1582-1591.
[33] April KT, Moher D, Stinson J, *et al.* Measurement of properties of questionnaires assessing complementary and alternative medicine use in pediatrics: A systematic review. PloS one 2012; 7(6): e39611.
[34] Feldman RH, Laura, R. The use of complementary and alternative medicine practices among Australian university students. Complementary Health Pract Rev 2004; 9: 173-179.
[35] Pilkington K, Kirkwood G, Rampes H, Richardson J. Yoga for depression: The research evidence. J Affective Disord 2005; 89: 13-24.
[36] Birdee SG, Legedza AT, Saper RB, Bertisch SM, Eisenberg DM, Phillips RS. Characteristics of yoga users: Results of a national survey. J Gen Intern Med 2008; 23(10): 1653-1658.
[37] Green CA, Pope CR. Gender, psychosocial factors and the use of medical services: A longitudinal analysis. Soc Sci Med 1999; 48(10): 1363-1372.
[38] Patwardhan B, Patwardhan A. Traditional medicine for global health. Tech Monitor 2006; Nov-Dec: 17-22.
[39] Dhananjai S, Sadashiv, Tiwari S, Dutt K, Kumar R. Reducing psychological distress and obesity through yoga practice. Int J Yoga 2013; 6(1): 66-70.
[40] Wardle J, Lui C, Adams J. Complementary and alternative medicine in rural communities: Current research and future directions. J Rural Health 2012; 28:101-112.
[41] Taylor MJ. Yoga therapeutics: An ancient, dynamic systems theory. Tech Orthop 2003; 18(1): 115-125.
[42] Garfinkel M, Schumacher HR. Yoga. Rheum Dis Clin North Am 2000; 26(1): 125-132.
[43] World Health Organization. Obesity and overweight 2012; [cited January 23, 2013]. Available from http://www.who.int/mediacentre/factsheets/fs311/en/.
[44] McEwen BS, Gianaros PJ. Central role of the brain in stress and adaptation: Links to socioeconomic status, health, and disease. Ann N Y Acad Sci 2010; 1186: 190-122.
[45] Peeke PM, Chrouso GP. Hypercortisolism and obesity. Ann N Y Acad Sci 1995; 771: 665-676.
[46] Rao T. Stress management through yoga and yogic diet. Intern J Multidis Educ Res 2012; 1(3): 123-130.
[47] Miller GE, Chen E, Zhou, ES. If it goes up, must it come down? Chronic stress and the hypothalamic-pituitary adrenocortical axis in humans. Psychol Bull 2007; 133(1): 25-45.

[48] Miller GE, Cohen S. Infectious disease and psychoneuroimmunology. In Vedhara K, Irwin M, editors. Human psychoneuroimmunology. New York: Oxford University Press 2005; 219-242.

[49] Van der Klink JL, Blonk RB, Schene AH, Van Dijk FH. The benefits of interventions for work-related stress. Am J Public Health 2001; 91: 270-276.

[50] Schoormans D, Nyklicek I. Mindfulness and psychologic wellbeing: Are they related to type of meditation technique practiced? Journal Alternat Complement Med 2011; 629-634.

[51] Brown RP, Gerbarg PL. Yoga breathing, meditation, and longevity. Ann N Y Acad Sci 2009; 1172, 54-62.

[52] Innes KE, Bourguignon C, Taylor AG. Risk indices associated with the insulin resistance syndrome, cardiovascular disease, and possible protection with yoga: A systematic review. J Am Board Family Pract 2005; 18(6): 491-519.

[53] Innes KE, Vincent HK, Taylor AG. Chronic stress and insulin resistance-related indices of cardiovascular disease risk, part 2:A potential role for mind-body therapies. Altern Ther Health Med 2007; 13(5): 44-51.

[54] Kiecolt-Glaser JK, Christian L, Preston H, Houts CR, Malarkey WB, Emery CF. Glaser, R. Stress, inflammation, and yoga practice. Psychosom Med 2010; 72: 113-121.

[55] Taylor AG, Goehler LE, Galper D.I., Innes KE, Bourguignon C. Top-down and bottom-up mechanisms in mind-body medicine: Development of an integrative framework for psychophysiological research. Explore 2010; (6)1: 29-41.

[56] Wu SD, Lo PC. Inward-attention meditation increases parasympathetic activity: A study based on heart rate variability. Biomed Res 2008; 29(5): 245-250.

[57] Bussing A, Michaelsen A, Khalsa SBS, Telles S, Sherman KJ. (2012). Effects of yoga on mental and physical health: A short summary of reviews. Evid Based Complement and Alternat Med, 1-7.

[58] Sharma R, Gupta N, Bijlani RL. Effect of yoga based lifestyle intervention on subjective well-being. Indian J Physiol Pharmacol 2008; 52(2): 123-131.

[59] Shankarapillai R, Nair MA, George R. The effect of yoga in stress reduction for dental students performing their first periodontal surgery: A randomized controlled study. Int J Yoga 2012; 5(1): 48.

[60] Innes KE, Selfe TK, Brown CJ, Rose KM, Thompson-Heisterman A. The effects of meditation on perceived stress and related indices of psychological status and sympathetic activation in persons with alzheimer's disease and their caregivers: A pilot study. Evid Based Complement Alternat Med 2012; 1-9.

[61] Yoshihara K, Hiramoto T, Sudo N, Kubo C. Profile of mood states and stress related biochemical indices in long-term yoga practitioners. Biopsychosoc Medic 2011; 5(6).

[62] Thompson WR. Worldwide survey of fitness trends for 2013. ACSM Health Fit J 2012; 16(6): 8-17.

[63] Roland KP, Jakobi JM, Jones GR. Does yoga engender fitness in older adults? A critical review. J Aging and Phys Act 2011; 19(1): 62-79.

[64] Arias AJ, Steinberg K, Banga A, Trestman RL. Systemic review of the efficacy of meditation techniques as treatment for medical illness. J Alternat Complement Med 2006; 12 (8): 817-832.

[65] Newberg AB, Iversen J. The neural basis of the complex mental task of meditation: Neurotransmitter and neurochemical considerations. Med Hypotheses 2003; 61(2): 282-291.

[66] Gokal R, Shillito L, Maharaj SR. Positive impact of yoga and pranayam on obesity, hypertension, blood sugar, and cholesterol: A pilot assessment. J Alternat Complement Med 2007; 13(10): 1056-1058.

[67] Telles S, Naveen VK, Balkrishna A, Kumar S. Short term health impact of a yoga and diet change program on obesity 2010. Med Sci Monit, 16(1): CR35-40

[68] Murthy SN, Rao NSN, Nandakumar B, Kadam A. Management of obesity through naturopathy and yoga interventions. Indian J Ancient Med Yoga 2010; 3(2): 73-78.

[69] Kristal AR, Littman AJ, Benitez D, White E. Yoga practice is associated with attenuated weight gain in healthy, middle-aged men and women. Altern Ther Health Med 2005; 11(4): 28-33.

[70] Manchanda SC, Narang R, Reddy KS, *et al.* Retardation of coronary atherosclerosis with yoga lifestyle intervention. J Assoc Physic India 2000; 48: 687-694.

[71] Sivasankaran S, Pollard-Quintner S, Sachdeva R, Pugeda J, Hoq SM, Zarich, SW. The effect of a six-week program of yoga and meditation on brachial artery reactivity: Do psychosocial interventions affect vascular tone? Clin Cardiol 2006; 29: 393-8.

[72] Yogendra J, Yogendra HJ, Ambardekar S, Lele RD, Shetty S, Dave M, Husein N. Beneficial effects of yoga lifestyle on reversibility of ischaemic heart disease: Caring heart project of International Board of Yoga. J Assoc Phys India 2004; 52: 283-9.
[73] Seo DY, Lee S, Figueroa A, Kim HK. Yoga training improves metabolic parameters in obese boys. Korean J Physiol Pharmacol 2012; 16(3), 175-180.
[74] Tamilselvi E, Hemamalini M, Swapna S, Haripriya D. Impact of short and intense yoga training on obesity risk factors in diabetic and hypertensive patients. J Pharmacy Research 2012; 5(8).
[75] Bacon L, Stern JS, Van Loan MD, Keim NL. Size acceptance and intuitive eating improve health for obese, female chronic dieters. J Am Diab Assoc 2005; 105(6): 925-936.
[76] Caldwell KL Baime MJ, Wolever RQ. Mindfulness based approaches to obesity and weight loss maintenance. J Ment Health Couns 2012; 34(3): 269-282.
[77] Greeson J. Mindfulness research update: 2008. Complement Health Pract Rev 2009; 14, 10-18.
[78] Kristeller JL, Baer RA, Quillian-Wolever R. Mindfulness-based approaches to eating disorders. In: Baer, RA, editor. Mindfulness-based treatment approaches: A clinician's guide to evidence base and applications. San Diego, CA: Academic Press 2006; p. 75-91.
[79] Dalen J, Smith BW, Shelley BM, Sloan AL, Leahigh L, Begay D. Pilot study: Mindful Eating and Living (MEAL): weight, eating behavior, and psychological outcomes associated with a mindfulness-based intervention for people with obesity. Complement ther med 2010; 18(6): 260-264.
[80] Tapper K, Shaw C, Ilsley J, Hill AJ, Bond FW, Moore, L. (2009). Exploratory randomised controlled trial of a mindfulness-based weight loss intervention for women. Appetite 2009; 52(2): 396-404.
[81] Daubenmier J, Kristeller J, Hecht FM, *et al.* Mindfulness intervention for stress eating to reduce cortisol and abdominal fat among overweight and obese women: an exploratory randomized controlled study. J Obes 2011; 1-13.
[82] Miller, CK, Kristeller JL, Headings A, Nagaraja H, Miser WF. Comparative effectiveness of a mindful eating intervention to a diabetes self-management intervention among adults with type 2 diabetes: A pilot study. J Acad Nutr Diet 2012; 112 (11): 1835-1842.
[83] Bulavin VV, Kliuzhev VM, Kliachkin LM, Lakshmankumar, Zulkhin ND, Vlasova, TN. Elements of yoga therapy in combined rehabilitation of myocardial infarction patients in the functional recovery period. Voprosy Kurortologii Fizioterapii I Lechebnoi Fizicheskoi Kultury 1993; 4:7-9.
[84] Telles S, Naveen, KV. Yoga for rehabilitation: An overview. Indian J Med Sci 1997; 51:123-127.
[85] Orme-Johnson DW, Barnes VA, Schneider RH. Transcendental meditation for primary and secondary prevention of coronary heart disease. In: Allan R, Fisher, J, editors. Heart & Mind: the Practice of Cardiac Psychology. Washington, D.C.: American Psychological Association 2011; pg. 365-379.
[86] Paul-Labrador M, Polk D, Dwyer J, *et al.* Effects of a randomized controlled trial of transcendental meditation on components of the metabolic syndrome in subjects with coronary heart disease. Arch Int Med 2006;166(11): 1218.
[87] Castillo-Richmond A, Schneider RH, Alexander CN, Cook R, Myers H, Nidich S, Salerno J. Effects of stress reduction on carotid atherosclerosis in hypertensive African Americans. Stroke 2000; 31(3): 568-573
[88] Jayadevappa R, Johnson JC, Bloom BS *et al.* Effectiveness of transcendental meditation on functional capacity and quality of life of African-Americans with congestive heart failure: A randomized control study. Ethnic Dis 2007; 17(1): 72-77.
[89] Schneider RH, Nidich S, Kotchen J, Kotchen T, Grim C, Rainforth M. Effects of stress reduction on clinical events in African Americans with coronary heart disease: A randomized controlled trial. Circ 2009; 120, S461.
[90] Sullivan MJ, Wood L, Terry J, Brantley J. The Support, Education, and Research in Chronic Heart Failure Study (SEARCH): A mindfulness-based psychoeducational intervention improves depression and clinical symptoms in patients with chronic heart failure. Amer Heart J 2009; 157(1): 84-90.
[91] Aljasir B, Bryson M, Al-shehri B. Yoga practice for the management of type II diabetes mellitus in adults: A systematic review. Evid based complement alternat med 2010; 7(4), 399-408.
[92] Rosenzweig S, Reibel DK, Edman JS, Jasser SA, McMearty KD, Goldstein BJ. Mindfulness-based stress reduction is associated with improved glycemic control in type 2 diabetes: A pilot study. Altern ther 2007; 13(5): 36-38.
[93] Birdee, G. S., Yeh, G. Complementary and alternative medicine therapies for diabetes: A clinical review. Clinical Diabetes 2010, 28(4), 147-155.

[94] Okonta, NR. Does yoga therapy reduce blood pressure in patients with hypertension?: An integrative review. Holist Nurs Pract 2012; 26(3), 137-141.

[95] Cohen D, Townsend RR. Yoga and hypertension. J Clin Hyperten 2011; 9(10): 800-801.

[96] Selvamurthy W, Sridharan K, Ray US, Tiwary RS, Hegde KS, Radhadrishan U, Sinha KC (1998). A new physiological approach to control essential hypertension. Indian J Physiol and Pharmacol 1998; 42(2): 205-213.

[97] Jayasinghe, S. Yoga in cardiac health (a review). Eur J Cardiovasc Prevent and Rehabil 2004; 11(5): 369-375.

[98] Goldstein CM, Josephson R, Xie S, Hughes JW. Current perspectives on the use of meditation to reduce blood pressure. Int J Hyperten 2012; 1-11.

[99] Anderson, JW, Liu C, Kryscio, RJ. Blood pressure response to transcendental meditation: A meta-analysis. Amer J Hyperten 2008; 21(3): 310-316.

[100] Cysarz D., Bussing A. Cardiorespiratory synchronization during Zen meditation. Eur J App Physiol 2005; 95(1): 88-95

[101] Nesvold, A., Fagerland, M. W., Davanger, S. Increased heart rate variability during nondirective meditation. Eur J Prev Cardiol 2012; 19(4): 773-780.

[102] Bijlani RL, Vempati RP, Yadav RK. A brief but comprehensive lifestyle education program based on yoga reduces risk factors for cardiovascular disease and diabetes mellitus. J Alternat Complement Med 2005; 11(2), 267-274.

[103] Mahajan AS, Reddy KS, Sachedeya U. Lipid profile of coronary risk subjects following yogic lifestyle. Indian Heart J 1999; 51: 37-40.

[104] Vyas R, Dikshit N. Effect of meditation on respiratory system, cardiovascular system and lipid profile. Indian J Physiol Pharmacol 2002; 46(4): 487-491.

[105] Vyas R, Raval KV, Dikshit, N. Effect of raja yoga meditation o the lipid profile of post-menopausal women. Indian J Physiol Pharmacol 2008; 52(4): 420-424.

[106] Yang, K. A review of yoga programs for four leading risk factors of chronic diseases. Evid Based Complement Alternat Med.2007; 4(4), 487-491.

[107] Amita S, Prabhakar S, Manoj I, Harminder S, Pavan T. Effect of yoga-nidra on blood glucose level in diabetic patients. Indian J Physiol Pharmacol, 2009; 53: 97-101.

[108] Agte VV, Tarwadi K. Sudarshan Kriya yoga for treating Type 2 Diabetes: A preliminary study. Altern Complement Ther, 2004; 10: 220-222.

[109] Chaiopanont, S. Hypoglycemic effect of sitting breathing meditation exercise on type 2 diabetes at Wat Khae Nok Primary Health Center in Nonthaburi Province. J Med Assoc Thailand 2008; 91(1): 93-98.

[110] Gordon LA, Morrison EY, McGrowder DA, *et al.* Effect of exercise therapy on lipid profile and oxidative stress indicators in patients with type 2 diabetes. Complement Alternat Med 2008; 8(21): 1-10.

[111] Ershow AG, Ortega A, Baldwin JT, Hill JO. Engineering approaches to energy balance and obesity: Opportunities for novel collaborations and research. J Diab Sci Tech 2007; 1(1), 95-105.

[112] Pomeranz JL, Teret SP, Sugarman SD, Rutkow L, Brownell KD. Innovative legal approaches to address obesity. The Milbank Quarterly 2009; 87(1).

[113] Unnikrishnan AG, Kalra S, Garg MK. Preventing obesity in India: Weighing the options. Indian J Endocrinol Metabol 2012; 16(1): 4-6.

[114] Kuttner L, Chambers CT, Hardial J, Israel DM, Jacobson K, Evans, K. A randomized trial of yoga for adolescents with irritable bowel syndrome. Pain Res Manag 2006; 11(4): 217-223.

[115] Sirven JI, Drazkowski JF, Zimmerman RS, Bortz JJ, Shulman DL, Macleish M. Complementary/alternative medicine for epilepsy in Arizona. Neurol 2003; 61(4): 576-577.

[116] Steiner NJ, Sidhu TK, Pop PG, Frenette EC, Perrin EC. Yoga in an urban school for children with emotional and behavioral disorders: A feasibility study. J Child Family Studies 2012; Advance online publication.

[117] Gura, S. T. Yoga for stress reduction and injury prevention at work. Work 2002; 19(1): 3-7.

[118] Wadsworth EJK, Simpson SA, Moss SC, Smith AP. The Bristol Stress and Health Study: Accidents, minor injuries and cognitive failures at work. Occupational Medicine 2003; 53(6): 392-397.

[119] Ilgen DR. Health issues at work: Opportunities for industrial/organizational psychology. The American Psychologist 1990; 45(2): 273-283.

[120] Wolever RQ, Bobinet KJ, McCabe K, Mackenzie ER, Fekete E, Kusnick CA, Baime M. Effective and viable mind-body stress reduction in the workplace: A randomized controlled trial. J Occupat Health Psychol 2012; 17(2), 246-258.
[121] Cryer B, McCraty R, Childre D. Pull the plug on stress. Harvard Business Review 2003; 81(7): 102-107.
[122] Manocha R, Black D, Sarris J, Stough C. A randomized, controlled trial of meditation for work stress, anxiety and depressed mood in full-time workers. Evid Based Complement Alternat Med 2011; 1-8.
[123] Deshpande, RC. A healthy way to handle work place stress through yoga, meditation and soothing humor. Int J Environment Sci 2012; 2(4): 2143-2154.
[124] Himelstein S, Hastings A, Shapiro S, Heery, M. (2012). Mindfulness training for self-regulation and stress with incarcerated youth: A pilot study. Prob J 2012; 59(2): 151-165.
[125] Sumter, MT, Monk-Turner E, Turner C. The benefits of meditation practice in the correctional setting. J Correct Health Care 2009; 15(1): 47-57.

CHAPTER 15

Prescribing Medications for Older Adults: Dealing with Obesity, Misuse, Polypharmacy and Adverse Drug Events!

T.S. Dharmarajan[*,1,2] and S. Davuluri[3]

[1]Vice Chairman, Department of Medicine, Clinical Director, Geriatrics, Montefiore Medical Center (Wakefield Campus), Bronx, New York, USA; [2]Professor of Clinical Medicine, Albert Einstein College of Medicine, USA; and [3]Fellow in Geriatric Medicine, Montefiore Medical Center (Wakefield Campus), Bronx, New York, USA

Abstract: Aging trends reflect an older population characterized by increasing life expectancy. Aging is characterized by diminished physiological reserves and increasing co-morbidity, with outcomes tending to be worse in overweight and obese individuals. Older adults and especially the obese are on a large number of medications; these include prescribed and over the counter drugs. Providers require an understanding of the principles of appropriate prescribing for alterations in age related pharmacokinetics and pharmacodynamics. Body characteristics that influence drug actions include leaner body mass and changes in fluid and lipid compartment status; overweight and obese individuals therefore have altered kinetics and dynamics. Medications can cause both weight gain and weight loss. Polypharmacy is a common issue in the older population. The consequences of inappropriate prescribing and polypharmacy include adverse drug events and reactions, likely resulting in unwanted outcomes and hospitalizations. Prescribing medicines for obese individuals imposes challenges. Medication management must adopt principles to ensure adherence, surveillance, reconciliation and cost containment, with the aim to maintain quality of health care as well as safety.

Keywords: Adverse drug events, adverse drug reactions, drug interactions, drug-drug interactions, drug-nutrient interactions, drugs and weight changes, medication adherence, medications and metabolic syndrome, obesity and medication effects, pharmacodynamics, pharmacokinetics, pharmacology of aging, polypharmacy, potentially inappropriate medications (PIMs) potentially inappropriate medications, principles of prescribing, renal function and prescribing.

***Corresponding author T.S. Dharmarajan:** 31 Pheasant Run, Scarsdale, NY 10583, USA; Tel: (718) 920-9889; Fax: (914)723-4297; E-mail: dharmarajants@yahoo.com

Judith Wylie-Rosett & Sunil S. Jhangiani (Eds)

INTRODUCTION

The cost of prescription drugs, often used to treat older adults including overweight or obese individuals, is a burden to health care expenditure in the United States (U.S.). Data suggest that 30% of the U.S. population over 65 years old are on multiple medications, including alternative medicines such as herbs and supplements [1]. Over a fifth of the geriatric population (generally considered over 65 years) are on five or more medications, and of these, some are on an excess of ten. The geriatric age group comprises only 13% of the population, but consumes a third of the prescription medications; in another three decades, this population will become 25% of the U.S. population and account for half of the prescription medications.

Along with aging of society, there has been a less noticed but bothersome increase in the prevalence of overweight and obese adults in the United States and all over the world. Based on the "body mass index" (BMI), derived by dividing the weight in kilograms by height in meters squared, an individual can be categorized as underweight (< 18.5 kg/m^2), healthy weight (18.5-24.9 kg/m^2), overweight (25-29.9 kg/m^2) and obese (> 30 kg/m^2). Excessive accumulation of fat in overweight and obese adults poses health risks [2]. Besides BMI, which has limited reliability as an indicator of body fat (as it does not directly measure body fat), waist circumference, skin fold thickness and waist to hip circumference ratio are additional measures used to assess body fat [3]. Obesity results from an energy imbalance between calorie consumption and expenditure, genetics, disease and may include medication adverse effects [4].

More than a third of adults in the U.S. are obese; the prevalence in adults remains a significant problem and remained stable between 2003-4 and 2009-2010 [5]. The prevalence of high BMI (overweight and obesity) is 69 for all adults over 20 years, with the number even higher over the age of 60 years, calling for a continued need for surveillance [5]. Obesity, as a contributor to chronic diseases has become a public health challenge. New obesity guidelines address the challenges faced by primary care physicians. The approaches to tackle the issue include: identification of patients who need to lose weight and counseling them regarding the benefits of weight loss; dietary therapy for weight loss; lifestyle interventions and counseling; and bariatric surgery [6]. The medical costs of obesity related illnesses in the U.S. are over $200 billion annually; this includes a huge cost of medications used for obesity-related disorders such as diabetes, calling for interventions with long term efficacy [7].

In a background of an aging society that includes many who are overweight or obese, health care providers including physicians, nurses, pharmacists and others have a role and responsibility to ensure appropriate prescribing without compromising quality. This chapter addresses the pharmacologic effects of medications with regards to preventing adverse effects in older adults.

PHARMACODYNAMICS AND PHARMACOKINETICS

A pharmaceutical drug is a chemical used to prevent, diagnose, treat and cure disease [8]. Herbal medicine or botanical medicine refers to the use of plant sources for medicinal purposes. Various plant components possess distinguished chemical properties that offer therapeutic effects [9].

Pharmacodynamics in simple terms refers to the action of a drug in the body, at cellular, molecular, sub molecular and tissue levels. *Pharmacodynamics* firstly includes, the desired effects, *i.e.,* therapeutic and beneficial effects, and secondly, the undesired and adverse effects (or toxicity) [10]. While providers and patients desire only the beneficial effects, adverse effects cannot be totally avoided. The term *pharmacokinetics* refers to the course of a drug within the body or what the body does to the drug; including absorption, bioavailability, distribution, protein binding and elimination of the drug from the body through a variety of routes, following administration through any route [11].

Both pharmacokinetics and dynamics are heavily influenced by several physiological changes that occur with aging. Physiological changes pertinent to body composition vary from person to person, differ with gender and are influenced by age, nutritional status, physical activity and hormonal influences [12-15].

Body weight undergoes alteration with aging. A decline occurs in bone and muscle mass; the latter referred to as sarcopenia. Lean body mass, comprised of muscle, bone and non-fatty tissue, declines significantly as one ages. While body water accounts for 60% or more of body weight in young to middle age adult, the water compartment declines as one gets older and is closer to 50% of body weight in a 65 or 70 year old. The fat compartment increases through life to about 30% of the body weight, with the increase being relatively higher in women as compared to men; fat is largely central in distribution. The overall decline in body water and increase in fat significantly influences kinetics and dynamics of water and lipid soluble drugs. Therefore, obesity has an impact on pharmacokinetics and dynamics. A decline in body water increases serum concentration of water soluble drugs (*e.g.*, digoxin, diuretics, aminoglycosides, vancomycin, theophylline and lithium) as well as alcohol, altering their effects favorably or adversely. This is one reason that older people (should they consume alcohol) are advised to consume lesser quantities; the blood levels for a given drink of alcohol are higher in the old as compared to the young. On the contrary, the larger fat stores retain lipid soluble drugs (*e.g.*, benzodiazepines) for a longer than usual period of time, increasing their half-life, with resultant adverse effects on gait, balance and cognition; the adverse effects continue long after the drug is discontinued, as lipid soluble drugs are retained for longer periods by the fat depots [16-22].

Age-related sarcopenia is relevant to drug kinetics; a decline in skeletal muscle mass results in a lower serum creatinine level. Typically, renal function declines with age; however, the expected increase in serum creatinine does not occur because of sarcopenia. It must be recognized that the serum creatinine level is likely to be lower than expected, giving a false impression of a better than true renal function. Renal blood flow declines with age. In many older people, the glomerular filtration rate (GFR) may decline at the rate of about 8.0 ml/min/1.73 m^2/decade (or about 0.8-1% annually) after the third decade; based on longitudinal studies, the rate of decline is highly variable, ranging from zero to over 1% [15, 23-26]. Tubular secretion also tends to decline by about 0.7 to 1% annually [23-26]. However, the expected rise in creatinine level is offset by the decline in the synthesis of creatinine from muscle. As the serum creatinine level is a poor reflector of renal function, one must utilize an acceptable formula such as the Cockroft-Gault equation (CGF) or the Modification of Diet in Renal Disease Study equation to assess kidney function [23-26]. Discrepancies between these equations and the newer Chronic Kidney Disease Epidemiology Collaboration (CKD-EPI) equation occur with age, as demonstrated by a study comparing the equations [26]. The effect of age on renal function has a major influence on the dosing of drugs that are excreted by the kidneys; a reduction in dose is recommended for these medications. In fact, many commonly utilized medications fall under this category.

Additionally, hepatic function may be affected in the elderly, commonly by a disease rather than by age. Drug absorption in the gastrointestinal tract is not appreciably altered as one gets older. If a drug is consumed, failure of absorption is seldom an issue in the absence of gastrointestinal disease or a history of resection of gastro-intestinal tract segments [27, 28]. Hepatic influence on drugs occurs largely through a complex cytochrome p450 system, with various inhibitors and inducers of medications. Table **1** summarizes physiological age related changes, while Fig. (**1**) schematically explains the drug pathway.

Table 1. Physiological changes with aging: Influence on drug metabolism [12-20].

Body Water
Declines with age, more pronounced in females
Water soluble drugs and alcohol levels tend to attain higher levels Examples: lithium, aminoglycosides, digoxin, warfarin, and vancomycin levels are higher
Body Fat
Relative increase in body fat with age, more pronounced in females
Large fat stores accommodate and retain the lipid soluble drugs In addition, obesity is common in the old Examples: benzodiazepines, especially intermediate and long acting forms stay longer in the body; vitamin D and certain hormones are sequestrated in lipid depots
Skeletal Muscle
Muscle mass declines with age (sarcopenia)
Muscle derived serum creatinine does not increase as much as expected in spite of a decline in renal function
Necessitates an estimate of renal function through use of an acceptable formula
Serum Albumin
Levels remain normal in spite of aging
However, levels decline with disease: renal glomerular disease, malnutrition, malabsorption and liver disease
Protein bound drugs have altered sensitivity from changes in the free drug level
Examples: warfarin, diuretics and digoxin
Renal Function
GFR and tubular secretion decline variably with aging (range 0% to 1%)
Decreased elimination of drugs is dependent on removal through glomerular filtration and tubular secretion.
Dosage of drugs excreted by the kidney must be adjusted to renal function: *e.g.,* digoxin, meperidine, aminoglycosides, vancomycin, penicillins, amantadine, dabigatran and oseltamivir

Adverse Drug Reaction and Adverse Drug Event

An adverse drug reaction (ADR) is defined by the International Conference on Harmonization as "a response to a drug that is noxious and unintended, which occurs with doses administered to modify physiological function for prophylaxis, diagnosis or therapy of disease" [29]. An adverse drug event [ADE] is defined broadly as "harm resulting from use of a drug, and includes all adverse drug

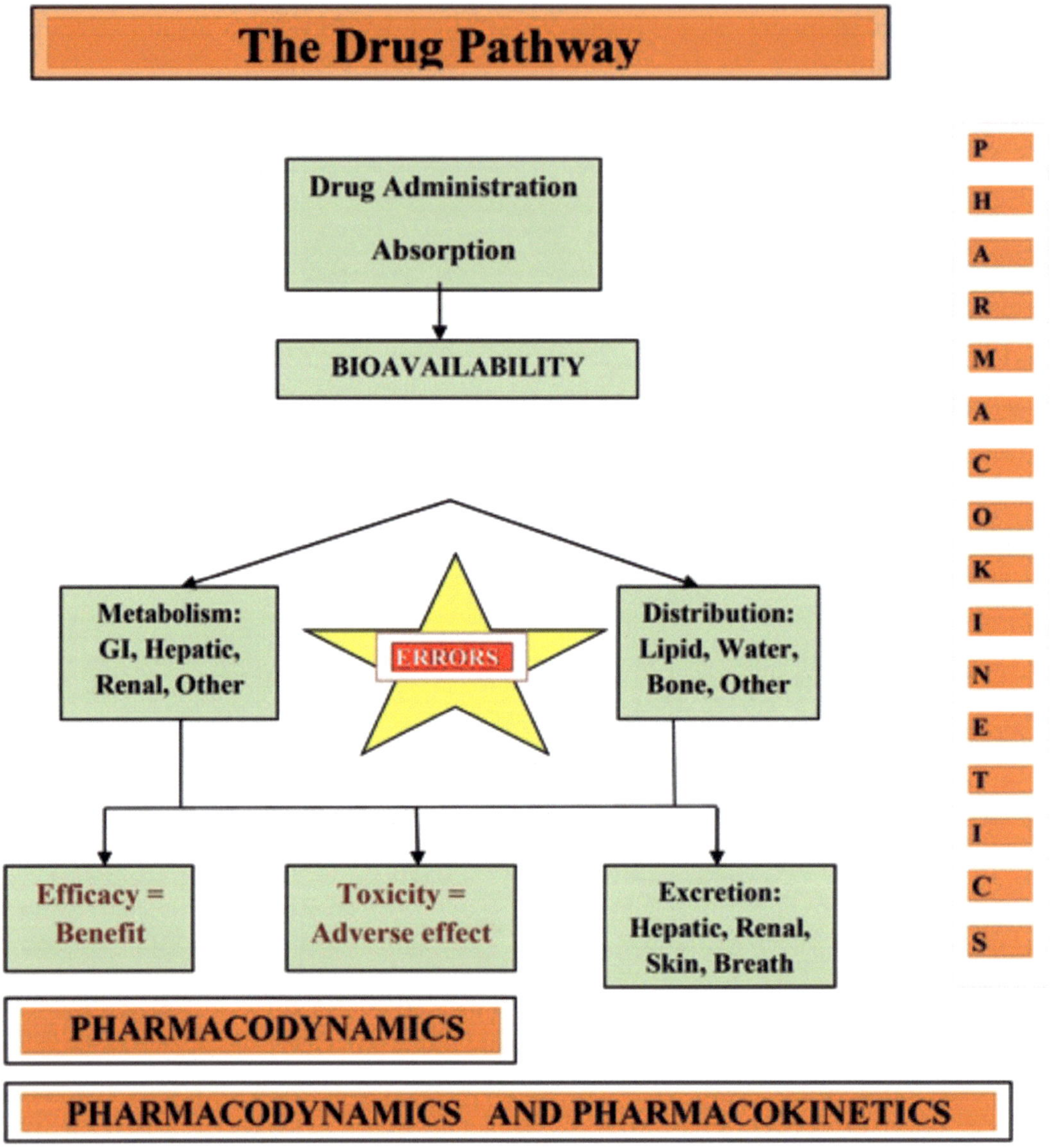

Fig. (1). The drug pathway: Kinetics and dynamics.

reactions, resulting from overdose, dose reduction and discontinuation of drug therapy" [30]. While the terms may be confusing, and are often used interchangeably, adverse drug reactions (ADRs) are really a category of adverse drug events (ADEs). ADRs result in up to 10% of hospitalizations. They are of two types, A and B. Type A is related to the pharmacological actions of the drug and is predictable, resulting from dosing and interactions. Type B is unrelated to the drug's pharmacological actions, is unpredictable and results largely from idiosyncracy or an immunological cause. The use of the term "side-effects" is not recommended any further [30]. Over a quarter of hospital admissions in older adults have been attributed directly or indirectly to adverse drug events. Fig. (**2**) provides a schematic concept of ADEs and ADRs. The term "medication error" includes near misses, close calls and potential adverse events; medication errors are preventable events that cause or lead to inappropriate medication use and patient harm, although medication control is largely in the hands of the health care professional, patient or consumer [30].

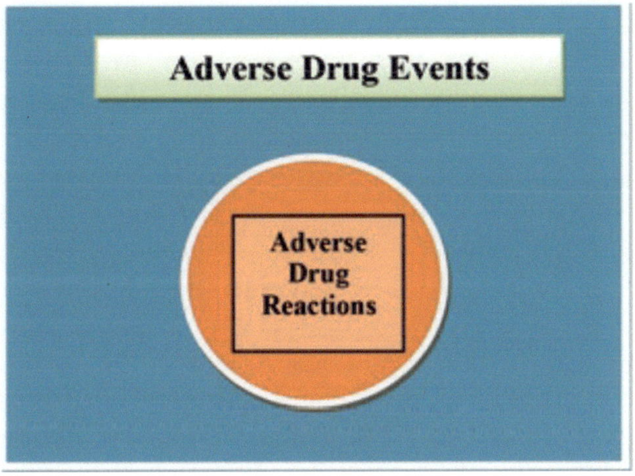

Fig. (2). Adverse drug reactions are a component of adverse drug events (adapted from ref. [30]).

POLYPHARMACY

Polypharmacy refers to prescription of multiple medications for a patient; the exact number of medications that define polypharmacy is debatable, and range from a definition of over three (by the WHO) to four, five or more on a continued basis [31, 32]. More than the number, it is the inappropriate, often excessive or unwarranted prescription of multiple medications that characterize polypharmacy. Older adults are particularly vulnerable to the adverse effects of polypharmacy, rendering them prone to high rates of adverse drug reactions [33]. Often, multiple medications are prescribed by different doctors for a patient with one or more health problems, resulting in duplicate medications, with some patients getting the same medication in different forms. Polypharmacy increases the prescription drug related health expenditure, and renders the patient more vulnerable to drug interactions [34]. Clinical judgment of the primary health care physician to screen for polypharmacy is expected on a routine basis since there are no validated tools for the purpose; the typical approach is to question the patient periodically regarding all prescribed and non-prescribed medications in a non-threatening manner. Patients must be encouraged to bring all their medications in a bag for verification at the time of office visit. The process not only offers an opportunity for a review of the list, but also uncovers several unnecessary medications and duplication between generic and brand names. Avoiding potentially inappropriate medications (PIMs) is of paramount importance in view of the consequences or adverse drug events that may be avoided by a review [35]. Polypharmacy in the elderly is associated with frailty, falls, syncope, delirium, falls, fractures and mortality [36, 37]. Adverse drug events account for a large number of hospitalizations; in fact, any new manifestation in a person on multiple medications should entertain the possibility of an ADE before embarking on a laborious and expensive evaluation. An adverse drug event often begets a second adverse drug event, as the first manifestation is treated with yet another unnecessary drug, rather than withdrawal of the first agent (Table **2**).

Adverse Drug Event Begets Another Adverse Drug Event

A prescription cascade is the phenomenon where the adverse event from a prescribed drug is interpreted as a new and additional health problem for which more medications are prescribed. This scenario creates a broader scope for drug-drug interactions and more adverse drug events. Polypharmacy may play a vital role in the initiation of the prescription cascade (Table **2**). A screening tool for potentially inappropriate medication use is one approach to minimize polypharmacy.

Table 2. Case scenario: Adverse drug event begets another adverse drug event!

• **Drug A** (pioglitazone) is initiated for glucose intolerance.
○ Edema develops as an adverse drug event from the medication.
○ But edema is mistaken for fluid overload, **Drug B** (hydrochlorothiazide) is added.
• Edema persists; patient now develops hyponatremia (from the thiazide).
○ As edema persists, a more potent diuretic **Drug C** (furosemide) is added.
• Hyponatremia becomes worse; edema continues to persist.
○ Patient becomes hypotensive from intravascular volume depletion and develops syncope.
○ Hospitalization is required; pioglitazone, thiazide and furosemide are all discontinued.
• The patient improves upon discontinuing all three medications and is discharged home.

The Screening Tool of Older Persons' Potentially Inappropriate Prescriptions (STOPP) criteria from Europe, developed in 2006, has similarities and differences from the Beers criteria [38-40]. Many drugs at high risk for ADEs and drugs to avoid for reasons of drug interactions are consistent in both Beers' and STOPP criteria, with a higher proportion of hospitalizations noted to result from adverse drug events relating to the STOPP criteria [40]. Common selected examples of Potentially Inappropriate Medications (PIMs) suggested by the STOPP criteria are provided in the table below; these medications nevertheless continue to be prescribed despite proof for poor outcomes [40, 41]. Tables **3**, **4** and **5** provide information on the inappropriate use of drugs in certain situations; disorders where certain medications are best avoided; and the over and under use of medications.

Table 3. Inappropriate use of drugs by disorder - STOPP 2006 criteria [38-41].

• Anticholinergic medications for extrapyramidal adverse effects of antipsychotic medications
• Antihistamines of the first generation type for insomnia or movement disorders
• Antipsychotic drug use in presence of Parkinson's disease or seizures
• Aspirin use with no history of coronary, cerebral or peripheral vascular disease
• Antispasmodic medications, except for short term palliative care
• Benzodiazepines prescribed for those with a history of falls in the prior 3 months
• Digoxin used in a dose over 0.125 mg/day for heart failure
• Neuroleptics for agitation, long term
• Use of any NSAIDs for long term, in the presence of chronic kidney disease or heart failure
• Non-selective NSAIDs for long term or with a history of peptic ulcer
• Nitrofurantoin for long term suppression of urinary infection in CKD (GFR <60 ml/min)
• Loop diuretics for edema (without heart failure), or as initial monotherapy for hypertension
• Antipsychotics, hypnotics, antihistamines and opioids with a history of falls/fractures

The Beers Criteria, originally developed by Mark Beers in 1991, was updated by the American Geriatrics Society in 2012. The list, revised several times over the years, provides examples of inappropriate drug use and various drug-disease interactions (as outlined in Table **4**) with the potential for poor outcomes in practice.

Table 4. 2012 American Geriatrics Society Beers Criteria for potentially inappropriate medication use (PIMS) in selected disorders in older adults [39-41].

Heart failure, chronic kidney disease and edema
• Avoid NSAIDs, COX-2 inhibitors and glitazones
Chronic kidney disease and hyperkalemia
• Caution with use of ACE inhibitors, angiotensin receptor blockers and spironolactone
Constipation
• Caution with use of anticholinergics, opioids, antihistamines and TCAs
Syncope and Orthostatic Hypotension
• Avoid or minimize the use of cholinesterase inhibitors and tricyclic antidepressants
Seizures and Involuntary Movements
• Avoid or minimize the use of bupropion, tramadol, meperidine and antipsychotics
Delirium
• Avoid anticholinergics, benzodiazepines and antipsychotics
Falls and Fractures by History
• Avoid antipsychotics, hypnotics, TCAs, SSRIs and opioids
Insomnia
• Avoid decongestants, caffeine, stimulants and theophylline
Parkinson's Disease
• Avoid antipsychotics and metoclopramide
Stress Incontinence
• Avoid alpha blockers
Benign Prostatic Hyperplasia
• Avoid anticholinergics, calcium channel blockers and antihistamines

COMMON MEDICATION CLASSES WITH RELEVANT PRESCRIBING INFORMATION

Antibiotics

Antibiotics are lifesaving medications when used in appropriate situations with adequate information about the cause of infection, and where relevant results of specimen culture and sensitivity are required. Upper respiratory symptoms, often from benign conditions such as viral syndromes are common grounds for inappropriate use of antibiotics [43]. Overprescribing antibiotics also occurs in

Table 5. Examples of inappropriate prescribing (Beers and STOPP Criteria) [38-42].

Over Prescribed Medications
Anti-infective agents
Anti-cholinergic drugs
Anti-psychotic drugs
Benzodiazepines
Laxatives and stool softeners
Proton pump inhibitors
Sedating antihistamines
Non-steroidal anti-inflammatory agents
Vitamins and minerals
Opioids for musculoskeletal disorders
Under Prescribed Medications
ACE inhibitors for heart failure or diabetes
Angiotensin receptor blockers for heart failure
Anticoagulants in atrial fibrillation
Antihypertensives for hypertension
Diuretics (thiazides) for hypertension
Beta blockers for heart failure
Proton pump inhibitors with NSAIDs
Statins for hyperlipidemia
Vitamin D and calcium for osteoporosis

accordance to patients expectations during visits to a physician and the fear on part of the patient that the doctor may be overlooking an infection [44]. Complications of inappropriate prescribing of antibiotics include development of resistance, increased organism virulence and pathogenicity due to resistance [45]. Antibiotic associated diarrhea and *Clostridium difficile* diarrhea are well recognized consequences of antibiotic use; the latter is the only condition resulting from antibiotic use that subsequently requires another course of antibiotics for its treatment.

Significant interactions may follow antibiotic courses following the inhibition of microsomal enzymes in the CYP450 system. When fluoroquinolones, metronidazole, macrolides and imidazole antifungals are prescribed along with drugs with a narrow therapeutic index (*e.g.,* theophylline, digitalis, warfarin and phenytoin), the potential for high drug levels of the latter with resultant adverse effects, many serious, is high [46]. Penicillin, cephalosporins, clindamycin and sulfonamides, used without justification, may even be associated with psychiatric and neurological manifestations, necessitating emergency room visits [47].

Anticholinergic Medications

Several medications possess variable degrees of anticholinergic activity. Chronic use of these medications is generally associated with constipation, xerostomia, urinary retention and more importantly, with a decline in memory and cognition. Use of medications for appropriate indications (such as urge incontinence) requires careful follow up for associated adverse effects. Thus, a risk benefit ratio and individualization of therapy is called for. Use of anticholinergics (*e.g.*, diphenhydramine) to promote sleep is strongly discouraged, as also their use in patients with benign prostatic hyperplasia where the drugs can predispose the patient to urinary retention. Patients with mild cognitive impairment may worsen following use of anticholinergic medications. Many anticholinergic drugs have reduced clearance with age.

Antipsychotics

There is considerable evidence in the literature detailing adverse effects from long-term use of anti-psychotic agents, now strongly discouraged except for rare indications. Both first generation (conventional) and second generation (atypical) drugs in this class are associated with increased risk of metabolic syndrome, cardiovascular and cerebrovascular adverse events. Chronic use is associated with higher mortality. Extrapyramidal movement disorders, which develop following their use, may not reverse upon discontinuation of the medications. Chronic use carries an association with falls and fractures [48].

Sedative Hypnotics

In view of their fat soluble properties, and an increase in size of the lipid compartment with age, the drugs remain in the fat depots with much slower clearance as one ages. Use of sedative hypnotics is associated with an increase in falls, fractures, accidents and worsening confusion. Barring the settings of seizure disorders, alcohol withdrawal with delirium tremens and severe anxiety disorder, their use is discouraged. Sedative hypnotics are not even recommended to promote sleep in chronic insomnia or for the management of delirium. Their pharmacokinetics varies based on whether the drug action is short, intermediate or long acting; additionally, the half-life increases with aging.

Warfarin and Novel Anticoagulants

As hypercoagulable disorders increase in prevalence in older adults, accordingly, indications for use of anticoagulants become higher with age. Their use is indicated in several situations, but caution must be exercised in view of their high adverse effect profile. Most novel anticoagulants (such as dabigatran) do not have an antidote when bleeding occurs, and dosage needs to be adjusted for renal function. Warfarin is titrated based on the International Normalized Ratio, but more important is the need for awareness of the drug's interactions with nutrients or herbals (*e.g.,* green leafy vegetables, garlic, ginseng, feverfew, ginkgo biloba, saw palmetto and ginger), medications (NSAIDs, antibiotics, aspirin) and the effect of disease on its kinetics and dynamics (thyroid function, liver status); dosing does not need to be adjusted for renal function. Close monitoring is called for sick in-patients on warfarin, as the ill are subjected to major medication regimen changes, especially when hospitalized [49].

Proton Pump Inhibitors

FDA labeled indications for proton pump inhibitors include active duodenal ulcer, Helicobacter pylori duodenal ulcer, erosive esophagitis to maintain healing, gastroesophageal reflux disease, gastric ulcer and stress ulcer prophylaxis. However, proton pump inhibitor use is associated with the increased incidence of Clostridium Difficile Associated Diarrhea (CDAD) [50], a higher risk of spinal, hip and wrist fractures secondary to osteoporosis (when PPIs are used for over a year), and a higher likelihood for infection (*e.g.,* pneumonia) with resistant organisms [51, 52]. Proton pump inhibitors are now listed as a class of PIMs in the STOPP criteria.

MULTIPLE EFFECTS: INTENDED AND UNINTENDED

Medication Induced Hypertension

Several drugs used over time have been documented to cause elevations in blood pressure. Chemically induced hypertension needs to be recognized and tackled by withdrawing the medication rather than adding yet another antihypertensive. Medications or ingredients implicated include glucocorticoids, NSAIDs, phenylephrine and other nasal decongestants, cyclosporine, erythropoietin, caffeine and licorice (mineralocorticoid-like) amongst others [53].

Medications and Weight Changes

Allopathic Drugs Promoting Weight Gain or Weight Loss

Either as intended or unintended effects, medication use may result in weight changes. Several medications cause undesired weight gain. Most anti-hypertensives tend to cause some degree of salt retention, readily reversed by the use of diuretics. The thiazolidinediones, used in the management of type 2 diabetes, contribute to weight gain and edema, even at times precipitating heart failure; the effects are not always readily reversible on discontinuing the drug.

The classical example of diuretics meant to cause sodium and water excretion along with weight loss is a perfectly intended use, and well utilized in heart failure, hypertension or any other state with salt and water retention (such as in hepatic or renal failure). Metformin, on the other hand, is modestly effective in reducing weight and other risk factors for cardiovascular disease in clinically stable overweight patients. Weight loss was demonstrated in overweight patients with chronic schizophrenia over a 16-week period, demonstrating that metformin could play a significant role in decreasing the adverse outcomes of obesity and metabolic syndrome [54].

Among the antidepressants, paroxetine (but not all serotonin reuptake inhibitors) has been noted to effect weight gain. Valproic acid, used for epilepsy, affects appetite and through a complex process involving protein utilization, causes weight gain. Mirtazapine, an antidepressant, improves appetite through an enhancing effect on serotonin and norepinephrine, and produces an often welcome weight gain in those who previously had lost weight. An adverse effect of the long-term use of antipsychotic drugs is weight gain and development of the metabolic syndrome; chronic use of several antipsychotic agents (such as clozapine, risperidone, quetiapine, olanzapine) is associated with the increase in risk for vascular events and mortality. A study suggests that antipsychotic drug-induced changes in metabolic indices may be evident as early as after 2 weeks of treatment, reaching a maximum at 3 months of treatment, and are higher in those receiving second generation antipsychotics [55]. The findings warrant a need to sensitize health care providers about the need to screen and monitor patients receiving antipsychotics for the metabolic syndrome [55]. Thus, treatment of schizophrenia requires attention towards the psychiatric condition and additionally also to the medical conditions such as metabolic syndrome, which are highly prevalent in these individuals who may be receiving antipsychotics [56].

Other drugs associated with weight gain include selective serotonin reuptake inhibitors (SSRIs), amitriptyline, lithium, valproic acid, carbamazepine, gabapentin and valproic acid [57]. Medication associated weight gain may influence outcomes in a weight management program; this aspect is often overlooked in obese patients trying to lose weight [58].

A variety of drugs are available for the long-term drug treatment of obesity. Medications, when utilized as an adjunct to life style intervention, lead to a greater mean weight loss and an increased likelihood of achieving meaningful weight loss at the end of a year [59]. The medications should be discontinued if a weight loss of at least 5% fails to occur, thereby reducing the opportunity for adverse effects with little benefit [59]. No obesity medication has been demonstrated by well-designed studies to lower cardiovascular morbidity and mortality [59].

Supplements and Weight Loss

Several herbs and supplements are presented with claims to boost metabolism and cause weight loss [60]. Based on a randomized controlled trial, herbal caffeine (at about 192 mg/day) and ephedra (about 90 mg/day) demonstrated a beneficial effect in lipid profile and favored weight loss [61]. The combination of ephedrine and caffeine has not been proven to be better than either supplement studied individually. The combination of ephedra and caffeine is associated with adverse effects related to autonomic hyperactivity (anxiety and palpitations) and gastrointestinal effects (nausea and vomiting) [62]. The effects of caffeine (*Coffea arabica*) are highly variable and individualized based on daily intake, metabolism and body weight. "Caffeinism" is a syndrome seen in long-term excessive users of caffeine, characterized by depression, restlessness, anxiety, palpitations and poor performance [63]. The FDA considers a toxic caffeine dose as over 1000 mg daily. Withdrawal from caffeine can result in drowsiness, insomnia, irritability, headache and fatigue, beginning a day or two after withdrawal, lasting up to a week [64].

Ginseng (*Panax quinquefolius)* is used with claims for improving cognitive and physical performance. Scientific evidence is inconclusive based on trial data [65]. Ginseng may have effects on serum leptin and neuropeptide Y to cause a reduction in food intake [66]. Devil's backbone (*Cissus quadrangularis)* extract and supplement have been shown to control appetite by increasing serotonin levels and alleviating cardiovascular risk by diminishing serum glucose, lipids and weight in a randomized controlled trial [67]. Peanut (*Arachis hypogea*) shell extracts can inhibit intestinal lipases and increase lipid excretion through a decrease in fat absorption in the gut [68].

The use of complementary and alternative medicine is common among the elderly overweight and obese persons with knee osteoarthritis [69]. It is worth emphasizing that promotion of energy expenditure by physical activity and adherence to an exercise program, along with appropriate diets remain the crux of weight management health programs [69].

Other Considerations in Obesity

An interesting study of over 11,000 adults assessed the pattern of opioid medication use for non- cancer pain in these individuals before and after bariatric surgery. Over three quarters of patients were chronic opioid users before surgery; the use of opioids was greater post-operatively than pre-operatively, suggesting the need for better, more judicious pain management in obese persons in the post-operative period [70].

Although we recognize that lifestyle modification rather than drugs remains the most effective and prudent way to prevent and manage overweight or obesity states, the approach may not always be clear or straightforward. The dilemma may be apparent when certain disorders coexist with obesity, for example, hard to control hypertension or diabetes; the choice of management in such individuals may range from weight loss by addressing diet and exercise, use of weight loss medications and / or bariatric surgery [71]. A meaningful discussion between provider and patient on the recommended options is called for.

Drug - Drug Interactions

Older adults on multiple prescribed and over-the-counter medications, are more likely to develop drug interactions. These can be drug-drug, drug-nutrient and drug-disease interactions. Polypharmacy clearly compounds the likelihood. Key factors leading to interactions are: patient factors include age, consumption of multiple drugs, the vehicle and comorbidity; nutrient factors include fasting or postprandial state and delivery modality; drug factors include kinetics and narrow therapeutic index [72, 73]. A combination of factors is usually operative. Drug-drug interactions have become recognized in the past few decades as significant, in that, many can be avoided through knowledge of these reactions, by adopting steps for prevention [74]. The frequency and nature of potential drug-drug interactions even in settings such as the intensive care unit warrant attention [75].

Several examples are worthy of mention. Tricyclic antidepressants can cause QTc prolongation and cardiac arrhythmias. Even innocuous over the counter medications used for a common cold, such as antihistamines, may result in QTc prolongation, the effects compounded in the patient on antidepressants and antihistamines [76]. Amiodarone inhibits CYPC29, which metabolizes warfarin, thereby enhancing the anticoagulant effect of warfarin with increased bleeding risk [77]. The addition of NSAIDs to a patient on ACE inhibitors for heart failure will antagonize the beneficial effects of the latter and cause sodium retention, increase blood pressure and accentuate the effects on renal potassium handling thus increasing the likelihood for hyperkalemia. The use of ACE inhibitors along with spironolactone warrants close monitoring for hyperkalemia. The combined use of alpha adrenergic blockers for benign prostatic hyperplasia along with anticholinergics such as diphenhydramine, negate the beneficial effects of alpha blockers on the internal sphincter and may lead to urinary retention. Erythromycin, commonly used for respiratory infections, can induce carbamazepine toxicity by inhibiting the cytochrome p450 enzymes and enhancing the adverse drug effect [78]; the drug also interacts with valproic acid resulting in hepatotoxicity.

Drug - Nutrient Interactions

Drug-food or drug-nutrient interactions are defined as "alterations of pharmacokinetics or pharmacodynamics of a drug or nutritional element, or a compromise in nutritional status, resulting from the addition of a drug" [79]. Essentially, there may be an alteration in the drug effect and/or altered nutrient availability. Careful drug selection in association with patient counseling reduces the risk [80]. The implications for practice are enormous [81].

Grape fruit juice, popular in the U.S., inhibits intestinal CYP3A4 and transporter glycoprotein P, thereby causing an increase in drug levels (and systemic effects) of certain medications metabolized by the enzyme. Examples of medications in this category include certain statins, calcium channel blockers and cyclosporine [82]. Guava leaf tea, which contains polyphenols, only weakly inhibits CYP, with low likelihood for drug interactions [83].

As older patients are on a large number of medications, they are at the highest risk for drug interactions [84]. Dietitians and pharmacists have a role to focus on drug-food interactions and patient counseling [85]. Drug-nutrient interactions can enhance effects of the drug or cause treatment failure by altering the bioavailability of the drug besides leading to deficiency of the nutrient [86]. Examples are decreased bioavailability of alendronate or levothyroxine when taken with food; both these medications must be taken on empty stomach with plain water. Carbidopa, used in Parkinson's disease, loses some bioavailability when taken with food protein. On the other hand, vitamin D is best absorbed after meals, with dietary fat facilitating its absorption. Isoniazid and cycloserine can cause B6 and niacin deficiency. Supplementation of folate is recommended with anticonvulsants as the medications act as folate antagonists. Fat soluble vitamins K and D malabsorption can result from cholestyramine use [87]. Chronic metformin therapy for diabetes can cause deficiency of vitamin B12, by interfering with the intrinsic factor complex absorption at the ileal cell surface; the process is calcium dependent and restored to normal by calcium supplementation [88-90] as summarized in Table **6**.

Table 6. Examples of drug-nutrient interactions.

Medication and Food or Nutrient	Consequences
Alendronate and food or beverages	Decreased bioavailability of alendronate
Grapefruit juice and certain statins	Increased bioavailability of statins
Calcium carbonate and food	Better absorbed in the presence of gastric acid pH
Calcium citrate and gastric acid	Absorbed with or without gastric acid
Cholestyramine and food	Decrease absorption of fat soluble vitamins
Levothyroxine and food	Food hampers absorption
Metformin and vitamin B12	Decrease absorption of B12 in ileum
Milk and cations in dairy products	Chelate iron, tetracyclines, fluoroquinolones
Proton pump inhibitors and vitamin B12	Lower B12 absorption by decreasing gastric acidity
Proton pump inhibitors and H2 blockers	Impair absorption of iron, calcium, zinc, folic acid
Phenytoin and effect on hepatic CYP450	Inhibit the system and causes vitamin D deficiency
Warfarin and green leafy vegetables	Lower the effect of warfarin (and decreases INR)
Warfarin and ginger or garlic	Increase the effect of warfarin (and raises INR)
Fatty food on Vitamin D	Increase bioavailability of vitamin D

Prescription Management: Adherence, Medication Reconciliation, Costs

Physiological changes with aging, as stated earlier, influence pharmacokinetics and pharmacodynamics, requiring alterations in drug dosing to avert adverse reactions [91]. Additionally, there is the influence of disease; a third of the population over 65 years may have chronic kidney disease, stage 3 or worse, altering kinetics of drugs from the decline in renal function. As a general rule in the elderly, the approach is to 'Start Low-Go Slow'; the exceptions are for anticancer agents and antibiotics, where it should be to 'Go fast – Hit Hard' [92].

During patient visits, a 'brown bag review' of all medications must be conducted by the primary physician; these include over the counter or non-prescription medications in addition to those prescribed; herbals and supplements must be included in the review process. A thorough review helps minimize polypharmacy, the discontinuation of unnecessary medications and an opportunity to lower prescription related expenditure [93]. On the clinic visit day, the brown bag review provides the most accurate record of medications the patient is taking compared to pharmacy records [94]. Medication therapy management (MTM) sessions help review prescriptions, over the counter drugs and inactive medications, besides going a long way in lowering medication errors, duplications of drugs and non-adherence. Relevant family input is important in that it helps oversee medication adherence in the elderly [95]. Medication adherence in the cognitively impaired can be improved by frequent communication reminders [96].

Medication Reconciliation is a process enforced in hospitals by the Joint Commission in the U.S. The process includes developing a list of current medications, comparing them with prior lists and reconciliation with the new list that will be compiled. Medication reconciliation is a must during transfer of patients across settings within the hospital and outside such as community or other institutions. The current list must be communicated to the patient, caregiver where relevant and the providers of care. Prevention of adverse drug events in those discharged from hospitals and improvement of monitoring to prevent iatrogenic risk is a priority process in the prevention of hospital readmissions [97].

The American Geriatrics Society, in conjunction with the American Board of Internal Medicine, recently introduced an initiative titled "Choose Wisely"; four of the five listed items to be chosen relate to precautions with medication use. The suggestions include avoidance of the use of benzodiazepines for insomnia, delirium and agitation; avoidance of antipsychotics for behavioral manifestations in dementia; avoidance of tight diabetic control to lower HbA1c below 7.5 in those aged over 65 years; and avoidance of the use of antimicrobials for bacteruria in the absence specific urinary symptoms.

"Should the choice of prescribed medications be generic or brand", is a question often asked. Compared to the past, we are more cost conscious today. The use of generics is very much on the increase; in most cases, they cost less than the brand. Optimal care is often possible at lower cost. For example, evidence supports the choice of generic statins for cardiovascular risk reduction [98]. The goal is to maintain health care quality at the lowest cost; promoting generic drug use is a key for this effort [99]. The influence of industry on prescribing practices or physician behavior in yielding to the request of brand name prescriptions from the patient are areas that require further study [100].

Appropriate prescribing should also include consideration for life expectancy and goals of care [101]. In the final analysis, the prescription must be specifically tailored to each patient, based on requirements or indications, patient preferences and socioeconomic factors; the success for appropriate prescribing is largely in the physician's hands.

Table 7. Principles of appropriate prescribing in older adults [27, 28, 39, 42, 102].

• "Start low, go slow" in the older adults (exceptions include antibiotics, diuretics for fluid overload, anti-seizure medications, chemotherapy).
• Prescription medications must not be initiated without a true indication. Non-pharmacological measures must gain precedence over pharmacological measures.
• Prescription medication is only provided for the desired duration and must be promptly stopped once the indicated duration is successfully completed.
• The primary care physician should be the nexus of all medication prescribing, oversee the specialty prescriptions and must practice a 'brown bag' review of all medications at visits.
• Polypharmacy is more prevalent in older adults; every effort should be made during clinic visits to address the matter and revise the regimen.
• Where possible, more than one (*i.e.* multiple) disorders can be addressed by one drug.
• Newly approved drugs may best wait before use, until the safety profile is established.
• New patient manifestations may be a clue to an adverse drug effect warranting a careful review of current and recent medications given to the patient.
• Dosing of drugs must be adjusted to renal function, following a GFR estimate by using an acceptable formula.

CONCLUSION

Aging is accompanied by several physiological changes in body composition, hepatic and renal function, significantly impacting pharmacokinetics and dynamics. Older people consume the largest proportion of prescribed medications and require dosage adjustments based on their organ function. Overweight and obese individuals have altered pharmacokinetics posing unique challenges to prescribing medications in this group. Polypharmacy refers to the prescription of multiple medications for a single patient on a continued basis, often inappropriate and unwarranted. Polypharmacy is associated with adverse drug events and increase in health care cost. Potentially inappropriate medications (PIMs) continue to be prescribed in spite of available proof of poor outcomes; examples include proton pump inhibitors [103], anticholinergic agents, benzodiazepines, hypnotics, antipsychotics and neuroleptics. Drug-drug interactions, drug-nutrient interactions and drug-disease interactions are all potential consequences of medication intake, warranting consideration before prescribing. Physicians need to practice the 'brown bag' review of all medications during patient visits. Medication reconciliation must be implemented in all settings based on the Joint Commission recommendations in the United States. The prescribing responsibility and its consequences are largely in the doctor's hands.

ACKNOWLEDGEMENTS

Declared none.

CONFLICT OF INTEREST

The authors confirm that this chapter contents have no conflict of interest.

REFERENCES

[1] Foster, DF, Phillips RS, Hamel MB, Elsenberg DM. Alternative medicine use in older Americans. J Am Geriatr Soc 2000; 48(12): 1560-5.
[2] Health topics - obesity. [Cited March 3 2014]. Available at http://www.who.int/topics/obesity/en/.
[3] Overweight and obesity. [Cited March 3 2014]. Available at http://www.cdc.gov/obesity/adult/defi ning.html.
[4] Overweight and Obesity. Causes and consequences. [Cited March 3 2014]. Available at http://www. cdc.gov/obesity/adult/causes/index.html.
[5] Ogden CL, Carroll MD, Kit BK, Flegal KM. Prevalence of childhood and adult obesity in the United States, 2011-2012. JAMA, 2014; 311(8): 806-14.
[6] Jensen MD, Ryan DH. New obesity guidelines. Promise and potential. JAMA 2014; 311(1): 23-24.
[7] Apovian CM. The clinical and economic consequences of obesity. Am J Managed Care 2013; 19(10Suppl): s219-28.

[8] US Federal Food, Drug, and Cosmetic Act, SEC. 210., (g)(1)(B) 2012.
[9] Cambridge Advanced Learners' Dictionary & Thesaurus, Cambridge University Press: headword "Herb" Online version. [Updated 2012, Cited March 3 2014].
[10] Lees P, Cunningham FM, Elliott J. Principles of pharmacodynamics and their applications in veterinary pharmacology. J Vet Pharmacol Ther, 2004. 27(6): 397-414.
[11] Benet LZ, Zia-Amirhosseini P. Basic principles of pharmacokinetics. Toxicol Pathol, 1995. 23(2): 115-23.
[12] Taffet GE. Age related physiological changes. In Cobbs EL, Duthie EH Jr., Murphy JB eds.Geriatrics Review Syllabus: A Core Curriculum in Geriatric Medicine, 4th ed. Iowa: Kendall/Hunt publishing 1999: 10-23.
[13] Dharmarajan TS, Ugalino JT. The physiology of aging. In Dharmarajan TS, Norman RA, eds. Clinical Geriatrics. 1st ed. Boca Raton. CRC Press/Parthenon Publishing 2001; 9-22.
[14] Fedarko NS. Biology. In Pacala JT, Sullivan GM.eds. Geriatrics Review Syllabus: A Core Curriculum in Geriatric Medicine, 7th ed. New York. American Geriatrics Society 2010: 9-19.
[15] Dharmarajan TS. Physiology of Aging. In Pitchumoni CS, Dharmarajan TS. Eds. Geriatric Gastroenterology. New York, Springer 2012; 17-31.
[16] Buffa R, Floris GU, Putzu PF, Marini E. Body composition variations in ageing. Coll Antropol 2011; 35(1): 259-65.
[17] Zamboni M, Zoico E, Scartezzini T, *et al.* Body composition changes in stable-weight elderly subjects: the effect of sex. Aging Clin Exp Res 2003; 15(4): 321-7.
[18] Sonati JG, Modeneze DM, Vilarta R, Maciel ES, Boccaletto EM. Body weight as an indicator of fat-free mass in active elderly women. Maturitas 2011; 68(4): 378-81.
[19] Caskey CI, Zerhouni EA, Fishman EK, Rahmouni AD. Aging of the diaphragm: ACT study. Radiology 1989; 171(2): 385-9.
[20] Iannuzzi-Sucich M, Prestwood KM, Kenny AM. Prevalence of sarcopenia and predictors of skeletal muscle mass in healthy, older men and women. J Gerontol A Biol Sci Med Sci 2002; 57(12): M772-7.
[21] Chan LN. Drug-nutrient interaction in clinical nutrition. Curr Opin Clin Nutr Metab Care, 2002. 5(3): 327-32.
[22] Lourenco R. Enteral feeding: drug/nutrient interaction. Clin Nutr, 2001. 20(2): 187-93.
[23] Cockcroft DW, Gault MH. Prediction of creatinine clearance from serum creatinine. Nephron.
[24] Levey AS, Bosch JP, Lewis JB, Greene T, Rogers N, Roth D. A more accurate method to estimate glomerular filtration rate from serum creatinine: a new prediction equation. Modification of Diet in Renal Disease Study Group. Ann Intern Med 19991976; 16(1): 31-41.; 130(6): 461-470.
[25] Levey AS, Stevens LA, Schmid CH, *et al.* A new equation to estimate glomerular filtration rate. Ann Intern Med., 2009; 150: 604-612.
[26] Dharmarajan TS, Yoo J, Russell RO, Norkus EP. Chronic Kidney Disease staging in nursing home and community older adults: Does the choice of Cockcroft-Gault, Modification of Diet in Renal Disease Study, or the Chronic Kidney Disease Epidemiology Collaboration Initiative Equations Matter? J Am Med Dir Assn 2012; 13: 151-5.
[27] Haumschild RJ. Pharmacokinetics of aging. In Pitchumoni CS, Dharmarajan TS. Eds. Geriatric Gastroenterology. New York, Springer 2012; 83-87.
[28] Jain V, Dharmarajan TS, Pitchumoni CS. Drug effects on the gastrointestinal tract. In Pitchumoni CS, Dharmarajan TS. Eds. Geriatric Gastroenterology. New York, Springer 2012; 73-81.
[29] "Adverse Drug Events, Adverse Drug Reactions and Medication Errors". VA Center for Medication Safety. [Updated 2012, Cited on November 3 2012].
[30] Nebeker JR, Barach P, Samore MH. Clarifying adverse drug events: a clinician's guide to terminology, documentation, and reporting. Ann Intern Med, 2004. 140: 795-801.
[31] Rambhade, Chakraborty A, Shrivastava A, Patil UK, Rambhade A. A survey on polypharmacy and use of inappropriate medications. Toxicol Int, 2012. 19(1): 68-73.
[32] Heuberger R. Polypharmacy and food-drug interactions among older persons: a review. J Nutr Gerontol Geriatr, 2012. 31(4): 325-403.
[33] Takane AK, MD Balignasay, CR Nigg. Polypharmacy reviews among elderly populations project: assessing needs in patient-provider communication. Hawaii J Med Public Health, 2013. 72(1): 15-22.

[34] Hovstadius B, Petersson G. The impact of increasing polypharmacy on prescribed drug expenditure-a register-based study in Sweden 2005-2009. Health Policy, 2013. 109(2): 166-74.
[35] Gokula M, Holmes HM. Tools to reduce polypharmacy. Clin Geriatr Med, 2012. 28(2): 323-41.
[36] Kojima T, Akishita M, Nakamura T, *et al.* Polypharmacy as a risk for fall occurrence in geriatric outpatients. Geriatr Gerontol Int, 2012. 12(3): 425-30.
[37] Gnjidic D, Hilmer SN, Blythe FM, *et al.* Polypharmacy cutoff and outcomes: five or more medicines were used to identify community-dwelling older men at risk of different adverse outcomes. J Clin Epidemiol, 2012. 65(9): 989-95.
[38] Hamilton H, Gallagher P, Ryan C, *et al.* Potentially inappropriate medications defined by STOPP criteria and the risk of adverse drug events in older hospitalized patients. Arch Intern Med, 2011. 171(11): 1013-9.
[39] Marcum ZA, Hanlon JT. Commentary on the new American Geriatrics Society Beets Criteria for potentially inappropriate medication use in older adults. Am J Geriatric Pharmacotherapy 2012; 10: 151-159.
[40] Gallagher P, O'Mahony D. STOPP (Screening Tool of Older Persons' potentially inappropriate Prescriptions): application to acutely ill elderly patients and comparison with Beers' criteria. Age and Ageing 2008; 37: 673-9.
[41] American Geriatrics Society Updated Criteria for Potentially Inappropriate Medication Use in Older Adults. The American Geriatrics Society 2012 Beers Criteria Update Expert Panel [cited on March 3rd, 2014]; Available from http://www.ncbi.nlm.nih.gov/pmc/articles/PMC3571677/.
[42] Fick D, Semla T, Beizer J, *et al.* American Geriatrics Society Beers Criteria Update Expert, P., American Geriatrics Society updated Beers Criteria for potentially inappropriate medication use in older adults. J Am Geriatr Soc, 2012. 60(4): 616-31.
[43] Chretien JH, Mc Garvey M, De stwolinski A, Esswein JG. Abuse of antibiotics. A study of patients attending a university clinic. Arch Intern Med, 1975. 135(8): 1063-5.
[44] Hamilton-Miller JM. Use and abuse of antibiotics. Br J Clin Pharmacol, 1984. 18(4): 469-74.
[45] Dancer SJ. How antibiotics can make us sick: the less obvious adverse effects of antimicrobial chemotherapy. Lancet Infect Dis 2004. 4(10): 611-9.
[46] Zebrowska-Lupina I, Szymczyk G, Wrobel A. Adverse effects of interactions of antibiotics with other drugs. Pol Merkur Lekarski, 2000. 9(51): 623-6.
[47] Shehab N, Patel PR, Srinivasan A, Budnitz DS. Emergency department visits for antibiotic-associated adverse events. Clin Infect Dis, 2008. 47(6): 735-43.
[48] Chatterjee S, Chen H, Johnson ML, Aparasu RR. Risk of falls and fractures in older adults using atypical antipsychotic agents: A propensity score-adjusted, retrospective study. Am J Geriatric Pharmacotherapy 2012; 10: 83-94.
[49] Dharmarajan L, Dharmarajan TS. Prescribing warfarin appropriately to meet National Patient Safety Goals. American Health and Drug Benefits 2008: 1 (6): 26-32.
[50] Dalton BR, Lye-Maccanell T, Henderson EA, Maccannell DR, Louie TJ. Proton pump inhibitors increase significantly the risk of Clostridium difficile infection in a low-endemicity, non-outbreak hospital setting. Aliment Pharmacol Ther, 2009. 29(6): 626-34.
[51] Fraser LA, Leslie WD, Targownik LE, Papaioannou A, Adachi JD, CaMos Research Group. The effect of proton pump inhibitors on fracture risk: report from the Canadian Multicenter Osteoporosis Study. Osteoporos Int 2013; 24(4): 1161-8.
[52] Hines LE, Murphy JE. Potentially harmful drug-drug interactions in the elderly: A review. Am J Geriatric Pharmacother 2011; 9: 364-77.
[53] Grossman, E, Messerli FH. Drug-induced hypertension: An unappreciated cause of secondary hypertension. Am j Med 2012; 125: 14-22.
[54] Jarskog LF, Hamer RM, Catellier DJ, *et al.* Metformin for weight loss and metabolic control in overweight outpatients with schizophrenia and schizoaffective disorder. Am J Psychiatry 2013; 170 (9): 1032-40.
[55] Chadda RK, Ramshankar K, De KS, Sood M. Metabolic syndrome in schizophrenia: Differences between antipsychotic-naïve and treated patients. J Pharmacol Pharmacother 2013. 4(3): 176-186.
[56] Ko YK, Soh MA, Kang SH, Lee JI. The prevalence of metabolic syndrome in schizophrenic patients using antipsychotics. Clin Psychopharmacol Neurosci 2013; 11(2): 80-8.
[57] Ness-Abramof R, Apovian CM. Drug induced weight gain. Drugs Today (Barc), 2005.41(8): 547-55.

[58] Malone MI, Alger-Mayer SA, Anderson DA. Medication associated with weight gain may influence outcome in a weight management program. Ann Pharmacother 2005. 39(7-8): 1204-8.
[59] Yanoski SZ, Yanosvski JA. Long term drug treatment for obesity. A systematic and clinical review. JAMA 2014: 311(1): 74-86.
[60] Hasani-Ranjbar S, Nayebi N, Larijani B, Abdollahi, M. A systematic review of the efficacy and safety of herbal medicines used in the treatment of obesity. World J Gastroenterol, 2009. 15(25): 3073-85.
[61] Boozer CN, Daly PA, Homel P, *et al*. Herbal ephedra/caffeine for weight loss: a 6-month randomized safety and efficacy trial. Int J Obes Relat Metab Disord, 2002. 26(5): 593-604.
[62] Shekelle PG, Hardy ML, Morton SC, *et al*. Efficacy and safety of ephedra and ephedrine for weight loss and athletic performance: a meta-analysis. JAMA, 2003. 289(12): 1537-45.
[63] Gilliland K, Bullock W. Caffeine: a potential drug of abuse. Adv Alcohol Subst Abuse, 1983. 3(1-2): 53-73.
[64] Hughes JR, Oliveto AH, Helzer JE, *et al*. Should caffeine abuse, dependence, or withdrawal be added to DSM-IV and ICD-10? Am J Psychiatry, 1992. 149(1): 33-40.
[65] Vogler BK, Pittler MH, Ernst E. The efficacy of ginseng. A systematic review of randomised clinical trials. Eur J Clin Pharmacol, 1999. 55(8): 567-75.
[66] Kim, JH, Hahm DH, Yang DC, Kim JH, Lee HJ, Shim I. Effect of crude saponin of Korean red ginseng on high-fat diet-induced obesity in the rat. J Pharmacol Sci, 2005. 97(1): 124-31.
[67] Oben JE, Enyegue DM, Fomekong GI, Soukontoua YB, Agbor GA. The effect of Cissus quadrangularis (CQR-300) and a Cissus formulation (CORE) on obesity and obesity-induced oxidative stress. Lipids Health Dis, 2007. 6: 4.
[68] Moreno DA, Ilic, N, Poulev A, Raskin I. Effects of Arachis hypogaea nutshell extract on lipid metabolic enzymes and obesity parameters. Life Sci, 2006; 78(24): 2797-803.
[69] Lapane KL, Yang S, Jawahar R, McAlindon T, Eaton CB. CAM use among overweight and obese persons with radiographic knee osteoarthritis. BMC Complementary and Alternative Med 2013; 13: 241.
[70] Raebel MA, Newcomer SR, Reifler LM, *et al*. Chronic use of opioid medications before and after bariatric surgery. JAMA 2013; 310(13): 1369-1376.
[71] Bioch MJ, Viera AJ. Should patients with obesity and hypertension be treated differently from those who are not obese? Curr Hypertens Rep 2014; 16 (3): 418.
[72] Gunturu SG, Dharmarajan TS. Drug nutrient interactions. In Pitchumoni CS, Dharmarajan TS. Eds. Geriatric Gastroenterology. New York, Springer 2012; 89-97.
[73] Hines LE, Murphy JE. Potentially harmful drug-drug interactions in the elderly: A review. Am J Geriatric Pharmacother 2011; 9: 364-77.
[74] Hanlon JT. How important are drug-drug interactions to the health of older adults? Am J Geriatric Pharmacother 2011; 9: 361-2.
[75] Askari M, Eslami S, Louws M, *et al*. Frequency and nature of drug-drug interactions in the intensive care unit. Pharmacoepidemiol Drug Saf 2013; 22(4): 430-7.
[76] Stillman MJ, Tepper DE, Tepper SJ, Cho L. QT Prolongation, Torsade de Pointes, myocardial ischemia from coronary vasospasm, and headache medications. Part 2: Review of headache medications, drug-drug interactions, QTc Prolongation, and other arrhythmias. Headache 2013. 53(1): 217-24.
[77] Shirolkar SC, Fiuzat M, Becker RC. Dronedarone and vitamin K antagonists: a review of drug-drug interactions. Am Heart J 2010; 160(4): 577-82.
[78] Zitelli BJ, Howrie DL, Altman H, Maroon TJ. Erythromycin-induced drug interactions. An illustrative case and review of the literature. Clin Pediatr (Phila) 1987; 26(3): 117-9.
[79] Genser D. Food and drug interaction: consequences for the nutrition/health status. Ann Nutr Metab, 2008; 52 Suppl 1: 29-32.
[80] Leibovitch ER, Deamer RL, Sanderson LA. Food-drug interactions. Careful drug selection and patient counseling can reduce the risk in older patients. Geriatics 2004; 59(3): 19-33.
[81] Boullata JI, Hudson LM. Drug-nutrient interactions: a broad view with implications for practice. J Acad Nutr Diet 2012; 112: 506-17.
[82] Dahan A, Altman H. Food-drug interaction: grapefruit juice augments drug bioavailability--mechanism, extent and relevance. Eur J Clin Nutr 2004; 58(1): 1-9.

[83] Kaneko K, Suzuki K, Iwadate-Iwata E, Kato I, Uchida K, Onoue M. Evaluation of food-drug Interaction of guava leaf tea. Phytother Res 2013: 27(2): 299-305.

[84] GenserD. Food and drug interaction: consequences for the nutrition/health status. Ann Nutr Metab 2008; 52 Suppl 1: 29-32.

[85] Wix AR, Doering PL, Hatton RC. Drug-food interaction counseling programs in teaching hospitals. Am J Hosp Pharm, 1992. 49(4): 855-60.

[86] Dharmarajan TS, Kumar A, Pitchumoni CS. Drug - nutrient Interactions in older adults. Practical Gastroenterology 2002; 26 (4): 37-55.

[87] Matsui MS, Rozovski SJ. Drug-nutrient interaction. Clin Ther, 1982. 4(6): 423-40.

[88] Kumthekar AA, Gidwani HV, Kumthekar AB. Metformin associated B12 deficiency. J Assoc Physicians India, 2012. 60: 58-60.

[89] Mazokopakis EE, Starakis IK. Recommendations for diagnosis and management of metformin-induced vitamin B12 (Cbl) deficiency. Diabetes Res Clin Pract, 2012. 97(3): 359-67.

[90] Bauman WA, Shaw S, Jayatilleke E, Spungen AM, Herbert V. Increased intake of calcium reverses vitamin B12 malabsorption induced by metformin. Diabetes Care, 2000. 23(9): 1227-31.

[91] Sera LC, McPherson ML. Pharmacokinetics and pharmacodynamic changes associated with aging and implications for drug therapy. Clin Geriatr Med, 2012. 28(2): 273-86.

[92] Aymanns C, Keller F, Maus S, Hartmann B, Czock D. Review on pharmacokinetics and pharmacodynamics and the aging kidney. Clin J Am Soc Nephrol, 2010. 5(2): 314-27.

[93] Nathan A, Goodyer L, Lovejoy A, Rashid A. 'Brown bag' medication reviews as a means of optimizing patients' use of medication and of identifying potential clinical problems. Fam Pract, 1999. 16(3): 278-82.

[94] Caskie GI, Willis SL, Warner Schaie K, Zaniani FA. Congruence of medication information from a brown bag data collection and pharmacy records: findings from the Seattle longitudinal study. Exp Aging Res 2006; 32(1): 79-103.

[95] Martinez ML, Vande Griend JP, Linnebur SA. Medication management: a case of brown bag-identified medication hoarding. Consult Pharm, 2012. 27(10): 729-36.

[96] Campbell NL, Boustani MA, Skopeljia EN. Medication adherence in older adults with cognitive impairment: A systematic evidence-based review. Am J Geriatr Pharmacother 2012; 10: 165-77.

[97] Bonnet-Zamponi B, d'Arailh L, Konrat C, *et al.* Drug-related readmissions to medical units of older adults discharged from acute geriatric units; Results of the Optimization of medication in AGEd multicenter Randomization Controlled Trial. J Am Geriatr Soc 2013; 61: 113-21.

[98] Green JB, Ross JS, Jackevicius CA, Shah ND, Krumholz HM. When choosing statin therapy. A case for generics. JAMA Intern Med 2013; 173: 229-32.

[99] Alldredge BK, Kayser SR. Bending the curve toward increase use of generic drug. JAMA intern Med 2013; 173: 233-4.

[100] Campbell EG, Pham-Kanter G, Vogeli C, Lezzoni LI. Physician acquiescence to patient demands for brand-name drugs: results of a National Survey of Physicians. JAMA intern Med 2013; 173: 237-9.

[101] Bopara MD, Korc-Grodzicki B. Prescribing for older adults. Mt. Sinai J Med 2011; 78(4): 613-26.

[102] Semla T. Pharmacotherapy. In Pacala JT, Sullivan GM. eds. Geriatrics Review Syllabus: A Core Curriculum in Geriatric Medicine, 7th ed. New York. American Geriatrics Society 2010: 83-91.

[103] Maggio M, Corsonello A, Ceda GP, *et al.* Proton pump inhibitors and risk of 1-year mortality and re-hospitalization in older patients discharged from acute care hospitals. JAMA Intern Med 2013; 173(7): 518-23

CHAPTER 16

Using Systems Thinking to Understand the Dynamics of Obesity in Low and Middle Income Countries

David William Lounsbury*, Judith Wylie-Rosett and Beth A. Conlon

Department of Epidemiology and Population Health, Albert Einstein College of Medicine of Yeshiva University, 1300 Morris Park Avenue, Belfer Building, 13th Floor, Bronx, NY 10461 USA

Abstract: The current chapter applies a systems thinking approach to define and study the dynamics underlying increased rates of obesity in Low and Middle Income Countries (LMICs). Systems thinking and dynamics modeling belong to the rapidly evolving, interdisciplinary field of system science research. This field adds value to more traditional public health research methods by contributing to the design and testing of integrated models of change, to examine how key factors interact with each other and with health status. We frame the problem of obesity for LMICs as an aggregate, chronic energy imbalance of the population as a whole, due in large part to increased consumption of highly processed foods. To begin to explore the dynamically complex nature of global obesity, we develop a causal loop diagram, supported by the extant literature, showing a comprehensive qualitative model of the dynamics underlying increased rates of obesity in LMICs. Eighteen endogenous factors, or constructs, make up these seven distinct loops. In addition, selected exogenous factors are shown, representing the effect of policies by foreign governments, global corporate entities, and other institutions that explain obesity dynamics in LMICs. We suggest that there are two major points of intervention to curb current increasing obesity rates: the first is to sustain or grow healthy food production capacity and the second is public health education.

Keywords: Complex public health problems, exercise, fitness, global health, low and middle income countries, nutrition, obesity, overweight, processed foods, risk, systems thinking, wellness.

INTRODUCTION

In the realm of public health, one can use systems thinking to pose complex, non-linear hypotheses about how social, economic, and cultural forces impact public

***Corresponding author David William Lounsbury:** 1300 Morris Park Avenue, Belfer Building, 13th Floor, Bronx, NY 10461, USA; Tel: (718) 920-5490; Fax: (718) 652-1343;
E-mail: David.Lounsbury@einstein.yu.edu

Judith Wylie-Rosett & Sunil S. Jhangiani (Eds)

health [1-3]. The hallmark of the system dynamics approach is the study of feedback mechanisms, or cybernetics, which can be used to explain how things change over time [4-7]. Systems thinking can make explicit the interdependent relationships among these forces and how they interact over time to generate a health problem and, moreover, can identify gaps in current knowledge as well as robust policies for change [8].

Systems thinking and dynamics modeling belong to the rapidly evolving, interdisciplinary field of system science research. This field adds value to more traditional public health research methods by contributing to the design and testing of integrated models of change, to examine how key factors interact with each other and with health status. In addition to system dynamics modeling, social network analysis, agent-based modeling, micro-simulation, discrete event analysis, Markov modeling, and many operations research and engineering methods constitute systems science approaches that show great promise for public health research and policy studies [3, 9]. For example, the first author and colleagues used systems thinking to illustrate the utility of a system dynamics approach to promoting quality of life research in chronic disease, using diabetes as an example [10].

Systems thinking and system dynamics modeling has also been used to examine health care quality improvement [9, 11-16]; community-based systems of care [17-20]; epidemiology and disease surveillance [21-25]; global health care management [26-28]; behavioral health interventions in tobacco [25, 29-32], substance abuse [33-36], and mental health [37, 38]; as well as in managing chronic illness [20, 39, 40]. In addition, a system dynamics model called *HealthBound*, originally developed for the Centers for Disease Control and Prevention (CDC), is currently being used in a project called *ReThink Health*, to help people understand the critical relationship between "upstream" efforts to prevent illness and the demand for the relationships between a community's access to care, health status, and socioeconomic level [41].

OBESITY EPIDEMIOLOGY IN LMICs

Worldwide obesity has nearly doubled since 1980, with more than 1.4 billion adults overweight and approximately 200 million men and nearly 300 million women obese [42]. Prior research has show that, in low-income countries, obesity mostly affects middle-aged adults (women more than men) from wealthy, urban environments. In contrast, in high income countries (HICs) obesity affects both sexes and all ages, but is disproportionately higher among groups with lower socio-economic status (SES) [43].

Current epidemiology shows that the fastest growth in obesity is occurring in LMICs. A recent review of the global obesity epidemiology by Popkin and Slining [44] concluded that LMICs are experiencing a rapid increase in overweight and obesity prevalence, increased body mass index (BMI) levels among overweight and obese persons, and a potential change of obesity phenotypes-*i.e.*, increasing waist circumference at each BMI level in some countries (namely China and Mexico). Similarly, using nationally representative data from 1990 through 2010 (or the most recent year available) for all Demographic Health Survey (DHS) countries, Popkin and Slining [45] also showed that over two-thirds of women in North Africa and the Middle East were overweight or obese, followed by Latin America and the Caribbean, where approximately half of the women are overweight or obese.

SYSTEMS THINKING: A TOOL FOR UNDERSTANDING OBESITY TRENDS IN LMICs

The increasing prevalence of obesity in LMICs is a complex and dynamic problem that appears to stem from steadily increasing rates of consumption of sugary beverages and processed foods containing a high volume of fat and sugar [46-50]. In addition, there is evidence that increased access to tobacco products and alcoholic beverages is associated with increased consumption of sugary beverages and processed foods [47]. Since World War II, effective corporate strategies of manufacturing and marketing these unhealthy food commodities has served to increase average childhood and adult BMIs [51, 52], resulting in both obesity and, paradoxically, under-nutrition as persons consume energy dense foods that are low in other nutrients [44, 53-58]. To provide greater insight into the drivers of this problem, we propose using systems thinking to show the dynamic links between obesity rates and increased consumption of unhealthy commodities in LMICs.

Researchers and other obesity experts [48, 56, 57] have offered a variety of theories and perspectives about the drivers of these trends in LMICs. The nutrition transition model posits that food preferences are shifting away from traditional foods in favor of high-energy, low-nutrient foods [48], driven by the problematic role of easier access to processed foods and decreased physical activity levels, which are attributed to urbanization and other factors that characterize rapidly globalized economies [57]. Subsequently, these dynamics are ushering in a parallel increase in the global prevalence of non-communicable diseases, including diabetes, cardiovascular conditions, cancer [49, 59-64].

A Hypothesis of the Causal Structure of the Obesity Problem

The hallmark of the system dynamics approach is the study of feedback structures, or cybernetics [5-7, 65]. What we present below is a generic conceptualization of the hypothesized underlying cybernetic 'structure' of the obesity problem in LMICs, expressed in terms of multiple causal loops. Causal loop diagramming is a useful technique for illustrating how specified constructs are linked together and how they change over time, with respect to a given problem. Causal loop diagrams capture the qualitative nature of relationships among key constructs.

The objective was to design causal loops that illustrate general observations about the causes of overweight and obesity in LMICs based on the published reviews, empirical reports [44, 46, 50, 66, 67], and white papers [42, 59, 68] examined in this chapter. Collectively, these loops form a comprehensive qualitative model of the dynamics underlying increased rates of obesity in LMICs (see Fig. **1**). In total, eighteen endogenous factors, or constructs, make up these seven loops, which have been labeled A-G. In addition, four exogenous factors are shown. By definition, they are theoretically controlled (or specified) by external forces, such as a foreign government, a global corporate entity, or some other institution independent of the LMIC itself. Note that one could argue a way to make one or more of these exogenous factors part of the endogenous structure. However, for our purposes, that would move beyond the scope of the current chapter. The two exogenous factors shown in red (*Direct Foreign Investment in LMIC* and *LMIC population growth rate*) are hypothesized to have direct impact on 'Per capita productivity' within the LMIC. The two shown in green (*Healthy food production capacity* and *Public health education*) are policy levers, or intervention points that are hypothesized to be a means through which constructive impact on population obesity rates in LMICs could be achieved.

Interpreting Causal Loops

Table **1** provides a glossary of these key terms, to assist with interpretation of the loop diagrams. Note that linking arrows between variables infer causality, not correlation. Every causal link has a polarity, either positive (+) or negative (-). A positive (+) link indicates that an incremental increase in the input (antecedent) variable causes the output (dependent) variable to also increase (by some specified amount over each increment of time). Similarly, an incremental decrease in the input variable would cause the output variable to decrease (by some specified amount over each increment of time). A negative (-) link indicates the opposite relationship between two variables, such that an incremental increase in the input variable causes the output variable to decrease (by some specified amount over each increment of time) and *vice versa*.

Each feedback loop has postulated polarity that is either reinforcing (+) or balancing (-). Reinforcing loops tend to promote or accelerate the growth, often generating instability in the system. In contrast, balancing loops are stabilizing, or goal-seeking, creating a homeostatic (steady-state) condition. Depending on the postulated purpose of the loop, the resultant dynamics could generate a policy trend that either promote/fuels obesity or that slows/curbs its, over time. Keep in mind that the overall dynamics of the problem are the outcome of the interactive effects of the loops over time. For example, two reinforcing loops may interact to bring a particular construct into a steady state, or, alternatively, may generate an oscillating pattern over time, with one loop dominating the other in an alternating manner.

Table 1. A glossary of systems thinking terms.

Term	Definition
Dynamics	The behavior over time of a system or any of its components.
Systems Thinking	A non-linear approach to studying the dynamics of social problems in terms of causally linked, closed chains of variables.
Causal Loop Diagram	A visual representation of problem of interest expressed in terms of causally linked, closed chains of variables; a hypothesis of the dynamics underlying a given problem of interest.
Balancing Loop	A closed chain of variables that serves to stablize a system, over time, by forcing a correction, or a reversal, of whatever direction of change is imposed; a negative feedback structure.
Reinforcing Loop	A closed chain of variables that serves to destabilize a system over time, by amplification of whatever direction of change is imposed; a positive feedback structure.
Exogenous Factors	Any variable that changes due to conditions external to the looped (endogenous) dynamics of a social problem of interest; any contextual characteristic or environmental condition that is not influenced by the system dynamics of focus.

In Table **2** we have listed each of the seven loops shown in our model (Fig. **1**) by its corresponding letter (A-G) and a brief label. In addition, each loop is

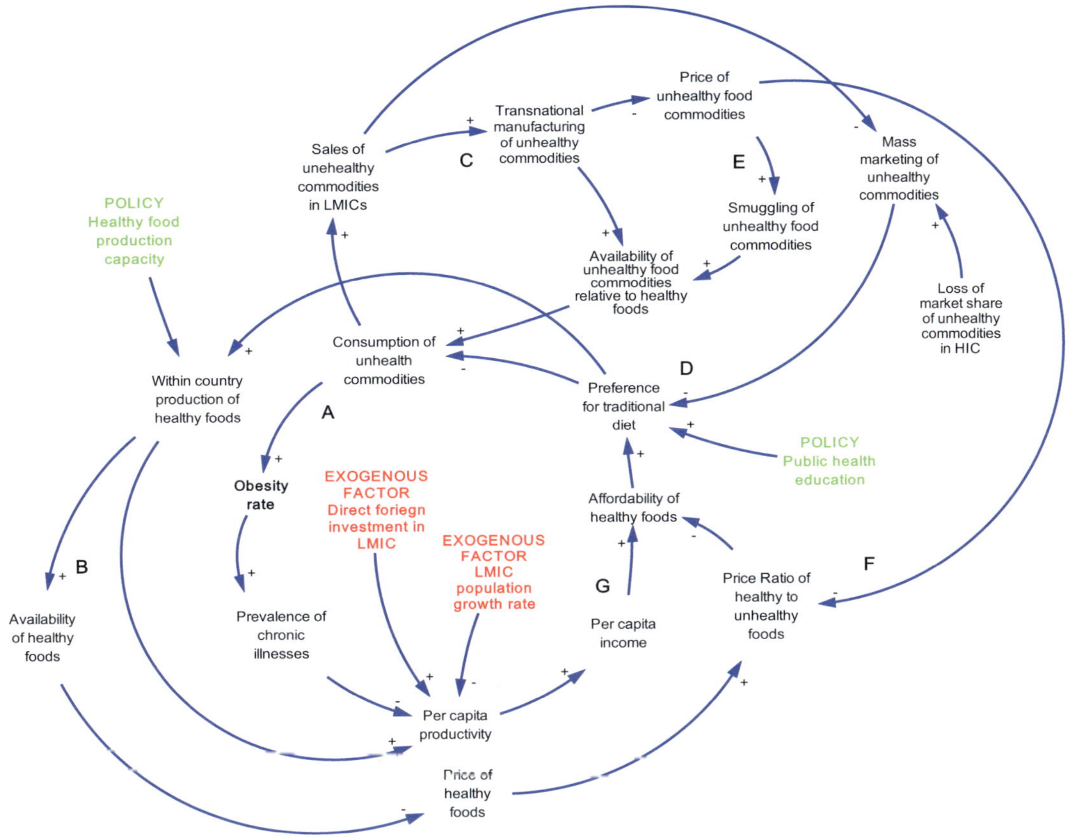

Fig. (1). Postulated model of the dynamics of obesity in low and middle income countries.

categorized by type (*i.e.*, Reinforcing or Balancing) and by predicted effect (*i.e.*, Fuels obesity or Curbs obesity). This assessment of the loop's effect is a value judgment based on whether the loop is expected to further exasperate or serve to mitigate the problem of overweight and obesity at the population level in a LMIC.

Loop A-Consumption of Unhealthy Commodities (Reinforcing, Fuels Obesity)

This loop is arguably the heart of our model, as it includes obesity rate, representing the pace at which the problem of overweight and obesity grows in LMICs. Estimates of current overweight and obesity rates range from 0.31% per year to 0.92% per year for Latin America and the Caribbean and for the Middle East and North Africa, respectively [44]. Results are similar for rural and urban settings, except for South Asia and sub-Saharan Africa, where higher underweight status was associated with rural communities [44].

Table 2. Index to the model's causal loops.

Loop ID	Descriptive Label	Dynamics	
		Type of Loop	Trend
A	Consumption of Unhealthy Commodities	Reinforcing	Fuels obesity
B	Within Country Production of Healthy Foods	Reinforcing	Curbs obesity
C	Transnational Manufacturing of Unhealthy Commodities	Reinforcing	Fuels obesity
D	Preference for Traditional Diet	Balancing	Curbs obesity
E	Smuggling Unhealthy Commodities	Balancing	Fuels obesity
F	Price Ratio of Healthy to Unhealthy Commodities	Reinforcing	Fuels obesity
G	Per Capita Productivity	Reinforcing	Curbs obesity

Tracing through Loop A, one can determine that it is a reinforcing loop comprised of seven variables. Consistent with the literature summarized here, this loop hypothesizes that increases in consumption of unhealthy commodities, defined as soft drinks, and processed foods that are high in salt, fat, and sugar, as well as tobacco and alcohol [47], will contribute to the obesity rate, the rate at which persons in a given LIMC meet objective criteria of obesity. Assuming that current trends will persist, this loop's dynamics serve to fuel, or increase the obesity rate in these countries.

Loop A represents the hypothesis that a higher obesity rates will eventually add to the prevalence of chronic illnesses, mainly non-communicable diseases such as diabetes, cardiovascular diseases, and cancers. Although the burden of chronic illness is still ramping up in LMICs, the level of compromised quality of life, reduced per capita productivity-both in terms of lost family income (per capita income) and social costs of delivering care to the sick-it has been described as a "a slow-motion disaster," as noted by Dr. Margaret Chan, Director-General of the World Health Organization [53].

Loop B-Within Country Production of Healthy Foods (Reinforcing, Curbs Obesity)

This loop taps the LMIC's potential to make more or to sustain levels of production of healthy foods. This is a reinforcing process with a potentially favorable impact on overweight and obesity prevalence. Loop B shares two variables with Loop A, namely affordability of healthy foods and preference for traditional diet. To the extent that the LMIC's preference for traditional diet is sustained or, ideally, expanded, we hypothesize that farmers and producers will be motivated to increase their production of these healthy foods, such as whole grains, vegetables, fresh poultry, fish and meats, and other natural products. Greater production means greater availability to healthy foods. Additionally, per commonly accepted economic theory, greater supply of these healthy foods should push their price lower. At the market then, the price ratio of healthy to unhealthy foods would favor the purchase of cheaper, healthy foods. Over time, within country production of healthy foods would be expected to expand to meet this demand, which is a good outcome, though not one that is hypothesized to directly impacting a LMIC's obesity rate.

However, Loop B could also reinforce an undesirable scenario, where the availability of health foods is decreased over time, driven by a shrinking level of within country production of health foods. Under these circumstances, we would expect the price of healthy foods to rise. This would, in turn, dampen preference for traditional diet, as it would require procurement of healthy foods, which are comparatively expensive [43, 47, 56, 57]. Then, a dampened preference for traditional diet would likely promote consumption of unhealthy commodities, which further increases the obesity rate [43, 47].

Loop C-Transnational Manufacturing of Unhealthy Commodities (Reinforcing, Fuels Obesity)

Another problematic, reinforcing dynamic concerns global corporations that profitably market unhealthy commodities to LMICs. Increasingly easier access to processed foods and out-of-home fast-food franchises are facilitating unhealthy dietary patterns, a direct result of the role of global corporate producers in the manufacturing, marketing, sale, and distribution of unhealthy commodities in these settings [51, 52, 69, 70]. From the perspective of these global corporations, sales of unhealthy commodities in these markets are profitable to the investing entity, as they can be produced at low cost, have a long shelf-life (minimizing waste), and support a high retail value [56-58]. Some of the largest multi-national producers include major soft drink and candy companies [52]. Arguably, they can exert substantial market control over the global supply of many of these unhealthy commodities [50, 51, 69].

Thus, Loop C represents the hypothesis that increasing consumption of unhealthy commodities will drive up sales of unhealthy commodities in LMICs. In turn, as sales increase, transnational manufacturing of unhealthy commodities rises to meet the demand, which increases the availability of unhealthy food commodities relative to healthy foods. Stuckler *et al.* [47] have performed analyses that showed growth in sales of unhealthy commodities has increased in many LMICs and has decreased in HICs. Moreover, they project that the pace of consumption of unhealthy commodities is expected to occur faster in LMICs than in HICs, and that transnational companies have as strong a presence in middle-income countries as they do in HICs.

Researchers have observed that higher intake of unhealthy foods correlates strongly with higher tobacco and alcohol consumption, suggesting use of common strategies in marketing and distribution across these industries [50-52, 69]. Higher levels of direct foreign investment and the implementation of free-trade agreements have been associated with rising income in some LMICs, but these economic policies have also been correlated with higher consumption of unhealthy commodities [56, 57]. However, economic growth is not always associated with higher unhealthy commodity consumption, which suggests that growth-oriented policies that are grounded in public health goals can promote healthy food choices and curb obesity trends.

Loop D-Preference for Traditional Diet (Balancing, Curbs Obesity)

Sales of unhealthy commodities in LMICs also drives *mass marketing of unhealthy commodities*. As hypothesized in Loop D, to the extent that demand for transnational processed food commodities is flat or dropping in HICs, they would invest more in the mass marketing of unhealthy commodities. Marketing of these unhealthy commodities, by billboard, radio, TV or internet, or by direct marketing in the form of free samples, would serve to decrease preference for traditional diet [43, 51, 57, 71]. Note that the causal influences of 'good' Loops B and G, and bad Loop C will also serve to affect preference for traditional diet. Yet, to the extent that preference for traditional diet is sustained or even enhanced, made possible through policies that limit unhealthy commodity marketing and keep healthy food relatively cheap (affordability of health foods), consumption of unhealthy commodities would drop, which would help slow, or ideally even reverse obesity rates. For example, this effect is evident in the rapidly declining consumption of tobacco in the United States, where the national adult smoking prevalence, estimated by the National Health Interview Survey, has reached a record low of 18.0% in 2013 [72]. In turn, this type of loss of market share has encouraged major investment in the marketing of tobacco to Africa and Latin American [69].

Loop E-Smuggling Unhealthy Commodities (Balancing, Fuels Obesity)

Another dynamic to take note of is the potential impact of smuggling unhealthy food commodities. Here we hypothesize that, to the extent that the price of unhealthy food commodities remains high and preference for traditional diet is dampened by suppressed effects of 'good' Loops B, D and G), smuggling will be more lucrative [47]. In turn, this contributes directly to the availability of unhealthy food commodities relative to healthy foods, and would drive up consumption of unhealthy commodities, over time. However, while the distinct possibility of smuggling exists, there are limited data to gauge such an effect on commodity availability in a given LMIC, and the effect may result in higher priced contraband products, which would likely include tobacco and alcohol.

Loop F-Price Ratio of Healthy to Unhealthy Commodities (Reinforcing, Fuels Obesity)

The matter of changes in the price ratio of healthy to unhealthy goods is of great concern. We believe that price will influence day-to-day food purchase decisions. There is a need for further study of price elasticity in LMICs, to explain, for example, how a consumer would change purchasing patterns given a price hike in fresh fruits and vegetables relative to processed fruits and vegetables, of how a fast food meal would be preferred over a home cooked one, if the fast food meal is perceived to be as cheap, or cheaper.

It has been relatively well established that global change in overweight status of a population is correlated with SES, using indices for educational level, income, or both. For example, using cross-sectional data, Subramanium *et al.* found a robust positive correlation between SES and overweight status [73]. Monteiro *et al.* [74] found that a lower SES was a protective factor against obesity, although countries with GNP per capita above $2,500 had a greater risk of obesity among lower SES women.

Jones-Smith *et al.* [75] studied national trends in overweight burden using both indices of wealth and education, and found that 27 of 37 countries showed a positive association between SES and overweight prevalence, but that higher per capita GNP and narrower income inequity were both linked to a higher proportion of overweight in lower SES subpopulations. The work of Monteiro *et al.* [74] and Jones-Smith *et al.* [75] also found that increased national wealth drives the burden of overweight and obesity to lower SES subpopulations. These results provide some context for understanding the effect of changes in price ratio of healthy goods to unhealthy goods.

Loop G-Per Capita Productivity (Reinforcing, Curbs Obesity)

Our final feedback structure, or loop, examines the impact of per capita productivity on per capita income. We hypothesize that new capacity for within country production of healthy foods will directly translate to increased per capita productivity. New jobs and wage increases will be generated, and this will make healthy foods more affordable, which is hypothesized to support a preference for traditional diet [47].

Moreover, higher prevalence of chronic illnesses will have profound impacts on per capita productivity, affecting population health and health economics in the long run [49, 76-78]. However, where external policies pump up direct foreign investment in an LMIC, per capita income will be buffered, which we hypothesize to increase consumption of unhealthy commodities [56]. Notably, careful data analyses suggest that rising income levels are a significant correlate of increasing exposure to unhealthy foods in LMICs [47, 56].

Note, here, that two exogenous effects, both shown to directly impact per capita productivity. The first is direct foreign investment in LMIC. More investment from overseas is welcomed, as it typically fosters growth in government institutions and business enterprises, which creates jobs and contributes to per capita productivity. The second is the country's population growth rate. The majority of LMICs are experiencing high population growth rates [42, 58, 74, 79]. Rapidly rising population growth rates tend to increase unemployment, which directly diminishes per capita productivity.

PUBLIC HEALTH POLICIES

Curb Consumption of Unhealthy Commodities and Obesity Rates in LMICs

Our model of obesity dynamics in LMICs identifies postulated feedback structures about the main drivers of the obesity epidemic in LMICs (Fig. **1**, Loops A-G). Given the complexity and the scale of the problem, what can be done to address it? The prevalence of obesity has been increasing worldwide for more than 30 years, in countries rich and poor [78, 80]. Our model helps identify multiple points of leverage, places where empowered stakeholders can intervene, to begin to stem the rate of obesity and all of the undesirable externalities that come with it, including increased prevalence of chronic illnesses and the resultant decrease in per capita productivity and income.

While governments and responsible public health institutions have the potential power and knowledge to curb obesity rates in LMICs, which policies and programs can be developed, effectively implemented, and sustained, is less clear. Government strategies to control tobacco and alcohol provide a potentially useful model, but arguably curbing obesity poses a more complex challenge. In short, management of the overweight and obesity problem requires multiple types of interventions that are staged at multiple levels. An ecological framework to guide effective interventions is necessary [81], to understand and effectively promote health-positive attitudes and behaviors at the individual level, as well as to organize and change social and built environments, such that choosing to eating healthfully and to exercise regularly are embedded in a dominant, continually reinforced feedback loop.

Having framed the problem for LMICs as a chronic energy imbalance of the population as a whole, due in large part to increased consumption of highly processed foods, we suggest that there are two major points of intervention. The first is to sustain or grow healthy food production capacity and the second is public health education.

Healthy Food Production Capacity

It is evident that, over time, the globalization of the world economy is changing systems of food production and distribution. In traditional societies, individuals managed the production of most of their food through family-based, community-level husbandry, which in market-based economies is being replaced by mass production methods, using vast networks of corporate farms and processing facilities. The result of this shift has been a reduction in the "time price" of food, making it cheaper and more accessible to simply purchase what was once grown, harvested, and prepared by individuals or families [66].

Promoting sustainable agriculture for healthy food production and distribution is a potentially robust policy for addressing overweight and obesity rates in LMICs. Sustainable agriculture systems in LMICs have the potential to produce whole foods conveniently and affordably. The major goal of sustainable agriculture is to develop technologies and practices that protect the environment while fostering improvements in food productivity. Arguably, there is a balance to be struck, as progress in agricultural productivity in the past 50 to 60 years has come *via* increased use of fertilizers, irrigation water, agricultural machinery, pesticides, and land. What is called for is a resumption of old (traditional) approaches that integrate biologically and ecologically sustainable processes into food production, and that promote healthier food consumption.

Our CLD model suggests that investment in policies that build healthy food capacity would support Loops A, B and G, all of which impact LMIC obesity rates. *Via* Loop A, to the extent that sustainable agriculture translates into jobs and more affordable healthy foods, we hypothesize that a preference for traditional diet (which is, in most instances, a working definition of healthy eating), would drive down consumption of unhealthy commodities. This dynamic would, over time, serve to decrease importation and sales of unhealthy commodities to the LMIC. Over time, these dynamics would help to build important assets in the form of well managed natural resources and an infrastructure for farming, processing and distribution of healthy foods that generate both financial capital and 'natural' capital [82].

For example, drawing on recent scientific literature, the United Nations General Assembly highlighted the utility of 'agroecology' as a mode of agricultural development that can effectively support the human right to healthy food, particularly for vulnerable communities within LMICs. Well implemented agroecology is complementary to better known conventional farming approaches in many LMICs and strongly contributes to community-level economic development [68, 83]. In fact, there is growing support by the international community [68] for interventions that are consistent with 'agroecology' [83], a form of action-research that can enhance existing traditional LMIC agricultural systems and develop capacity to grow, process, and distribute healthy foods in a manner that generates achieves these goals.

Most efforts to foster greater agricultural production in LMICs have focused on improving seeds and ensuring that farmers are provided with a set of inputs that can increase yields, replicating the model of most industrialized countries. Alternatively, an agroecological approach can simultaneously increase farm productivity and food security, improve incomes and rural livelihoods, and reverse the trend towards species loss and genetic erosion [68, 82, 84].

An example of 'agroecological' policy intervention is evidenced in Uganda, where experiments in organic farming have been stimulated by farmers and consumers working in collaboration with private, foreign companies. In Uganda, organic farming has focused more on the crop sector than livestock sector and has primarily involved the private sector, such as organic products exported by companies and non-governmental organizations. Agriculture in Uganda and many African countries is 'traditional' in that it is less mechanized, uses a minimum of chemical fertilizers, pesticides, and drugs, thus the essential characteristics of an organic approach. Traditional farming, however, does not always meet principles of organic farming (*i.e.,* ecology, fairness, health, and care) [85]. These efforts, however, have met challenges of implementation, including problems of managing disease, organic feed insufficiency, and limited education of farmers. While promising, there is a need for more scientific research in Uganda and other LMICs, research that supports their local farming communities and institutions.

Public Health Education

Education at multiple levels is also a recommended policy for addressing the obesity problem in LMICs. Programs that foster education of the general population about healthy nutrition and providing information about health problems caused by overweight and obesity are important [84, 86]. Such programs can be mounted in communities *via* local organizations and institutions, such as public schools. They can also be mounted in mass media campaigns, using print, television, or radio, as well as the internet and social media sites [87].

In addition, national programs to ensure that all packaged food is labeled with clear, accessible nutrition information and calorie counts per serving will help educate the populous about energy intake. Similarly, restaurants could be directed to provide calorie counts for dishes served on menus, and advertisements of unhealthy foods could be taxed, while those promoting healthy food making among parents could come with tax break or other incentive [88]. Education for health care professionals who can advise their patients about healthy nutrition, exercise, smoking cessation, and moderating alcohol use, is also effective [89]. Notably, health professionals typically have greater access to women who are often mothers, so for these patients they can impart education about how to better ensure the healthy weight of their children, for instance by teaching about the benefits of breast feeding among newborn children to prevent weight gain.

Notably, an agroecological approach is knowledge-intensive, requiring the development of both ecological literacy and decision-making skills in farmer communities and, more broadly, in the population at-large. To address the educational needs of farmers, investments in agricultural extension and agricultural research would be essential. Investing in extension programs would likely serve to reduce poverty and agricultural productivity in developing countries. According to the International Food Policy Research Institute, agricultural extension research generates large dividends and has had "the largest impact on agricultural production and second-largest impact on poverty reduction (after rural education) in China, and the second-largest impact on poverty reduction in rural India (after investment in roads)" [90].

In addition, there is a need to further educate and foster critical policy analyses among multi-sectoral, multi-disciplinary experts in nutrition, medicine, economics, sociology, anthropology and other health-related fields. Here, international 'working groups,' like the *Global Forum on Agricultural Research* (GFAR; http://www.egfar.org/) and *Global System Dynamics and Policy* (GSDP; http://www.gsdp.eu/), are building new platforms for global exchange of ideas and perspectives on complex topics, including the global problem of overweight and obesity. Both of these groups seek to inform and shape better policy making to help solve complex and interrelated issues impacting health of diverse societies and the world today.

CONCLUSION

Using systems thinking, the qualitative model that has been presented shows the complex dynamics associated with the growing obesity epidemic in LMICs. Systems thinking is a precursory step toward the development of formal system dynamics models, which are formally defined sets of differential and algebraic equations. These mathematical models are used to conduct virtual experiments, *via* simulation analyses, to quantify the short and long term impact of alternative policies. Effective systems thinking informs a sort of 'blueprint' for the subsequent design and development of a quantitative system dynamics model or models [5, 10]; models that could be calibrated to examine a particular LMIC, integrating country-specific environmental, cultural, social, and economic factors. However, the quality of this 'blueprint' is a function of how well extant theory and evidence are used to articulate the 'structure' of the problem. The choice of constructs to be included in key constructs by extant sources of evidence and research and becomes the basis for simulation analyses that compare and contrast alternative strategies to find feasible, sustainable ways to address the problem of concern [2, 4, 7, 91-94].

In this model, we have generated a host of interdependent causal hypotheses, calling attention to two general recommended policy domains: grow *healthy food production capacity* and promote *public health education*. An agroecological approach, strongly endorsed by the United Nations and its affiliated partners in addressing global health, would likely foster gains in both of our recommended policy domains. However, for such an approach to have recognizable impact, the need for collaborative, multi-sector partnerships is evident. At this juncture in the global obesity epidemic, public authorities, experts and local organizations need to come together in long-term, constructive relationships that invest in ambitious programs and policies to scale up agroecological models in diverse settings. Although today no population is unaffected or unthreatened by the global forces currently driving the obesity epidemic, our model suggests that change is possible and that obesity rates in all countries can be slowed or reversed over time, with effective leadership and support for effective policies.

ACKNOWLEDGEMENTS

Declared none.

CONFLICT OF INTEREST

The authors confirm that this chapter contents have no conflict of interest.

REFERENCES

[1] Homer JB, Hirsch G. System dynamics modeling for public health: Background and opportunities. Am J Public Health 2006; 96(3): 452-8.

[2] Maani KE, Cavana RY. Systems Thinking and Modeling: Understanding Change and Complexity. Auckland, New Zealand: Pearson Education New Zealand Limited; 2000.

[3] Mabry P, Olster D, Morgan G, Abrams D. Interdisciplinarity and systems science to improve population health: A view from the NIH Office of Behavioral and Social Sciences Research. Am J Prev Med 2008; 35(S2): S211-S24.

[4] Forrester JW. The model *versus* a modeling process. System Dynamics Review 1987; 1(1): 133-4.

[5] Repenning NA. A simulation-based approach to understanding the dynamics of innovation implementation. Organization Science 2002; 13(109-127).

[6] Richardson GP. Feedback Thought in Social Science and Systems Theory. Waltham, MA: Pegasus Communications, Inc.; 1991.

[7] Richardson GP, Pugh III AL. Introduction to System Dynamics Modeling. Portland, Oregon: Productivity Press 1981.

[8] Luke DA, Stamatakis KA. Systems science methods in public health: dynamics, networks, and agents. Annu Rev Public Health 2012; 33: 357-76.

[9] Hirsch G, Immediato CS. Microworlds and generic structures as resources for integrating care and improving health. System Dynamics Review 1999; 15(3): 315-30.

[10] Lounsbury DW, Hirsch GB, Vega C, Schwartz CE. Understanding social forces involved in diabetes outcomes: a systems science approach to quality-of-life research. Qual Life Res 2013.

[11] Arboleda CA, Abraham DM, Lubitz R. Simulation as a tool to assess the vulnerability of the operation of a health care facility. Journal of Performance of Constructed Facilities 2007; 21(4): 302-12.

[12] Cavana RY, Davies PK, Robson RM, Wilson KJ. Drivers of quality in health services: Different worldviews of clinicians and policy managers revealed. System Dynamics Review 1999; 15(3): 331-40.
[13] Hirsch G, Miller S. Evaluating HMO Policies with a Computer Simulation Model. Medical Care 1974; 12(8): 668-81.
[14] Hovmand PS, Gillespie DF. Implementation of Evidence-Based Practice and Organizational Performance. Journal of Behavioral Health Services & Research 2010; 37(1): 79-94.
[15] Royston G, Dost A, Townshend J, Turner H. Using system dynamics to help develop and implement policies and programmes in health care in England. System Dynamics Review 1999; 15(3): 293-313.
[16] Wolstenholme E, Monk D, McKelvie D, Arnold S. Coping but not coping in health and social care: masking the reality of running organisations beyond safe design capacity. System Dynamics Review 2007; 23(4): 371-89.
[17] Braithwaite J, Westbrook JI, Ranmuthugala G, Cunningham F, Plumb J, Wiley J, *et al.* The development, design, testing, refinement, simulation and application of an evaluation framework for communities of practice and social-professional networks. BMC Health Services Research 2009; 9.
[18] Elf M, Poutilova M, Ohrn K. A dynamic conceptual model of care planning. Scandinavian Journal of Caring Sciences 2007; 21(4): 530-8.
[19] Taylor K, Dangerfield B. Modelling the feedback effects of reconfiguring health services. Journal of the Operational Research Society 2005; 56(6): 659-75.
[20] Homer J, Hirsch G, Minniti M, Pierson M. Models for collaboration: How system dynamics helped a community organize cost-effective care for chronic illness. System Dynamics Review 2004; 20(3): 199-222.
[21] Dangerfield BC, Fang YX, Roberts CA. Model-based scenarios for the epidemiology of HIV/AIDS: the consequences of highly active antiretroviral therapy. System Dynamics Review 2001; 17(2): 119-50.
[22] Flessa S. Decision support for AIDS control programmes in eastern Africa. OR Spectrum 2003; 25(2): 265-91.
[23] Lebcir RM, Atun RA, Coker RJ. System Dynamic simulation of treatment policies to address colliding epidemics of tuberculosis, drug resistant tuberculosis and injecting drug users driven HIV in Russia. Journal of the Operational Research Society 2010; 61(8): 1238-48.
[24] Roberts C, Dangerfield B. Modeling the epidemiologic consequences of HIV infection and AIDS: A contribution from operational research. Journal of the Operational Research Society 1990; 41(4): 273-89.
[25] Roberts EB, Homer J, Kasabian A, Varrell M. A systems view of the smoking problem: Perspective and limitations of the role of science in decision-making. International Journal of Bio-Medical Computing 1982; 13(1): 69-86.
[26] Chick SE, Mamani H, Simchi-Levi D. Supply Chain Coordination and Influenza Vaccination. Operations Research 2008; 56(6): 1493-506.
[27] Homer J, Ritchie-Dunham J, Rabbino H, Puente LM, Jorgensen J, Hendricks K. Toward a dynamic theory of antibiotic resistance. System Dynamics Review 2000; 16(4): 287-319.
[28] Thompson KM, Tebbens RJD. Using system dynamics to develop policies that matter: global management of poliomyelitis and beyond. System Dynamics Review 2008; 24(4): 433-49.
[29] Ahmad S. The cost-effectiveness of raising the legal smoking age in California. Medical Decision Making 2005; 25(3): 330-40.
[30] Ahmad S. Closing the youth access gap: The projected health benefits and cost savings of a national policy to raise the legal smoking age to 21 in the United States. Health Policy 2005; 75(1): 74-84.
[31] Cavana RY, Clifford LV. Demonstrating the utility of system dynamics for public policy analysis in New Zealand: the case of excise tax policy on tobacco. System Dynamics Review 2006; 22(4): 321-48.
[32] Tengs TO, Osgood ND, Chen LL. The cost-effectiveness of intensive national school-based anti-tobacco education: Results from the Tobacco Policy Model. Preventive Medicine 2001; 33(6): 558-70.
[33] Homer JB. A system dynamics model of national cocaine prevalence. System Dynamics Review 1993; 9(1): 49-78.

[34] Homer JB, StClair CL. A model of HIV transmission through needle sharing. Interfaces 1991; 21(3): 26-49.
[35] Smith PC, van Ackere A. A note on the integration of system dynamics and economic models. Journal of Economic Dynamics & Control 2002; 26(1): 1-10.
[36] Wakeland W, Schmidt T, Gilson AM, Haddox JD, Webster LR. System Dynamics Modeling as a Potentially Useful Tool in Analyzing Mitigation Strategies to Reduce Overdose Deaths Associated with Pharmaceutical Opioid Treatment of Chronic Pain. Pain Medicine 2011; 12: S49-S58.
[37] Huz S, Andersen DF, Richardson GP, Boothroyd R. A framework for evaluating systems thinking interventions: An experimental approach to mental health system change. System Dynamics Review 1997; 13(2): 149-69.
[38] Smits M. Impact of policy and process design on the performance of intake and treatment processes in mental health care: a system dynamics case study. Journal of the Operational Research Society 2010; 61(10): 1437-45.
[39] Homer J, Hirsch G, Milstein B. Chronic illness in a complex health economy: the perils and promises of downstream and upstream reforms. System Dynamics Review 2007; 23(2-3): 313-43.
[40] Siegel CA, Siegel LS, Hyams JS, Kugathasan S, Markowitz J, Rosh JR, *et al.* Real-time Tool to Display the Predicted Disease Course and Treatment Response for Children with Crohn's Disease. Inflammatory Bowel Diseases 2011; 17(1): 30-8.
[41] Milstein B, Homer J, Hirsch GB. Analyzing natinal health reform strategies with a dynamic simulation model. Am J Public Health 2010; 100(5): 811-9.
[42] World Health Organization. Obseity and Overweight Fact Sheet2013. [Cited March 3 2014] Available at: http://www.who.int/mediacentre/factsheets/fs311/en/.
[43] Swinburn BA, Sacks G, Hall KD, McPherson K, Finegood DT, Moodie ML, *et al.* The global obesity pandemic: Shaped by global drivers and local environments. Lancet 2011; 378(9793): 804-14.
[44] Popkin BM, Slining MM. New dynamics in global obesity facing low- and middle-income countries. Obes Rev 2013; 14 Suppl 2: 11-20.
[45] USAID. Demographic and Health Surveys. US Agency for International Development, 2013. [Cited March 3 2014] Available at: http://www.dhsprogram.com/
[46] Vandevijvere S, Monteiro C, Krebs-Smith SM, Lee A, Swinburn B, Kelly B, *et al.* Monitoring and benchmarking population diet quality globally: a step-wise approach. Obes Rev 2013; 14 Suppl 1: 135-49.
[47] Struckler D, McKee M, Ebrahim S, Basu S. Manufacturing epidemics: The role of global producers in increased consumption of unhealthy commodities, including processed foods, alcohol, and tobacco. PLOS Medicine 2012; 9(6): 1-8.
[48] Popkin BM, Adair LS, Ng SW. Global nutrition transition and the pandemic of obesity in developing countries. Nutr Rev 2012; 70(1): 3-21.
[49] Owen J, Reisin E. Non-Communicable Disease: A Welcome and Long Needed Addition to the WHO's 2012 World Heath Statistics. Curr Hypertens Rep 2012; 14(6): 475-7.
[50] Monteiro CA, Moubarac JC, Cannon G, Ng SW, Popkin B. Ultra-processed products are becoming dominant in the global food system. Obes Rev 2013; 14 Suppl 2: 21-8.
[51] Brezis M, Wiist WH. Vulnerability of health to market forces. Med Care 2011; 49(3): 232-9.
[52] Wiist WH. Public health and the anticorporate movement: rationale and recommendations. Am J Public Health 2006; 96(8): 1370-5.
[53] Chan M, editor Noncommunicable diseases damage health, including economic health. High-level meeting on noncommunicable diseases, United Nations General Assembly; 2011 September 19, 2011; New York, NY: WHO.
[54] Wells JC. Obesity as malnutrition: the dimensions beyond energy balance. Eur J Clin Nutr 2013; 67(5): 507-12.
[55] Doak C, Adair L, Monterio C, Popkin B. Overweight and underweight coexist within households in Brazil, China and Russia. Journal of Nutrition 2000; 130: 2965-71.
[56] Hawkes C. The role of foreign direct investment in the nutrition transition. Public Health Nutr 2005; 8(4): 357-65.
[57] Hawkes C. Uneven dietary development: linking the policies and processes of globalization with the nutrition transition, obesity and diet-related chronic diseases. Global Health 2006; 2: 4.

[58] Rigby NJ, Kumanyika S, James WP. Confronting the epidemic: the need for global solutions. J Public Health Policy 2004; 25(3-4): 418-34.
[59] Nishida C, Uauy R, Kumanyika S, Shetty P. The Joint WHO/FAO Expert Consultation on diet, nutrition and the prevention of chronic diseases: Process, product and policy implications. Public Health Nutrition 2004; 7(1A): 245-50.
[60] Glasgow R, Wagner E, Kaplan R, Vinicor F, Smith L, Norman J. If diabetes is a public health problem, why not treat it as one? A population-based approach to chronic illness. Annals of Behavioral Medicine 1999; 21(2): 159-70.
[61] Mittal S, El-Serag HB. Epidemiology of hepatocellular carcinoma: consider the population. J Clin Gastroenterol 2013; 47 Suppl: S2-6.
[62] Norrving B, Kissela B. The global burden of stroke and need for a continuum of care. Neurology 2013; 80(3 Suppl 2): S5-12.
[63] Subramanian S, Chait A. Hypertriglyceridemia secondary to obesity and diabetes. Biochim Biophys Acta 2012; 1821(5): 819-25.
[64] Wagner KH, Brath H. A global view on the development of non communicable diseases. Prev Med 2012; 54 Suppl: S38-41.
[65] Wiener N. Cynbernetics of Control Communications in the Animal and the Machine. New York: John Wiley; 1948.
[66] Fleischhacker SE, Evenson KR, Rodriguez DA, Ammerman AS. A systematic review of fast food access studies. Obes Rev 2011; 12(5): e460-71.
[67] Ng SW, Popkin BM. Time use and physical activity: a shift away from movement across the globe. Obes Rev 2012; 13(8): 659-80.
[68] Assembly UG. Report submitted by the Special Rapporteur on the right to food, Olivier De Schutter. In: Council HR, editor. New York2010.
[69] Wiist W. We must reclaim public health from private corporate interests. BMJ 2012; 345: e6160.
[70] Wiist WH. Citizens United, public health, and democracy: the Supreme Court ruling, its implications, and proposed action. Am J Public Health 2011; 101(7): 1172-9.
[71] Gearhardt AN, Grilo CM, DiLeone RJ, Brownell KD, Potenza MN. Can food be addictive? Public health and policy implications. Addiction 2011; 106(7): 1208-12.
[72] NCHS. Health, United States, 2012: In Brief2013. [Cited March 3 2014] Available at http://www.cdc.gov/nchs/data/hus/hus13_InBrief.pdf
[73] Subramanian SV, Perkins JM, Ozaltin E, Davey Smith G. Weight of nations: a socioeconomic analysis of women in low- to middle-income countries. Am J Clin Nutr 2011; 93(2): 413-21.
[74] Monteiro CA, Moura EC, Conde WL, Popkin BM. Socioeconomic status and obesity in adult populations of developing countries: a review. Bull World Health Organ 2004; 82(12): 940-6.
[75] Jones-Smith JC, Gordon-Larsen P, Siddiqi A, Popkin BM. Is the burden of overweight shifting to the poor across the globe? Time trends among women in 39 low- and middle-income countries (1991-2008). Int J Obes (Lond) 2012; 36(8): 1114-20.
[76] Forrester JW. Urban Dynamics. Portland, OR: Productivity Press; 1961.
[77] Gagliardino JJ, Aschner P, Baik SH, Chan J, Chantelot JM, Ilkova H, *et al.* Patients' education, and its impact on care outcomes, resource consumption and working conditions: Data from the International Diabetes Management Practices Study (IDMPS). Diabetes & Metabolism 2012; 38(2): 128-34.
[78] Gortmaker SL, Swinburn BA, Levy D, Carter R, Mabry PL, Finegood DT, *et al.* Changing the future of obesity: science, policy, and action. The Lancet.378(9793): 838-47.
[79] World Health Organization. World Population to Increase by 2.6 Billion Over Next 45 Years. In: Division P, editor. New York2005.
[80] Finucane MM, Stevens GA, Cowan MJ, Danaei G, Lin JK, Paciorek CJ, *et al.* National, regional, and global trends in body-mass index since 1980: systematic analysis of health examination surveys and epidemiological studies with 960 country-years and 9.1 million participants. Lancet 2011; 377(9765): 557-67.
[81] Lounsbury DW, Mitchell SG. Introduction to special issue on social ecological approaches to community health research and action. American Journal of Community Psychology 2009; 44(3-4): 213-20.

[82] Pretty J. Agricultural sustainability: concepts, principles and evidence. Philos Trans R Soc Lond B Biol Sci 2008; 363(1491): 447-65.

[83] Altieri MA, Farrell JG, Hecht SB, Liebman M, Magdoff F, Murphy W, *et al.* Agroecology: The Science of Sustainable Agriculture. Boulder, CO: Westview Press; 1995.

[84] Karnik S, Kanekar A. Childhood obesity: A global public health crisis. Int J Prev Med 2012; 3(1): 1-7.

[85] Nalubwama SM, Mugisha A, Vaarst M. Organic livestock production in Uganda: potentials, challenges and prospects. Trop Anim Health Prod 2011; 43(4): 749-57.

[86] Franceschi S, Wild CP. Meeting the global demands of epidemiologic transition - the indispensable role of cancer prevention. Mol Oncol 2013; 7(1): 1-13.

[87] Ramanadhan S, Mendez SR, Rao M, Viswanath K. Social media use by community-based organizations conducting health promotion: a content analysis. BMC Public Health 2013; 13(1): 1129.

[88] Farley TA. The role of government in preventing excess calorie consumption: the example of New York City. JAMA 2012; 308(11): 1093-4.

[89] Emery JD, Shaw K, Williams B, Mazza D, Fallon-Ferguson J, Varlow M, *et al.* The role of primary care in early detection and follow-up of cancer. Nat Rev Clin Oncol 2014; 11(1): 38-48.

[90] Fan S. Public expenditures, growth, and poverty: Lessons from developing countries. In: IFPRI, editor 2008.

[91] Forrester JW. Counterintuitive behavior of social systems. Technology Review 1971; 73(January): 52-68.

[92] Forrester JW. Principles of Systems. 2nd ed. Cambridge: Wright-Allen Press; 1971.

[93] Forrester JW. Lessons from system dynamics modelling. System Dynamics Review 1987; 3: 136-49.

[94] Forrester JW, Senge PM. Tests for building confidence in system dynamics models. TIMS Studies in the Management Science 1980; 14: 201-28.

CHAPTER 17

The Effectiveness of Wellness Program Incentives in Reducing the Burden and Cost of Obesity

Chloe Cheng[*,1] **and Richard H. Bernstein**[2]

[1]*Wellness Division, Frenkel Benefits LLC, USA; and* [2]*Preventive Medicine and Geriatric and Palliative Medicine, The Icahn School of Medicine at Mount Sinai, USA*

Abstract: Public health approaches to obesity have more recently been supplemented by incentive programs in the private sector. The experience in the U.S. and abroad will be discussed, including the reasons obesity has been a recalcitrant and increasingly common problem. The complex behavioral underpinnings and dynamics of over-eating will be described along with motivational strategies to change these by use of various incentive arrangements. Evaluating wellness programs and incentive schemes is difficult. To determine the return on investment in such initiatives will require well designed programs and evaluations which recognize potential biases and inherent ethical concerns. Further research will be crucial to bend the curve on rising obesity rates with their attendant costs.

Keywords: BMI, diet, exercise, fitness, global health, incentives, nutrition, obesity, overeating, overweight, risk, smoking cessation, wellness program, wellness, workplace.

INTRODUCTION

Overweight and obesity have risen to alarming rates in the United States. This epidemic in the U.S. resulted in the nation heading the list of the world's fattest industrialized countries every year prior to 2013 and is currently second to Mexico [1]. Excess weight may pose the greatest worldwide health risk and billions of healthcare dollars are being spent as a result. While the causes of obesity are complex, they may be influenced by genes [2], emotional stress, human gut microbiota, associating with others who are obese [3] and medications among other factors. In addition, an array of unhealthy behaviors, including poor diet and physical inactivity, contributes to obesity and a host of serious chronic

***Corresponding author Chloe Cheng:** Frenkel Benefits, LLC-Wellness Division, USA; Tel: (516) 554-7338; E-mail: chloe.cheng@mssm.edu conditions. Against this backdrop, proponents of public health have sought innovative methods to encourage changes in health-related behavior. One important approach involves financial incentives.

While the epidemic has been managed using traditional public health approaches (*e.g.*, public service announcements, advertisements, educational literature, use of the bully pulpit and legislation), the onus of finding solutions now also involves many employers, insurers, and various levels of government. These three private and public payers have often applied financial incentives to reduce the trend of subsequent medical complications and preventable costs related to obesity.

This chapter will assess multiple dimensions of wellness incentives to encourage weight loss. After a brief sketch of obesity trends, obesity-related health conditions, and a summary of their financial burden, the next section will discuss applied behavioral interventions along with the approach of behavioral economics that underpins most current incentive programs. Reference will also be made to the global impact of obesity and several international approaches to using incentives to influence obesity rates. Next, we will review the use of wellness incentives in the U.S., including the impact of the Patient Protection and Affordable Care Act (ACA) with its salient financial and ethical issues. The chapter will conclude with some areas of needed research and methodological considerations to establish the value of incentives for reducing obesity and the return on investment of incentive based programs.

THE EPIDEMIC OF OBESITY IN THE U.S. AND THE RISK OF CHRONIC DISEASE AND DISABILITY

Over the past half century, the United States has witnessed nearly a three-fold increase in the prevalence of adult obesity [4, 5]. In the early 1960s, the percentage of obese U.S. adults aged 20 years and older was roughly 13.4%; today, 35.9% are obese [6]. If both overweight and obese individuals are included in this statistic, that percentage is approximately double (69.2%) [7]. These numbers have sounded an alarm to the lay press, legislators and those within public health.

Overweight and obesity increase the risk of a plethora of diseases and health conditions including hypertension, type 2 diabetes, heart disease, and numerous cancers [8]. Not surprisingly, as the prevalence of overweight/obesity has risen, rates of the above health conditions have surged in tandem. According to a 2004

Centers for Disease Control and Prevention's (CDC) Morbidity and Mortality Weekly Report, there has been an epidemiological transition in leading causes of death from those of an infectious nature to those of a chronic nature [9]. In fact, seven out of ten deaths among Americans each year stem from chronic diseases, with heart disease, cancer and stroke accounting for more than 50% of all deaths each year [10]. Consistent with these statistics, 25.8 million people in the United States, or 8.3% of the population, have diabetes. If this trend continues, the CDC projects that one out of three adults in the U.S. will have diabetes by 2050 [11]. These types of chronic conditions can have a significant effect on an individual's daily life. Roughly 25% of obese individuals experience limitations in one or more activities of daily living [12]. Degenerative arthritis, which is the most common cause of disability, has been reported to hinder the activities of nearly 19 million Americans [13]. Meanwhile, diabetes has maintained its position as the leading cause of kidney failure, non-traumatic lower extremity amputations, as well as blindness among adults [14].

OBESITY GOES GLOBAL

While the U.S. is typically associated with obesity, rates of this condition are also soaring outside of the States. The World Health Organization has reported that the worldwide prevalence of obesity has increased roughly two-fold from 1980 to 2008 [15]. During 2008, more than 50% of both men and women in Europe were overweight and approximately 21% were obese. In England specifically, the prevalence of obesity in adults was roughly 26% in 2011, according to the National Obesity Observatory, an arm of England's Department of Health [16]. This represents a rapid increase in prevalence since 1993 when approximately 15% of adults were obese. The same 2011 survey revealed that 42% of English men and 32% of English women were classified as overweight. Like the United States, there are also significant costs associated with obesity in England. In 2007, direct National Health Service costs of treating overweight and obesity in England totaled £4.2 billion ($6.8 billion), and projected indirect costs may be as high as £27 billion by 2015. Comparable statistics are reflected in Eastern Mediterranean countries. Over 50% of women in this region were overweight compared with an obesity rate of 24% of women in 2008. The prevalence in Eastern Mediterranean men is roughly half than that of women [17]. Moreover, three countries in the Middle East and North Africa top the list of the world's highest diabetes prevalence—Saudi Arabia, Kuwait, and Qatar. These countries spent $13.6 billion on diabetes-related care in 2013, and among adults in these countries, rates of overweight and obesity are especially high (men: 70-85%, women: 75-88%) [18].

THE CHALLENGE OF CHANGING BEHAVIOR

Lifestyle choices are often at the heart of these chronic health conditions. While individuals have the ability to sustain or improve their health, their behavioral choices may adversely affect their well-being. Public health professionals and health providers alike advocate for the consumption of appropriate quantities of healthy foods, regular exercise, and abstinence from smoking. They also encourage obtaining preventive care and heeding physicians' advice [19]. Despite a long history of such public health messages, individuals often fail to follow through. As a result, population health has eroded, and health care costs have ballooned. Every year approximately 40% of all premature deaths are attributable to unhealthy personal behaviors (*e.g.*, physical inactivity, unhealthful food choices, substance abuse, non-adherence with medications) [20].

DEFINING AND MEASURING OVERWEIGHT AND OBESITY

There are various techniques for measuring obesity, and each has limitations [21]. Body fatness is most commonly measured by body mass index (BMI), which is calculated from an individual's mass and height: BMI = mass (kg)/height $(m)^2$ or [mass (lb)/height $(in)^2$] x 703. "Normal" BMI ranges from 18.5 to 24.9; "overweight" from 25.0 to 29.9; and "obese" from 30.0 upwards [22].

While BMI calculation is the most common technique for determining fatness or fitness, its clinical limitations should also be recognized (Fig. **1**). BMI is a surrogate measure of body fatness. It accounts for excess weight rather than excess body fat. As a result, factors including age, sex, ethnicity, and muscle mass are often overlooked in the relationship between BMI and body fatness. BMI also does not reveal the distribution of fat on an individual, nor does it discriminate between muscle, bone mass, and excess fat [24]. Other potentially more precise methods include waist circumference, waist-to-hip ratio, skinfold thickness, bioelectric impedance, underwater weighing, air-displacement plethysmography, dilution method, dual energy x-ray absorptiometry (DEXA), and computerized tomography (CT)/magnetic resonance imaging (MRI) scans [25]. While these other techniques will not be further explored, it is important to acknowledge that, although it is almost universally employed, BMI is an imprecise measure of obesity.

WEIGHT lbs	kg	4'8" 142cm	4'9" 145	4'10" 147	4'11" 150	5'0" 152	5'1" 155	5'2" 157	5'3" 160	5'4" 163	5'5" 165	5'6" 168	5'7" 170	5'8" 173	5'9" 175	5'10" 178	5'11" 180	6'0" 183	6'1" 185	6'2" 188	6'3" 191	6'4" 193	6'5" 196
260	118	58	56	54	53	51	49	48	46	45	43	42	41	40	38	37	36	35	34	33	32	32	31
255	116	57	55	53	51	50	48	47	45	44	42	41	40	39	38	37	36	35	34	33	32	31	30
250	113	56	54	52	50	49	47	46	44	43	42	40	39	38	37	36	35	34	33	32	31	30	30
245	111	55	53	51	49	48	46	45	43	42	41	40	38	37	36	35	34	33	32	31	31	30	29
240	109	54	52	50	48	47	45	44	43	41	40	39	38	36	35	34	33	33	32	31	30	29	28
235	107	53	51	49	47	46	44	43	42	40	39	38	37	36	35	34	33	32	31	30	29	29	28
230	104	52	50	48	46	45	43	42	41	39	38	37	36	35	34	33	32	31	30	30	29	28	27
225	102	50	49	47	45	44	43	41	40	39	37	36	35	34	33	32	31	31	30	29	28	27	27
220	100	49	48	46	44	43	42	40	39	38	37	36	34	33	32	32	31	30	29	28	27	27	26
215	98	48	47	45	43	42	41	39	38	37	36	35	34	33	32	31	30	29	28	28	27	26	25
210	95	47	45	44	42	41	40	38	37	36	35	34	33	32	31	30	29	28	28	27	26	26	25
205	93	46	44	43	41	40	39	37	36	35	34	33	32	31	30	29	29	28	27	26	26	25	24
200	91	45	43	42	40	39	38	37	35	34	33	32	31	30	30	29	28	27	26	26	25	24	24
195	88	44	42	41	39	38	37	36	35	33	32	31	31	30	29	28	27	26	26	25	24	24	23
190	86	43	41	40	38	37	36	35	34	33	32	31	30	29	28	27	26	26	25	24	24	23	23
185	84	41	40	39	37	36	35	34	33	32	31	30	29	28	27	27	26	25	24	24	23	23	22
180	82	40	39	38	36	35	34	33	32	31	30	29	28	27	27	26	25	24	24	23	22	22	21
175	79	39	38	37	35	34	33	32	31	30	29	28	27	27	26	25	24	24	23	22	22	21	21
170	77	38	37	36	34	33	32	31	30	29	28	27	27	26	25	24	24	23	22	22	21	21	20
165	75	37	36	34	33	32	31	30	29	28	27	27	26	25	24	24	23	22	22	21	21	20	20
160	73	36	35	33	32	31	30	29	28	27	27	26	25	24	24	23	22	22	21	21	20	19	19
155	70	35	34	32	31	30	29	28	27	27	26	25	24	24	23	22	22	21	20	20	19	19	18
150	68	34	32	31	30	29	28	27	27	26	25	24	23	23	22	22	21	20	20	19	19	18	18
145	66	33	31	30	29	28	27	27	26	25	24	23	23	22	21	21	20	20	19	19	18	18	17
140	64	31	30	29	28	27	26	26	25	24	23	23	22	21	21	20	20	19	18	18	17	17	17
135	61	30	29	28	27	26	26	25	24	23	22	22	21	21	20	19	19	18	18	17	17	16	16
130	59	29	28	27	26	25	25	24	23	22	22	21	20	20	19	19	18	18	17	17	16	16	15
125	57	28	27	26	25	24	24	23	22	21	21	20	20	19	18	18	17	17	16	16	16	15	15
120	54	27	26	25	24	23	23	22	21	21	20	19	19	18	18	17	17	16	16	15	15	15	14
115	52	26	25	24	23	22	22	21	20	20	19	19	18	17	17	16	16	16	15	15	14	14	14
110	50	25	24	23	22	21	21	20	19	19	18	18	17	17	16	16	15	15	15	14	14	13	13
105	48	24	23	22	21	21	20	19	19	18	17	17	16	16	16	15	15	14	14	13	13	13	12
100	45	22	22	21	20	20	19	18	18	17	17	16	16	15	15	14	14	14	13	13	12	12	12
95	43	21	21	20	19	19	18	17	17	16	16	15	15	14	14	14	13	13	13	12	12	12	11
90	41	20	19	19	18	18	17	16	16	15	15	15	14	14	13	13	13	12	12	12	11	11	11
85	39	19	18	18	17	17	16	16	15	15	14	14	13	13	13	12	12	12	11	11	11	10	10
80	36	18	17	17	16	16	15	15	14	14	13	13	13	12	12	11	11	11	11	10	10	10	9

HEIGHT (Feet/inches & centimetres)

Obese above 30 | Overweight above 25 | Healthy 18.5 to 24.9 | Underweight below 18.5

Fig. (1). Body mass index (BMI) chart for adults (adapted from ref. [23]).

THE FINANCIAL IMPACT OF OBESITY

The effects of excess weight extend beyond the individual. Besides increasing the risk of chronic conditions and decreasing life span, obesity and its sequelae are very expensive to treat. In an analysis of the direct and indirect costs of common obesity-related conditions, Colditz determined that 5.5%, or roughly $39 billion, of those costs could be credited to obesity in 1986 [26]. The direct costs of obesity-related spending have been steadily climbing during the intervening years. By one estimate, obesity accounted for close to 10% of medical expenditures in the U.S in 2006, totaling about $147 billion [27]. A more recent, and potentially more accurate, calculation by Cawley and Meyerhoefer revealed that obesity-related costs amounted to 21%, or $190 billion, of medical spending in 2005 [28].

These current figures are anywhere between three to five times the 1986 estimate. If the prevalence of obesity maintains this growth trajectory, researchers have predicted that medical spending on obesity alone may rise by $48 to $66 billion per year [29].

The magnitude of this economic and physical burden has compelled individuals, communities, states, and the nation to take a hard look at what has caused this epidemic, and what avenues to pursue to reverse or reduce its consequences. In acknowledging this need for effective interventions, public health advocates are exploring various techniques that are aimed at every level of disease prevention. On the primary level, the objective is to prevent the acquisition of high-risk behaviors among those who do not presently engage in them but are at risk for doing so. On the secondary level, the goal is to detect and manage obesity and its associated risk factors, such as hypertension. On the tertiary level, measures are focused on rehabilitation, including bariatric surgery and treatment of joint disease and skin complications to minimize the effect of obesity's complications and to restore function as much as possible.

BEHAVIORAL INTERVENTIONS AND FINANCIAL INCENTIVES

In 2009, the National Institutes of Health (NIH) convened the Science of Behavior Change meeting. Some of the main presentations stressed the acquisition and prevention of unhealthy behavior, changing existing unhealthy behaviors, as well as maintaining health promoting behavior. Discussion of these processes revealed there was a general consensus among public health experts: applying "the science of behavior change" may be the key to preventing health-related risk behaviors [30].

Although behavioral and health promotion studies have not always translated favorably into practice [31], there are compelling examples demonstrating that success is attainable. A study published in 2009 investigated the effectiveness of financial incentives in achieving smoking cessation at a multi-national company based in the United States. In this study, employees were either assigned to receive information about smoking cessation programs or to receive information along with financial incentives. Researchers found that the incentive group demonstrated significantly higher rates of smoking cessation than the information-only group. Moreover, those in the incentive group also had significantly higher rates of enrollment in smoking cessation programs, completion of smoking cessation programs, as well as smoking cessation within the first six months after program enrollment [32]. In the same vein, Topp *et al.* [33] recently published a study on the use of modest, per-dose financial incentives to increase hepatitis B vaccination completion in people who inject drugs. Compared to the control group, significantly more participants in the incentive condition received all three HBV vaccine doses. This indicates that financial incentives may be useful in certain groups to increase adherence to a multi-dose vaccine schedule in populations among whom poor adherence has consistently been reported [33]. These cases illustrate the potential health benefits that can be borne from thoughtfully developed prevention efforts.

MOTIVATIONAL PROCESSES UNDERLYING BEHAVIOR CHANGE

From a behavioral perspective, the use of incentives to target risky behaviors would appear appropriate. There are a few motivational processes that are integral to the acquisition and maintenance of risk behaviors. Literature on the topic points to reinforcement and operant conditioning as mechanisms that steer the adoption or rejection of healthy behaviors [34-36].

Neurobiological Reinforcement

Drug addictions tap into the brain reward pathway, which is also known as the mesolimbic system. When neurons in this circuit are stimulated, certain chemicals, namely dopamine, Gamma-Aminobutyric Acid (GABA), and serotonin, are released, resulting in a "high," or feelings of pleasure [37-40]. After consuming foods that are rich in sugar, salt, and fat, the same reward pathways are stimulated that are activated after drug use [41]. Because of this comparable dopaminergic response, an addictive-like consumption of foods can be triggered, contributing to excessive high-calorie food intake, and, as a corollary, obesity. In other words, frequently "abused" fatty, sugary, salty foods directly stimulate brain reward centers, which in turn condition individuals to repeat the same behaviors in the future.

To a large extent, this type of risk behavior is governed by the behavioral process of reinforcement. From an evolutionary standpoint, the palatability of foods was previously beneficial, since supplies were scarce in many environments. Thus, when "palatable," energy-dense foods containing fat and sugar were available, it was sensible to gorge on them to amass body fat reserves in anticipation of famines [42]. Since the days of hunting and gathering, the food landscape has transformed. High-calorie, high-fat foods are ubiquitous and abundant today, so the physiological mechanism underlying overeating no longer serves its function. However, the evolution of human survival instincts has not kept pace.

What was formerly a means to prevent starvation has laid the groundwork for eating for pleasure. Salty, sugary, fatty foods cause marked increases in dopamine release, which induces conditioned responses and elicits an incentive or motivation to procure them [43]. Owing to conditioning, neutral stimuli (food images/cues) that are linked to the reinforcer (food loaded with salt, sugar, and fat) acquire the ability of the reinforcer to elicit the same responses (increase dopamine in the mesolimbic system). When food cues activate the reward circuitry, food cravings ensue, transferring the reward value of food from food intake to *anticipated* food intake.

Anticipation is more powerful than the act of consumption. Once conditioning has occurred, food cues elicit increased firing of dopamine neurons, which amplifies the reward value, consequently strengthening one's motivation to perform and sustain the behaviors necessary to achieve the same result. Each time an individual eats hyper-stimulating, hyper-palatable foods, it strengthens the neuro-circuitry to consume that food again, driving the behavior [44]. As it turns out, the basic struggle of collecting enough to eat has begat a convoluted psychological and physiological system that influences the way humans approach food.

Operant Conditioning

The theoretical rationale for the use of wellness incentives also comes from B.F. Skinner's operant conditioning theory. Operant conditioning zeroes in on the relationship between active behaviors and the environment. This theory explains how individuals acquire a range of learned behaviors through two core components: reinforcement and punishment. Reinforcers are any events that increase the probability of repeating a behavior (*i.e.*, strengthen behavior), whereas punishers are any events that decrease the likelihood of repeating a behavior (*i.e.*, weaken behavior).

In a 1957 paper featured in *American Scientist*, Skinner mentioned a Harvard University study in which rats were conditioned to eat even when they were not hungry, leading to what he referred to as "behavioral obesity" [45]. This phenomenon is mirrored in humans. As previously discussed, the modern world is inundated with highly palatable, calorie dense foods as well as occasions to eat it. According to the learning theory, this kind of food environment lends itself to countless highly effective operant conditioning trials, or opportunities to associate food with voluntary behaviors that lead to it [46]. While the causes of overeating are multifold, the concepts of conditioning and extinction are key to understanding what fuels food-seeking behavior. Conditioning mechanisms have allowed humans to survive for thousands of years. Nonetheless, with the abundance of palatable food today, and the known effects of behavioral learning processes, it is not surprising that humans are tempted to consume, and do consume, in so many settings.

In theory, extinction should be able to counteract the behaviors learned through conditioning. It is defined as the reduction in strength of a learned behavior that occurs when a conditioned stimulus is presented without reinforcement [47]. In this scenario, extinction should be able to be produced through weight loss regimens or by naturally occurring extinction trials, but the existence of myriad fad diets suggests otherwise. In fact extinction does not entirely negate the effects of conditioning [39]. It does not even partially erase learned behaviors. Instead, extinction should be thought of as a new learned behavior that is partially dependent on environment. Whereas basic conditioning tends to distribute across contexts, extinction generalizes in a less sweeping manner. Thus, it is not atypical for previously extinguished conditioned responses to re-emerge.

Spontaneous recovery, renewal, resurgence, and the like indicate that the original association between a conditioned stimulus and unconditioned stimulus remains intact. Rather than erasing the original association, it appears that extinction learning entails the development of a novel inhibitory association with the conditioned stimulus, and the novel association vies with the original association for manifestation [40]. Being cognizant of these theories contributes to understanding why a learned behavior, in this case overeating, is so enduring.

BIG FOOD'S APPLICATION OF BEHAVIORAL THEORY

Big Food (*i.e.*, the multinational food and beverage industry) utilizes this same knowledge in its development of products and marketing strategies. Michael Moss, an investigative reporter for the *New York Times*, published a piece on the addictive nature of salt, sugar, and fat in February of 2013. According to his research, the optimization of this trifecta creates a "bliss point" that causes serotonin and dopamine to be released, cultivating a biologically habit-forming association [48].

From the Skinnerian perspective, Big Food has also used operant conditioning to modify behavior. The Institute of Medicine reviewed a battery of studies demonstrating the influence that advertisements have on the unhealthy food and beverage preferences, including those of children. The wellness incentives discussed in this paper are aimed at adults, but childhood obesity is still relevant as overweight and obese children are likely to carry their excess weight into adulthood [49].

One of the most contentious issues surrounding food and beverage marketing practices involves stages of discernment. Up until about 11 years of age, children lack the mental capabilities to discriminate between commercial *vs* non-commercial content and may fail to recognize the persuasive objective of advertising [50]. This suggests that children, and even teens, are especially vulnerable to the impact of food/beverage marketing and overeating. While food marketing is not the focus of this paper, awareness of reinforcement, conditioning, and Big Food's use of these techniques may enable public health experts to combat obesity on a more level playing field.

BEHAVIORAL ECONOMICS RESEARCH

According to the *homo economicus* model underlying behavioral economics, people are rational, self-interested agents who are generally able to judge and decide on the means necessary to achieve subjectively defined goals [51]. Health behavior appears to challenge this theory. Despite wanting to lose weight, drink less alcohol, or stop smoking, people often fail to act in ways that bring them closer to these goals. In the case of weight loss, health care professionals highlight food restriction and exercise to patients [52]. Individuals are aware of what they must do to lose weight, yet they neglect to follow this advice.

Behavioral economics researchers have emphasized ***hyperbolic discounting*** and ***present preference*** as fundamental biases in the way that humans choose between different options [44]. These biases increase vulnerability to high-risk behaviors. Both are related to the tendency for people to choose a smaller reward sooner over a larger reward later. It also refers to the preferences of lower over higher initial costs even when the longer-term gain is greater in the higher-initial-cost option. In other words, people usually prefer tangible rewards in the present to ones that are less definite and occur much later [53-55]. These concepts clearly apply to the challenge of sustained weight loss. When presented with dessert, the pleasure obtained from a second helping of chocolate cake may overpower the pleasure of being healthier later. Similarly, the initially more taxing but healthier long-term effects of going for a run will often surrender to the comfort and minimal exertion of watching television on the couch.

Another principle of behavioral economics that has demonstrated relevance in incentivizing weight loss is loss aversion or prospect theory. In loss aversion, people disproportionately prefer to avoid losses rather than making gains of the same value [56]. As stated by Yale Law professor Ian Ayres, "What we know about incentives is that people work a lot harder to avoid losing $10 than they will work to gain $10. So something that's framed as a loss is really effective at changing behavior" [57]. These underlying mechanisms contribute to procrastination and inactivity, but it is also possible to capitalize on this knowledge by providing immediate, concrete feedback and rewards for behavior change.

WELLNESS INCENTIVES IN THE UNITED STATES

Employee wellness programs are not a new idea. They have been in existence in the U.S. for decades. Under federal law, employers are afforded wide latitude in the development and implementation of workplace wellness programs, provided that the programs are completely separate from health plans offered to employees. It becomes a more complicated situation when the programs are run as a component of an employer-sponsored health plan. In those circumstances, the program must conform to federal rules prohibiting workplace discrimination [58].

Interestingly, it may be regulations from the Health Insurance Portability and Accountability Act of 1996 (HIPAA) that have brought wellness programs to the forefront. Not only does HIPAA bar group health plans from charging workers different premiums based on health status, it also limits the range of financial incentives that employers can offer to workers who participate in certain health promotion programs [59]. The total percentage of differential premium prices allowed by HIPAA was 20% until May 2013 [60]. Now, under the final rules released by the Obama administration, employers are allowed to increase the limit to 30%, and the maximum permissible reward is further increased to 50% for programs designed to prevent or reduce tobacco use. For instance, if a base insurance premium cost $1000, the lowest insurance premium permitted for wellness program incentives would have been $800 through 2013. After 2013, if the base premium costs $1000, the lowest premium would drop to $700, or potentially as low as $500, if a tobacco cessation program were implemented.

In 2006, regulations delineating two categories of wellness programs were also passed. One category consists of ***participatory programs***. In this type of program, rewards and penalties are not dependent on an individual meeting a health-related standard. Examples of participatory activities include paying for gym membership, attending a nutrition seminar, or undergoing a diagnostic test. The outcomes of the programs or exams have no bearing on receipt of the reward.

The other category, which has drawn more controversy, is comprised of ***health-contingent programs***. These programs are further partitioned into activity-only programs and outcome-based programs. ***Activity-only programs*** extend rewards to those who perform or complete an activity, such as running or dieting. Penalties can also be imposed on those who do not partake in these programs. ***Outcome-based programs*** reward employees who attain or maintain a specific outcome, such as a certain BMI or blood pressure, cholesterol, or glucose control level. These programs usually require workers to submit screening results so that only those who meet the standard are provided with rewards. Those who fail to reach or maintain their goals must fulfill additional requirements to receive the reward. Otherwise, they may have to pay a penalty depending on the structure of the program [61]. In keeping with ACA, employers must offer an alternative standard for employees for those for whom it is unreasonably difficult or ill advised to participate in a wellness program [62].

WILL WELLNESS INCENTIVE PROGRAMS CONTRIBUTE TO OR DETRACT FROM THE ACA'S GOALS?

Wellness Incentives in the ACA

Among the primary objectives of the Affordable Care Act is the Triple Aim of health improvement, cost control and enhanced access to care. Wellness programs touch upon all three. The ACA urges employers to develop wellness programs to help them contain costs through improved employee health. Advocates of wellness programs recognize that while providing excellent care is of vital importance, preventing chronic diseases through health promotion provides individuals with a better quality of life along with a more cost-effective approach to disease prevention for employers and the nation altogether.

Workplace Wellness Programs

Employers have become increasingly concerned with health insurance costs and employee productivity. To address these concerns, workplace wellness programs have become an attractive solution. Wellness programs encourage employees to lose weight, scale back or cease smoking and reduce overall health risks. In order to gauge their health statuses, employees are asked to report information like their body weight, blood pressure, waist circumference, and smoking habits. These numbers can either be used to reward workers with "carrots" or penalize them with "sticks" as described below.

Wellness Programs in Practice

The RAND Corporation reported that in 2009, 92% of employers with 200 or more employees offered wellness programs, with exercise, smoking and weight loss listed as the most frequently targeted behaviors [63]. The popularity of wellness programs can partly be attributed to Safeway, the second largest North American supermarket chain. In 2009, the *Wall Street Journal* featured an article on Safeway's Healthy Measures Program [64]. In this article, Safeway's Chief Executive Officer (CEO) Steve Burd announced that the company's per-capita health care expenditures remained level since the implementation of its program in 2005, providing a stark contrast to the 40% increases of its corporate peers over the four years prior. Although the program is voluntary and is only available to non-unionized workers, 74% of its non-union work force participated in the program. Healthy Measures tests for smoking status, weight, blood pressure and cholesterol. For each field that employees pass, their premiums can be reduced up to $780 for individuals and $1560 annually for families.

On the whole, Safeway's plan is a translation of the automobile insurance model [65]. Driving behavior is associated with a risk for accidents. This, in turn determines different levels of premiums among drivers. Personal responsibility is the basis of establishing insurance premiums, and premiums of reckless drivers are not bankrolled by premiums of safe drivers. The Healthy Measures program essentially shifts some responsibility from employers to employees, since it is known that many health care costs are associated with individuals' behaviors [66, 67]. With Burd's assertions of the program's effectiveness, Healthy Measures became the foundation of the informally named Safeway amendment, which raises the maximum permissible reward or penalty under a health-contingent wellness program from 20% to 30%.

Safeway has taken a ***"carrot" approach*** to wellness programs, and many other employers have followed suit. IBM, the multi-national technology corporation, has also adopted a carrots-only program. Employees are offered up to two $150 payments per year if they complete internet-based assessments on healthy eating, exercise, overall health and children's health. To obtain these rewards, employees must meet specific requirements in each option. Options include healthy eating (*e.g.*, food tracking, meal planning, goal setting), physical activity (*e.g.*, walking, swimming, aerobics), preventive care (*e.g.*, preventive care recommendations, maintenance of personal health records), children's health rebate (*e.g.*, educational resources for employees to establish healthy eating/exercise routines for their children) and the new hire rebate (new employees can complete an online health assessment and visit an internet health resource) [68]. In 2008, IBM spent $1.3 billion on health care for its employees, dependents, and retirees. To determine the return on investment (ROI) for its rebate program, the company recruited the Health Management Research Center at the University of Michigan. IBM's director of well-being reported that IBM saved roughly $80 million in reduced health claims [69]. Smoking rates among company workers were also roughly half of the national average, and participants in the exercise rebate program spent about 20% less on out-of-pocket health costs than other employees, or about $70 per year [70].

Many programs also integrate ***both carrots and sticks*** as indicated in Table **1**. For instance, the state of Alabama gives employees a $25 monthly discount on their premiums if they do not use tobacco. They are given an additional $25 monthly wellness discount if they meet standards for blood pressure, cholesterol, glucose, and BMI. Those whose test results do not meet their goals but are taking steps towards these goals are still eligible to receive the discounts. The $50-per-month sticks of Alabama's program are used on tobacco users and individuals who do not take health risk assessments and/or steps to reduce their health risks. While the Alabama State Employees Insurance Board (ASEIB) has yet to publicize an evaluation of the wellness component of its program, information on its tobacco component has been released, which may be indicative of the wellness program's financial impact. According to 2008 figures from the ASEIB, Alabama estimated that carrots and sticks of the tobacco portion saved the state more than $2.7 million in 2004 and around $2.9 million from 2006-2007 [71].

Another well-known example of a corporation with an extensive wellness program is Scotts Miracle-Gro Company. Scotts incorporates both incentives and disincentives, but emphasizes disincentives. The carrots of the LiveTotal Health Initiative include a $10 monthly fitness center membership fee, which is reimbursable after 120 uses of the center, free health coaching, free medical services for employees and covered dependents and free prescriptions for generic drugs. Scotts employed a voluntary health-risk appraisal tool called *Health Quotient*. Workers who opt out of completing the assessment must pay a $40 per month premium surcharge. Moreover, if employees take the appraisal and are categorized as a mid- to high-risk, they can choose to consult a health coach and devise a plan to lower risks. If those employees choose not to take action, they will be penalized $67 per month [61]. Scotts' Maryville headquarters employs 1,100 individuals. Since its wellness initiative took effect in 2005, the percentage of overweight or obese workers dropped by 8%, and those with high or borderline high total cholesterol decreased by 12%. Those with moderate to high-risk blood pressure declined 10% [72]. Scotts has yet to determine the ROI on LiveTotal Health, but according to the Principal Financial Well-Being Index, 59% of employees reported having increased energy to be productive at work as a result of their participation in the wellness program [65].

AmeriGas Propane, a national propane distributor, has taken a ***strictly sticks approach***. After a stretch of steeply rising premiums, the company turned to a few voluntary wellness programs to promote healthy behaviors among employees. However, according to the Vice President of Human Resources, optional programs did not bring about any results [73]. At the start of 2008, AmeriGas mandated that employees have physical exams as well as blood pressure, cholesterol and glucose testing. Women were also expected to get Pap smears and mammograms if they were aged 40 years and older. These tests were entirely covered, but if employees and their dependents did not complete the tests, they would lose their coverage. During the first year of implementation, over 90% of employees underwent the required tests. Use of cholesterol medication increased by 13.6%, diabetes drugs by 7.7%, asthma medications by 7.4%, and blood pressure medications by 2.5%. Though these are steps toward improved health, health costs at AmeriGas were 3% higher that year than they would have been without the program. The escalated spending was associated with the cost of additional exams and follow-up care [66].

THE FINANCIAL IMPACT OF PROGRAMS

Cost Containment

According to a 2010 meta-analysis of literature on the costs and savings of workplace wellness programs, wellness interventions generated $358 in savings through reduced health spending per employee annually and cost the employer $144 per employee annually. 22 studies were included in this analysis. Of the 15 studies that reported program costs, $3.37 was saved for every dollar spent [74].

In terms of absenteeism, average program savings were more modest. $294 was saved per employee per year, while program costs amounted to $132 per employee per year. Based on these numbers and the absenteeism program costs reported by twelve programs, the average ROI totaled $3.27 for each dollar spent [67].

Table 1. An overview of carrot-, stick-, and carrot-and-stick programs.

Carrots *Incentives intended to increase participation in wellness program*	***Sticks*** *Penalties for nonparticipation in wellness program*	***Carrots & Sticks*** *Use of both incentives and penalties*
Safeway's Health Measures Program If employees meet conditions for tobacco use, weight, blood pressure, and cholesterol levels; annual premiums for employees are reduced up to $780 for individuals and $1560 for families.	***AmeriGas Propane's Operation Save-A-Life*** Employees must undergo preventive testing, otherwise they may not receive medical benefits in the future.	***State of Alabama's Wellness Program*** Employees who do not use tobacco receive a $25 monthly discount on premiums. Those who do are penalized $50 per month.
IBM's Healthy Living Rebate Programs Employees can enroll in several rebate programs (*e.g.*, Personal Vitality, Physical Activity-Nutrition, Children's Health, New Hire) during annual benefits enrollment. Successful completion of the requirements results in a $150 rebate per rebate program.	***CVS/Caremark's Wellness Review*** Employees who do not participate in a "wellness review" (*e.g.*, weight, blood pressure, body fat) face an annual penalty of $600.	***Scotts Miracle-Gro's LiveTotal Health*** Employees receive a heavily discounted monthly fitness center membership fee and free health coaching among other incentives. Those who do not participate in the voluntary health-risk appraisal must pay a monthly $40 premium surcharge.

Dr. Kenneth Pelletier conducted a six-part series reviewing clinical and cost-effectiveness studies of corporate worksite wellness programs. In his latest review published in 2005, he drew a major conclusion that the majority of more than 122 studies to date indicated positive clinical and cost outcomes [75]. Osilla and her colleagues reported similar findings in 2012 [76]. Their analysis of 33 studies found improved health-related and cost outcomes. Roughly half of the studies showed improved diet- and exercise-related outcomes, but the effects were minor or not reported explicitly. As for calculations on health care costs and absenteeism, only five of the studies offered calculations of ROI. Returns ranged between $1.65 and $6.00 for every dollar invested [77-81]. Four of the 33 studies assessed the costs associated with absenteeism. These studies revealed a significant ROI of $15.60 per dollar spent [82], $1350 saved per employee in short-term disability costs [83], 0.1% point risk reduction in illness days [84] and $180 saved per enrollee per year with health care costs included [81].

Based on these reviews as well as most numbers referenced in the previous section, it appears that larger employers that utilize wellness programs reaped substantial positive returns. A 2012 meta-analysis of 62 studies estimated reductions in sick leave, health plan costs, workers' compensation, and disability insurance costs to be 25% [85]. The meta-review described previously reported an ROI of $358 per employee [67]. However, these figures are inconsistent with marketplace numbers.

If medical expenditures were reduced so drastically, one would expect that insurers would have also embraced wellness incentives from the outset. Since that has not occurred, it is possible that there is incomplete reporting of information on this subject, especially negative findings.

According to an article in *Health Affairs*, one reason for this divergence is that "unlike insurers who are immersed in this field and accustomed to hearing implausible outcomes claims, their employer counterparts who champion wellness programs typically rose through the corporate ranks in the non-quantitative HR (human resources) field" [86]. This suggests that HR departments of private employers should restructure their HR departments to match those of insurers if they intend to critically assess wellness programs.

There are also flaws inherent to the design of most program evaluations. Standards of comparison are often lacking. Showing only results for those who participated in the health risk questionnaires to acquire baseline risk would introduce participation bias or selection bias since those less likely to achieve desired clinical and cost outcomes would be excluded from the ROI estimate. Other methodological flaws also make it difficult to detect meaningful differences and to determine the true source of reduced costs [68, 69]. Confounding factors must be controlled to observe the cost and health-improvement changes of incentives alone. Sufficient follow-up poses an additional issue. It takes a few years for any true cost benefits to materialize, and, even with properly designed and executed programs, employers are more likely to see slower growth in health care costs than actual cost savings [61].

Safeway's program is a case in point. Its wellness program was unable to control costs or even keep costs flat. A 2010 follow-up piece by the *Washington Post* showed that while expenses did decrease by 12.5% in 2006, the decline was unrelated to their use of wellness incentives, since that element of their benefits program did not take effect until 2009 [87]. Costs began to climb again after 2006. Safeway forecasted that per-capita health costs for its employees would grow by 8.5% in 2009, but according to a survey of over 1,500 health plans by Aon Hewitt, the average national increase was 6.1% [80]. The economic ramifications of Safeway's incentives are unclear, but from a health outcomes standpoint, program participants did witness a 5% decline in obesity as well as improved blood pressure and cholesterol tests [80].

When looking at figures on program impact, it is important to keep in mind that study results must be examined with a certain amount of skepticism, and there are limitations to the generalizability of study findings. It is possible that large employers tend to adopt programs because they are more likely than their smaller peers to have the necessary resources to implement well-designed programs that might yield positive ROIs. Furthermore, companies that have the most to gain are the most likely to implement these programs.

There is also the possibility of publication bias [69]. Programs with the most sizeable returns will attract the most attention, and studies with significant findings of positive ROIs have the greatest probability of being published. Programs that had negative results would be less likely to be publicized, creating a false impression of the value of workplace incentives.

Incentives and Health Equity

Aside from cost containment, health equity is a defining desideratum of the Affordable Care Act and health policy in general. Access, which is one component of health equity, is addressed in wellness incentive schemes, and there are ethical considerations with each type of scheme.

Wellness programs are constructed to reward those who participate in activities or achieve targeted outcomes. Successful employees will receive greater financial benefit than their less successful coworkers. This differentiation is a genuine concern because it will be more difficult for certain individuals (*e.g.*, those in poor health or the socially disadvantaged) to meet the conditions linked to rewards. Programs tend to focus on changing the behaviors of high-risk individuals, and while there are numerous factors that contribute to their high-risk statuses, social determinants play an important role. This often means that people of low socioeconomic status are in worse health than those of a higher socioeconomic status [88, 89]. As mentioned earlier, wellness incentives are usually linked to BMI, cholesterol, blood pressure, glucose levels and smoking status. There is a social gradient in these health variables, which suggests that from the beginning, those from disadvantaged backgrounds are less likely to hit their health targets than their higher-income peers. Individuals living in low-income neighborhoods are reported to have less access to healthier food [90], fewer opportunities to exercise [91], and increased exposure to tobacco advertising [92].

Participatory and activity-only programs are often considered fairer than those that are outcome-based because they are aimed at behavioral processes [13]. However, these types of programs still have the potential to be discriminatory. Something as seemingly simple as keeping a doctor's appointment can prove to be more difficult for those whose employment offers minimal flexibility in determining work hours and who rely on public transportation to travel [93]. Participating in educational seminars or weight loss classes can even be susceptible to problems of access. Lower-income individuals may face greater burden in finding transport or paying for childcare services that allow for trips to the gym or other health-related activities. The strains of participating in time-consuming wellness programs are magnified for those who face greater demands on their time.

Environmental factors are germane to equitable access to rewards as well. Those who live near multiple supermarkets that offer healthy options will find it easier to obtain healthful foods. [94]. Neighborhood safety also makes a difference in whether one engages in exercise. Living in an unsafe area can be a barrier to regular physical activity [95]. In addition, health status at the time of program enrollment can influence program results. Healthy individuals may meet the targets from the start, and depending on the design of the program, they may be rewarded on this alone. Workers who have not met the targets may confront physical challenges to doing so (*e.g.*, having hip problems). Genetics, gut microbiota, or other physical disabilities may hinder weight loss and blood pressure, cholesterol and blood sugar reductions [96-98].

While wellness programs have a multitude of potentially discriminatory aspects, there are some ethical advantages to well-designed programs. One is that they can assist employees in surmounting obstacles they face in attempting to fend off disease and disability [13]. Those who have the largest hurdles to clear are likely to also have the most to gain from these programs.

Financial incentives can function as a tool to encourage health improvement efforts. They also help to offset some of the monetary costs of engaging in healthy behaviors, such as purchasing fresh produce, gym membership, or nutrition classes. Finally, programs can reward incremental improvements from a baseline rather than an all-or-nothing reward for attaining some ideal target. This would help those whose starting point might make achieving target goals less attainable.

Carrots and Sticks: Program Design

Wellness programs are voluntary in nature, so companies cannot mandate that employees participate as a prerequisite for employment. Privacy protection is an often-cited concern [13, 99], so employees who are worried about sharing health information with their employers, mixing their personal and professional lives and being exposed to employment discrimination should be permitted to refuse participation without jeopardizing their jobs. In keeping with HIPAA policies, medical data that is used to assign rewards and penalties should also be kept confidential.

Program designers must decide on the mix of carrots and sticks. Whichever blend they choose is likely to depend upon the objective the firm is trying to achieve. Carrots tend to be more popular among workers, so if their goal is to have a high participation rate, carrots would be the appropriate choice. On the other hand, if the goal is to have a more effective program, the answer is less clear. Efficacy appears to favor sticks because they target those who could benefit from changing their behaviors, whereas carrots may result in utilizing resources on already healthy individuals [100]. The literature suggests that loss aversion influences behavior more than making gains. But while penalties may be more effective in motivating behavior change, rewards foster a more positive and supportive wellness environment.

Ethics of Carrots

With programs that are designed to specifically target unhealthy individuals, the issue of undue inducement comes into question. For instance, if rewards were only offered to overweight individuals, achieving a target (*e.g.*, BMI $< 25 kg/m^2$) would put them ahead of their former selves as well as their current overweight and normal weight coworkers. Though most ethicists would not consider this coercive, they may categorize it as undue inducement [13, 101].

Ezekiel Emanuel, the respected American bioethicist, evaluated the ethical consequences of using financial incentives in human research. According to his exploration on the topic, "The core worry seems to be that individuals are offered some good that, against their better judgment, makes them assume substantial risks of harm that compromise their welfare" [102-104]. He identified four elements of undue inducement [102]:

1. "Individuals must be offered something that is valuable or desirable in order to do something.

2. The offered good must be so large in excess that it is irresistible in the context.

3. The offer leads individuals to exercise poor judgment in an important decision.

4. The individual's poor judgment leads to sufficiently high probability that he or she will experience a harm that seriously contravenes his or her interests [102]".

Under Emanuel's criteria, it is unlikely that a well-constructed rewards program would qualify as an undue inducement. It is possible that the prospect of gaining a reward may encourage poor judgment that violates self-interest. Running could pose a health risk for an obese individual with knee problems. Revealing exam results could lead to health-related discrimination. The size of financial incentives could also sway people's decisions to participate in the program. However, Halpern *et al*. demonstrated that participants are cognizant of varying risk levels regardless of payment amounts [105]. Cryder and her colleagues also found that while higher payments increase willingness to participate, individuals infer riskiness from payment amount [106].

Wellness programs might prompt enrollees to base decisions on short-term carrots rather than long-term gains. Nonetheless, more often than not, the long-term preference is to be healthier. Programs attempt to counteract dynamic inconsistency by using present preference to correct decision errors that undercut people's long-term interests. Therefore, it is improbable that wellness incentive programs will be charged with undue inducement.

Ethics of Sticks

Health-contingent programs that employ sticks are likely to be regressive in that they may discriminate against those with health problems and with fewer means. Wellness programs are directed at decreasing prevalence of unhealthy conditions among workers. The rates of those unhealthy conditions are highest among unhealthy employees who are also most likely to be low-income [81]. Penalties need to be carefully and fairly selected. Employers must keep in mind that the purpose of penalties is not to recover costs that stem from unhealthy behavior. They are meant to serve as incentives to encourage behavior change. If not implemented properly, penalty programs may disproportionately hurt low-income employees and possibly force high-risk employees out of health coverage.

The magnitude of penalties is also an aspect of programs that must be considered. If a single flat rate penalty is used, it may particularly harm low-income employees, while weakening the strength of the incentives for more highly compensated employees [91]. Some programs, like CVS/Caremark [107] and AmeriGas [66], penalize workers who do not submit to wellness screenings and other health reviews. It is conceivable that this use of sticks can exacerbate existing inequalities in the affordability of health care, making it more difficult for those with health issues to meet the expense of coverage. Depending on its implementation, a sticks-only strategy may reintroduce a form of medical underwriting masquerading as wellness incentives [108]. This type of cost-shifting may worsen inequalities based on health status or outcome.

Conversely, disincentive programs can restrict the ability of unhealthy workers to be rewarded for unhealthy personal behaviors. They also generate health improvements, which in turn diminish health disparities.

The Worldwide Wellness Experience: Incentives to Counter Obesity in Europe and Asia

To counter their increasing rates of obesity, many industrialized countries, namely those in the European Union, have attempted to levy taxes on unhealthful foods. In October of 2011, Denmark introduced a tax on saturated fat that added 16 kroner ($2.70) per kilogram of saturated fat in a product [109]. A year following implementation, the tax was repealed due to mounting administrative troubles facing food companies and supermarkets. It also appeared to transfer the tax entirely to consumers, impeding health equity [110].

Hungary imposed aggressive food taxes as well. In less than two years, the country instituted taxes on salt, sugar, and soft drink ingredients in an effort to force those consuming unhealthy foods to offset health care costs [111]. Hungarians viewed the taxes as a way for the government to recoup health expenses, but one of the consequences of this effort turned out to be product reformulation. Manufacturers wanted to avoid taxes, and consumers wanted to avoid purchasing these heavily taxed items. A solution to this problem was lowering the amounts of salt, sugar, and fats in packaged foods. This is an example of how taxation can facilitate substitution with healthier products and improved purchasing behavior.

Asian countries are not known for having a large overweight population, yet their rates of obesity and diabetes have also been climbing for the past three decades [112]. They have not reached levels comparable to those of Western nations, but the incidence of metabolic syndrome, a constellation of risk factors that increases one's chances of developing heart disease, stroke, and diabetes, has been on the rise. To respond to this burgeoning problem, Japan's Ministry of Health enacted the "metabo" law in 2008 to curb the rise of obesity and metabolic syndrome [113]. The law requires waist measurement during physical exams for those between 40 and 75 years-old, capping male waistlines at 33.5 inches and female waistlines at 35.4 inches [114]. Although individuals are not penalized when they cannot meet these guidelines, the law is actually aimed at companies and local governments. These entities must ensure a minimum of 65% participation, placing the responsibility into the hands of employers. If Japanese companies do not cut overweight/obesity rates of employees by 25% by 2015, they will face fines of close to 10% of their current health payments into the national health insurance program.

In addition to these illustrations, some governments are making radical moves to reverse the effects of excessive weight gain, ranging from a push for taxes on sugar-sweetened beverages in the UK [115] to paying for weight loss with gold in Dubai [116]. Widening waistlines and high BMIs carry significant physical and economic consequences, and each country's line of attack has policy implications for other countries facing similar problems.

CONCLUSION

Wellness incentives can function as a component of an effective public health or employer based program to respond to the burden and costs of obesity and other chronic diseases. Many employers embrace worksite wellness because it has great intuitive appeal: workers will identify health risks, take steps toward mitigating them and also save money for the companies through reduced use of medical care. However, the literature has revealed conflicting evidence that wellness programs result in cost reduction. If programs do generate cost savings, it is difficult to determine what factors are responsible for the accrued savings.

The overall efficacy of wellness incentives is unclear, and their use raises questions about distributional equity. Nevertheless, it appears that a behavioral approach to improving health outcomes and containing costs is gaining momentum. The ACA's final rules on incentives have reinforced this trend, but it is important to note that the effectiveness of each program is contingent on its design and implementation.

More rigorous and systematic evaluations of incentive programs must be performed. Such studies are the only way employers and public health professionals will develop a better understanding of how to achieve a defensible ROI, improve health and also craft programs that minimize discrimination and maximize equity.

ACKNOWLEDGEMENTS

Declared none.

CONFLICT OF INTEREST

The authors confirm that this chapter contents have no conflict of interest.

REFERENCES

[1] Food and Agriculture Organization of the United Nations. The state of food and agriculture: food systems for better nutrition 2013 report. Rome: Food and Agriculture Organization of the United Nations; 2013.

[2] Barabási A. Network medicine—from obesity to the "diseasome". N Engl J Med 2007; 357(4): 404-407.

[3] Christakis NA, Fowler JH. The spread of obesity in a large social network over 32 years. N Engl J Med 2007; 357(4): 370-379.

[4] Flegal KM, Carroll MD, Kit BK, Ogden CL. Prevalence of obesity and trends in the distribution of body mass index among US adults, 1999-2010. JAMA 2012; 307(5): 491-497.

[5] Ogden CL, Carroll MD. Prevalence of overweight, obesity, and extreme obesity among adults: United States, trends 1960-1962 through 2007-2008. National Center for Health Statistics 2010; 6: 1-6.

[6] Ogden C, Carroll M, Kit B, Flegal K. Prevalence of obesity in the United States, 2009-2010 data brief [Internet]. National Center for Health Statistics; c2012 [cited 24 August 2013]. Available from: http://www.cdc.gov/nchs/data/databriefs/db82.pdf

[7] Health, United States, 2012, Table 63. [cited 24 August 2013]. Available from: http://www.cdc.gov/nchs/data/hus/2012/063.pdf

[8] United States. Centers for Disease Control and Prevention. National Center for Chronic Disease Prevention and Health Promotion. At a glance 2010—Obesity: halting the epidemic by making health easier. Atlanta (GA): Centers for Disease Control and Prevention; 2008.
[9] Marks J, Harris V. Indicators for chronic disease surveillance. MMWR 2004 September 10; 53(11): 1-6.
[10] Kung HC, Hoyert DL, Xu J, Murphy SL. Deaths: final data for 2005. Natl Vital Stat Rep 2008 Apr 24; 56(10): 1-120.
[11] United States. Centers for Disease Control and Prevention. National Center for Chronic Disease Prevention and Health Promotion. Division of Diabetes Translation. At a glance 2011—Diabetes: successes and opportunities for population-based prevention and control. Atlanta (GA): Centers for Disease Control and Prevention; 2011.
[12] Anderson G. Chronic conditions: making the case for ongoing care. Baltimore, MD. Johns Hopkins University; 2004.
[13] Centers for Disease Control and Prevention. Prevalence of doctor-diagnosed arthritis and arthritis-attributable activity limitation--United States, 2003-2005. MMWR Morb Mortal Wkly Rep 2006 Oct 13; 55(40): 1089-1092.
[14] U.S. Department of Health and Human Services. National diabetes fact sheet, 2011 [fact sheet]. Washington, D.C.: Centers for Disease Control and Prevention; 2011 [cited 2014 February 13]. Available from: http://www.cdc.gov/diabetes/pubs/pdf/ndfs_2011.pdf
[15] World Health Organization. Obesity data and statistics [Internet]. c2013 [updated 2013; cited 2013 December 5]. Available from: http://www.who.int/topics/obesity/en/
[16] England. The NHS Information Centre, Lifestyles Statistics. Statistics on obesity, physical activity and diet, 2012 report. England: National Obesity Observatory; 2012 February 23: 26.
[17] World Health Organization. Global Health Observatory (GHO): Overweight [Internet]. c2013 [updated 2013; cited 2013 December 5]. Available from: http://www.who.int/gho/ncd/risk_factors/overweight_text/en/index.html
[18] Ng S, Zaghloul S, Ali H, Harrison G, Popkin B. The prevalence and trends of overweight, obesity and nutrition-related non-communicable diseases in the Arabian Gulf States. Obes Rev 2011; 12(1): 1-13.
[19] Madison KM, Volpp KG, Halpern SD. The law, policy, and ethics of employers' use of financial incentives to improve health. J Law Med Ethics 2011; 39(3): 450-468.
[20] Schroeder SA. We can do better—improving the health of the American people. N Engl J Med 2007; 357(12): 1221-1228.
[21] Yanovski SZ, Yanovski JA. Obesity prevalence in the United States—up, down, or sideways? N Engl J Med 2011; 364(11): 987-989.
[22] Centers for Disease Control and Prevention (CDC). About BMI for adults [Internet]. c2011 [updated 2011 September 13; cited 2013 August 2]. Available from: http://www.cdc.gov/healthyweight/assessing/bmi/adult_bmi/index.html
[23] Body mass index (BMI) chart for adults 2014;
Available at: http://www.cdc.gov/healthyweight/assessing/bmi/
[24] Centers for Disease Control and Prevention (CDC). Body Mass Index: considerations for practitioners [fact sheet]. Atlanta (GA): Centers for Disease Control and Prevention; [cited 2013 August 2]. Available from: http://www.cdc.gov/obesity/downloads/bmiforpactitioners.pdf
[25] Hu FB. Chapter 5: Measurements of adiposity and body composition. In Hu FB, editor. Obesity epidemiology. New York (NY): Oxford University Press, 2008; p. 53-83.
[26] Colditz GA. Economic costs of obesity. Am J Clin Nutr 1992 Feb; 55(2 Suppl): 503S-507S.
[27] Finkelstein EA, Trogdon JG, Cohen JW, Dietz W. Annual medical spending attributable to obesity: payer-and service-specific estimates. Health Aff 2009; 28(5): w822-w831.
[28] Cawley J, Meyerhoefer C. The medical care costs of obesity: an instrumental variables approach. J Health Econ 2012; 31(1): 219-230.
[29] Wang YC, McPherson K, Marsh T, Gortmaker SL, Brown M. Health and economic burden of the projected obesity trends in the USA and the UK. The Lancet 2011; 378(9793): 815-825.
[30] National Institutes of Health. NIH Science of Behavior Change: Meeting Summary, June 15-16, 2009 [conference summary]. Bethesda, MD: National Institutes of Health (NIH); 2009.

[31] Glasgow RE, Klesges LM, Dzewaltowski DA, Bull SS, Estabrooks P. The future of health behavior change research: what is needed to improve translation of research into health promotion practice? Ann Behav Med 2004; 27(1): 3-12.
[32] Volpp KG, Troxel AB, Pauly MV, Glick HA, Puig A, Asch DA, *et al.* A randomized, controlled trial of financial incentives for smoking cessation. N Engl J Med 2009; 360(7): 699-709.
[33] Topp L, Day CA, Wand H, Deacon RM, van Beek I, Haber PS, *et al.* A randomised controlled trial of financial incentives to increase hepatitis B vaccination completion among people who inject drugs in Australia. Prev Med 2013; 57(4): 297-303.
[34] Higgins ST, Heil SH, Lussier JP. Clinical implications of reinforcement as a determinant of substance use disorders. Annu Rev Psychol 2004; 55: 431-461.
[35] Bickel WK, Jarmolowicz DP, Mueller ET, Gatchalian KM. The behavioral economics and neuroeconomics of reinforcer pathologies: implications for etiology and treatment of addiction. Curr Psychiatry Rep 2011; 13(5): 406-415.
[36] Jeffery RW. Financial incentives and weight control. Prev Med 2012; 55: S61-S67.
[37] Lowinson JH. Substance abuse: A comprehensive textbook. Philadelphia (PA): Lippincott Williams & Wilkins; 2005.
[38] Ritz M. Chapter 6: Molecular mechanisms of addictive substances. In: Niesink R, Jaspers R, Kornet L, van Ree J, editors. Drugs of Abuse and Addiction: Neurobehavioral Toxicology. New York (NY): CRC Press; 1999; p. 150-189.
[39] Ritz M. Chapter 5: Reward Systems and Addictive Behavior. In: Niesink R, Jaspers R, Kornet L, van Ree J, editors. Drugs of Abuse and Addiction: Neurobehavioral Toxicology. New York (NY): CRC Press; 1999; p. 124-149.
[40] Koob G, Nestler E. The Neurobiology of Drug Addiction. J Neuropsychiatry Clin Neurosci 1997; 9: 482-497.
[41] Volkow N, Wang G, Tomasi D, Baler R. Obesity and addiction: neurobiological overlaps. Obes Rev 2013; 14(1): 2-18.
[42] Monteleone P, Piscitelli F, Scognamiglio P, Monteleone AM, Canestrelli B, Di Marzo V, *et al.* Hedonic eating is associated with increased peripheral levels of ghrelin and the endocannabinoid 2-arachidonoyl-glycerol in healthy humans. a pilot study. J Clin Endocrinol Metab 2012; 97(6): E917-E924.
[43] Owesson-White CA, Ariansen J, Stuber GD, Cleaveland NA, Cheer JF, Mark Wightman R, *et al.* Neural encoding of cocaine-seeking behavior is coincident with phasic dopamine release in the accumbens core and shell. Eur J Neurosci 2009; 30(6): 1117-1127.
[44] Adan RA, Kaye WH. Behavioral neurobiology of eating disorders. In: Adan R, Kaye W, editors. New York (NY): Springer; 2011; p. 82-83.
[45] Skinner B. The experimental analysis of behavior. Am Sci 1957; 45(4): 343-371.
[46] Bouton ME. Learning and the persistence of appetite: Extinction and the motivation to eat and overeat. Physiol Behav 2011; 103(1): 51-58.
[47] Hartley C, Phelps E. Extinction learning. In: Seel N, editor. Encyclopedia of the Sciences of Learning 2012th ed. New York (NY): Springer; 2011; p 1252.
[48] Moss M. The extraordinary science of addictive junk food. New York Times 2013 February 24; Sunday Magazine: MM34.
[49] World Health Organization. Childhood overweight and obesity [Internet]. c2013 [updated 2013; cited 2013 September 3]. Available from: http://www.who.int/dietphysicalactivity/childhood/en/
[50] McGinnis JM, Gootman JA, Kraak VI. Food marketing to children and youth: threat or opportunity? Washington (DC): National Academies Press; 2006; p. 1-16.
[51] Schmidt H, Asch DA, Halpern SD. Fairness and wellness incentives: What is the relevance of the process-outcome distinction? Prev Med 2012; 55: S118-S123.
[52] WebMD. Obesity - Treatment overview [Internet] 2011 April 23 [cited 2013 August 27]. Available from: http://www.webmd.com/diet/tc/obesity-treatment-overview
[53] Bickel WK, Marsch LA. Toward a behavioral economic understanding of drug dependence: delay discounting processes. Addiction 2001; 96(1): 73-86.
[54] Laibson D. Golden eggs and hyperbolic discounting. Q J Econ 1997; 112(2): 443-478.
[55] Frederick S, Loewenstein G, O'Donoghue T. Time discounting and time preference: A critical review. J Econ Lit 2002; 40(2): 351-401.

[56] Kahneman D, Tversky A. Prospect theory: An analysis of decision under risk. Econometrica 1979: 263-291.

[57] Aubrey A. Put your money where your girth is [Internet] 2008 [cited 2013 August 27]. Available from: http://www.npr.org/templates/story/story.php?storyId=87931325

[58] Volk J, Corlette S. Premium incentives to drive wellness in the workplace: a review of the issues and recommendations for policymakers report. Princeton (NJ): Robert Wood Johnson Foundation; 2012 February.

[59] Guaranteed availability of coverage. 42 U.S.C. 300gg-1(b)(2)(B). Washington, D.C.: United States Congress; 2010. cited 2013 August 27]. Available from: http://www.gpo.gov/fdsys/granule/USCODE-2010-title42/USCODE-2010-title42-chap6A-subchapXXV-partA-subpart1-sec300gg-1

[60] Appleby J. Final rule upholds increased rewards, penalties for wellness participation [Internet]. c2013 [updated 2013 May 29; cited 2013 September 3]. Available from: http://capsules.kaiserhealthnews.org/index.php/2013/05/final-rule-upholds-increased-rewards-penalties-for-wellness-participation/

[61] Jost T. Implementing Health Reform: Workplace Wellness Programs. c2013 [updated 2013 May 29; cited 2013 September 4]. Available from: http://healthaffairs.org/blog/2013/05/29/implementing-health-reform-workplace-wellness-programs/

[62] Pear R. Employers get leeway on health incentives. New York Times 2013 May 30: B3.

[63] Mattke S, Schnyer C, Van Busum KR. RAND Health Occasional Paper: A review of the US workplace wellness market. Santa Monica. (CA: RAND Corporation; 2012 July.

[64] Strassel K. Mr. Burd goes to Washington. The Wall Street Journal 2009 June 19; Opinion.

[65] Burd S. How safeway is cutting health-care costs. The Wall Street Journal 2009 June 12; Opinion.

[66] Sturm R. The effects of obesity, smoking, and drinking on medical problems and costs. Health Aff 2002; 21(2): 245-253.

[67] Martin D. Obesity, smoking add immense burdens to health care costs [Internet]. c2009 [updated 2009 August 10; cited 2013 September 5]. Available from: http://thechart.blogs.cnn.com/2009/08/10/obesity-smoking-add-immense-burdens-to-health-care-costs/

[68] Hand L. Employer health incentives: employee wellness programs prod workers to adopt healthy lifestyles [Internet]. c2009 [updated 2009; cited 2013 September 5]. Available from: http://www.hsph.harvard.edu/news/magazine/winter09healthincentives/

[69] Petrecca L. Cost-conscious companies re-evaluate wellness programs. USA Today [Internet] 2009 June 16 [cited 2013 September 5]. Available from: http://usatoday30.usatoday.com/money/workplace/2009-06-16-wellness-programs-companies_N.htm

[70] Parker-Pope T. Being Paid to Lose Weight. New York Times 2008 December 9.

[71] Conis E. Alabama's wellness premium discount program. Atlanta (GA): Health Policy Monitor; 2008 November. Report No.: (12) 2008.

[72] Tortora A. Healthiest Employers: A new spin on wellness. Columbus Business First 2013 March 29.

[73] Mathews A. When All Else Fails: Forcing Workers into Healthy Habits. The Wall Street Journal 2009 July 12; Your Money.

[74] Baicker K, Cutler D, Song Z. Workplace wellness programs can generate savings. Health Aff 2010; 29(2): 304-311.

[75] Pelletier KR. A review and analysis of the clinical and cost-effectiveness studies of comprehensive health promotion and disease management programs at the worksite: update VI 2000-2004. J Occup Environ Med 2005; 47(10): 1051-1058.

[76] Osilla KC, Van Busum K, Schnyer C, Larkin JW, Eibner C, Mattke S. Systematic review of the mpact of worksite wellness programs. Am J Manag Care 2012; 18(2): e68-e81.

[77] Henke RM, Goetzel RZ, McHugh J, Isaac F. Recent experience in health promotion at Johnson & Johnson: lower health spending, strong return on investment. Health Aff 2011 Mar; 30(3): 490-499.

[78] Merrill RM, Hyatt B, Aldana SG, Kinnersley D. Lowering employee health care costs through the Healthy Lifestyle Incentive Program. J Public Health Manag Pract 2011; 17(3): 225-232.

[79] Milani RV, Lavie CJ. Impact of worksite wellness intervention on cardiac risk factors and one-year health care costs. Am J Cardiol 2009; 104(10): 1389-1392.

[80] Naydeck BL, Pearson JA, Ozminkowski RJ, Day BT, Goetzel RZ. The impact of the highmark employee wellness programs on 4-year healthcare costs. J Occup Environ Med 2008; 50(2): 146-156.

[81] Yen L, Schultz AB, Schaefer C, Bloomberg S, Edington DW. Long-term return on investment of an employee health enhancement program at a Midwest utility company from 1999 to 2007. Int J Workplace Health Manag 2010; 3(2): 79-96.
[82] Aldana SG, Merrill RM, Price K, Hardy A, Hager R. Financial impact of a comprehensive multisite workplace health promotion program. Prev Med 2005; 40(2): 131-137.
[83] Gold DB, Anderson DR, Serxner SA. Impact of a telephone-based intervention on the reduction of health risks. Am J Health Promot 2000; 15(2): 97-106.
[84] Herman CW, Musich S, Lu C, Sill S, Young JM, Edington DW. Effectiveness of an incentive-based online physical activity intervention on employee health status. J Occup Environ Med 2006; 48(9): 889-895.
[85] Chapman LS. Meta-evaluation of worksite health promotion economic return studies: 2012 update. Am J Health Promot 2012; 26(4): TAHP-1-TAHP-12.
[86] Lewis A, Khanna V. Is It Time To Re-Examine Workplace Wellness 'Get Well Quick' Schemes? Internet]. c2013 [updated 2013 January 16 ; cited 2013 July 6]. Available from: http://healthaffairs.org/blog/2013/01/16/is-it-time-to-re-examine-workplace-wellness-get-well-quick-schemes/
[87] Hilzenrath DS. A success story that isn't shapes health-care debate. The Washington Post 2010 January 17; Business.
[88] Marmot M, Friel S, Bell R, Houweling TA, Taylor S. Closing the gap in a generation: health equity hrough action on the social determinants of health. The Lancet 2008; 372(9650): 1661-1669.
[89] McLaren L. Socioeconomic status and obesity. Epidemiol Rev 2007; 29: 29-48
[90] Powell LM, Slater S, Mirtcheva D, Bao Y, Chaloupka FJ. Food store availability and neighborhood characteristics in the United States. Prev Med 2007; 44(3): 189-195.
[91] Devine CM, Jastran M, Jabs J, Wethington E, Farell TJ, Bisogni CA. "A lot of sacrifices: " Work-amily spillover and the food choice coping strategies of low-wage employed parents. Soc Sci Med 2006; 63(10): 2591-2603.
[92] Yerger VB, Przewoznik J, Malone RE. Racialized geography, corporate activity, and health disparities: tobacco industry targeting of inner cities. J Health Care Poor Underserved 2007; 18(6): 10-38.
[93] Families USA. Reward/Penalty Plans for Wellness: Coming Soon to an Office Near You? [Internet]. c2008 [updated 2008 February; cited 2013 August 29]. Available from: http://www.familiesusa.org/assets/pdfs/wellness-plans.pdf.
[94] Inagami S, Cohen DA, Finch BK, Asch SM. You are where you shop: grocery store locations, weight, and neighborhoods. Am J Prev Med. 2006; 31: 10-17.
[95] Bennett GG, McNeill LH, Wolin KY, Duncan DT, Puleo E, Emmons KM. Safe to walk? Neighborhood safety and physical activity among public housing residents. PLoS Medicine 2007; 4(10): e306.
[96] Greenwood V. You Are Your Bacteria: How the Gut Microbiome Influences Health. Time Magazine 2013 August 29; Science and Space.
[97] Kolata G. In Gut Research's Latest Advance, Bacteria From Thin Humans Can Slim Mice Down. New York Times 2013 September 6: A15.
[98] Pollan M. Some of My Best Friends Are Bacteria. New York Times 2013 May 19; Sunday Magazine: MM36.
[99] Pearson SD, Lieber SR. Financial penalties for the unhealthy? Ethical guidelines for holding employees responsible for their health. Health Aff 2009; 28(3): 845-852.
[100] Volpp KG, Asch DA, Galvin R, Loewenstein G. Redesigning employee health incentives—lessons from behavioral economics. N Engl J Med 2011; 365(5): 388-390.
[101] Wertheimer A. Remarks on Coercion and Exploitation. Denv UL Rev 1996; 74: 889.
[102] Emanuel EJ. Undue inducement: Nonsense on stilts? Am J Bioeth 2005; 5(5): 9-13.
[103] Lemmens T, Elliott C. Guinea pigs on the payroll: The ethics of paying research subjects. Account Res.1999; 7(1): 3-20.
[104] Macklin R. On paying money to research subjects: 'due' and 'undue' inducements. IRB 1981 May; 3(5): 1-6.
[105] Halpern SD, Karlawish JH, Casarett D, Berlin JA, Asch DA. Empirical assessment of whether moderate payments are undue or unjust inducements for participation in clinical trials. Arch Intern Med 2004; 164(7): 801.

[106] Cryder CE, John London A, Volpp KG, Loewenstein G. Informative inducement: Study payment as a signal of risk. Soc Sci Med 2010; 70(3): 455-464.

[107] Tozzi J. Employers Love Wellness Programs. But Do They Work? Bloomberg Businessweek [Internet]. c2013 [updated 2013 May 6; cited 2013 September 6]. Available from: http://www.businessweek.com/articles/2013-05-06/employers-love-wellness-programs-dot-but-do-they-work

[108] Schmidt H, Stock S, and Doran T. Moving Forward with Wellness Incentives Under the Affordable Care Act: Lessons from Germany. The Commonwealth Fund 2012 May 29; 13.

[109] Khazan O. What the world can learn from Denmark's failed fat tax. The Washington Post [Internet]. c2012 [updated 2012 November 11; cited 2013 December 9]. Available from: http://www.washingtonpost.com/blogs/worldviews/wp/2012/11/11/what-the-world-can-learn-from-denmarks-failed-fat-tax/

[110] Smed S, Robertson A. Are taxes on fatty foods having their desired effects on health? BMJ 2012; 345(7882): 9.

[111] Daley S. Hungary Tries a Dash of Taxes to Promote Healthier Eating Habits. New York Times 2013 March 3: A6.

[112] Ghosh P. Japan Has Many Problems, But Obesity Isn't One Of Them. The International Business Times [Internet] 2013 January 25 [cited 2013 December 11]. Available from: http://www.ibtimes.com/japan-has-many-problems-obesity-isnt-one-them-1038090

[113] Onishi N. Japan, Seeking Trim Waists, Measures Millions. New York Times 2008 June 13; Asia Pacific.

[114] Japanese Ministry of Health, Labour, and Welfare. Order 159: Standard Concerning Implementation Special Health Examinations and Special Public Health Guidance 2008 April 1.

[115] Block JP. A substantial tax on sugar sweetened drinks could help reduce obesity. BMJ 2013; 347.

[116] Menon P. Dubai offers gold to fight obesity epidemic. Reuters 2013 July 19.

CHAPTER 18

Obesity Interventions: Integration with Community-Based Systems

Nichola Davis*,[1], Kristie Lancaster[2] and Marcelle Pigananelli[3]

[1]North Bronx Healthcare Network, Albert Einstein College of Medicine, USA; [2]Department of Nutrition, Food Studies & Public Health, New York University, USA; and [3]Universidad Iberoamericana, Santo Domingo, Dominican Republic, USA

Abstract: Obesity is a global health problem. Interventions that work beyond controlled, intensive settings are needed to combat the obesity epidemic. The default behavior in obesogenic environments leads toward unhealthy diets and minimal physical activity. Interventions conducted in community settings have the potential to reach a wider population of adults and children; targeting both the individual and the environment. Community health centers, recreation centers, churches, and schools are community settings in which obesity interventions have been successfully implemented. Within community health centers, newer models of obesity care including increased provider and nurse training, remote support for weight loss, utilization of weight loss coaches, and community health educators show promise. Diabetes Prevention Program group interventions have been successfully disseminated through recreation centers such as the Young Men's Christian Association (YMCA) and churches. In comparison to controlled intensive studies, the magnitude of weight loss and diabetes reduction in community settings yields more modest results. However, the impact of modest weight reductions disseminated at the population level can contribute to significant population level improvements. In targeting childhood obesity, changes in the school environment including changes to the food environment in schools, distribution of body mass index report cards to parents, and increasing physical activity in schools have all shown an impact in reducing obesity. Successful obesity treatment and prevention models that have been disseminated in community settings including healthcare, recreation, church, and schools will be reviewed.

Keywords: Behavior, community health centers, community, diabetes prevention, diet, global health, health care settings, insulin, lifestyle diseases, lifestyle intervention, nurse education, nutrition, obesity, overweight, risk, weight loss, wellness.

***Corresponding author Nichola Davis:** 3424 Kossuth Avenue, Bronx NY 10467, USA; Tel: (718) 519-3968; Fax: (718) 519-3141; E-mail: nichola.davis@nbhn.net

Judith Wylie-Rosett & Sunil S. Jhangiani (Eds)

INTRODUCTION

Obesity is a global health problem. Worldwide, over half a billion adults over the age of twenty are obese and over forty million children under the age of five are overweight [1]. In the U.S., which has among the highest rates of obesity, it is estimated that by the year 2030, 86% of adults will be overweight or obese [2]. There is a clear need for interventions to combat the obesity epidemic. Much of the obesity intervention literature is focused on intensive interventions conducted in controlled settings. Interventions that work beyond controlled settings are necessary to meet the global obesity crisis.

In its 2012 report, the Institute of Medicine conceptualized obesity within the socioecological framework. Within this framework, healthcare, communities, and schools are important settings that can influence the prevention and treatment of obesity [3]. These settings provide opportunities for various levels of intervention strategies to target obesity. In this chapter, we will discuss successful interventions that have been disseminated in community settings; including healthcare, recreation, church, and schools that show promise as obesity treatment and prevention models.

OBESITY TREATMENT IN HEALTH CARE CENTERS

Community health centers provide primary medical care for children and adults, and thus offer opportunities to provide long-term obesity prevention and treatment. Health care providers have the opportunity to identify weight-related health concerns and offer weight management services. However, only a minority of patients obtaining primary care receive weight loss counseling. Health care providers miss many counseling opportunities. Reasons such as provider lack of knowledge about obesity [4, 5], lack of reimbursement, and time barriers [6] have all been cited to explain the absence of obesity related prevention and treatment services within primary care clinical settings. Thus new models of care that involve the health center as a whole while expanding beyond the individual patient provider relationship have been tested as ways to improve obesity treatment.

The Counterweight Program in the United Kingdom (UK) attempted to transform primary care delivery such that weight loss treatment was an integral part of primary care [7]. The program was evaluated in 65 general practices throughout the UK. This model incorporated standardized treatment protocols, training materials, and patient education materials. General Practitioners received one hour of training where they reviewed the screening and treatment protocols. General Practitioners were also taught the importance of discussing weight with their patients and the benefits of modest (5-10%) weight loss. Nurses in the practice received 8 hours of training, which provided them with the skills to provide patients with education about weight management including teaching behavioral skills. Weight management advisers who were registered dietitians guided the implementation of the program at the different clinical sites, and provided mentorship to the nurses as they gained skills in weight management [7]. Patients were eligible to participate if they had a BMI>30 or BMI>28 with co-morbid conditions and were in the action or contemplative stages of change. The intervention focused on goal setting, patient education, behavioral change, relapse prevention and maintenance. If >5% weight loss was not achieved at 3 months, pharmacotherapy with orlistat or sibutramine could be incorporated. A program analysis that included 1,906 patients from 56 different practices demonstrated a mean weight change of -3.0 kilograms after 12 months, and -2.3 kilograms after 24 months [8]. 14% of patients after 12 months and 24 months lost >5% of their weight [8]. Some factors associated with greater weight losses included being male, having a higher baseline BMI, increased number of visits, absence of diabetes (co-morbidity), and absence of arthritis. Economic analysis of the counterweight program determined the interventions to be cost-effective [9]. The UK Counterweight Program is also the model of weight management being disseminated in primary care sites in Scotland [10].

In the United States, several models of weight management delivery in health care settings have been tested in clinical trials. In these studies, involvement of the health care providers ranged from supportive roles to actually providing the intervention. Appel *et al.* randomized 415 obese adults recruited from primary care practice sites to one of three treatment conditions: (1) remote support only with use of weight loss coaches *via* telephone; a study specific web site and e-mail, (2) in-person support with weight loss coach or (3) a control group who had one session with a weight loss coach at the time of randomization and received brochures and suggestions for weight loss promoting web sites [11]. In this study, primary care doctors received progress reports on their enrolled patients and played a supportive role by providing encouragement and motivation during routine scheduled visits. After 24 months of follow-up, both intervention arms had significant weight reduction (-4.6 kg in the remote only and -5.1kg in the in-person support), with minimal weight change in the control arm. Eligibility criteria for this study included having access to a computer and basic computer skills. Of note, enrolled participants were highly educated with 60% having greater than a college education, and 41% reporting annual household incomes >$100,000. This study importantly demonstrated that remote support may be an effective model for obesity treatment and the potential for disseminating this model is great. However, there may be challenges in disseminating this model to resource poor settings, where there may be less computer access and lower levels of education and literacy.

In a second study, Wadden *et al.* randomized 390 obese patients from 6 primary care sites to one of three models of care: usual care, brief counseling, and enhanced brief counseling [12]. In this study, health care providers played a more active role and received training in delivering the intervention. In the usual care arm, participants had quarterly visits with their primary care physicians, (PCPs) where the PCPs reviewed participants weight change and discussed handouts regarding achieving a healthy weight. The brief lifestyle arm received the usual care and had a 10-15 minute session each month with a medical assistant trained to deliver abbreviated lessons from the Diabetes Prevention Program. The third arm was the enhanced brief lifestyle counseling arm where participants had brief lifestyle counseling, quarterly PCP visits, and were given the option of using meal-replacements or taking medication (orlistat or sibutramine) based on consultation with their physician. Weight loss outcomes after 24 months demonstrated greater weight loss in the enhanced brief lifestyle arm (-4.6kg), compared to the brief lifestyle (-2.9kg) or the usual care (-1.7kg). 35% of participants in the enhanced brief lifestyle arm had a clinically significant (>5%) weight loss at 24 months.

Focusing on a socioeconomically disadvantaged population, Bennett *et al.* randomized 365 participants recruited from urban community centers to either usual care or an intervention focused on behavioral changes to promote weight loss [13]. Trained community health educators delivered the intervention and included monthly counseling phone calls for the first year and bi-monthly phone calls in the second year. The intervention was tailored to populations with low literacy and numeracy skills, and included community resources for healthy eating and physical activity. The usual care group received a brochure about healthy weight. Primary care providers in this study delivered a standard message about the importance of participating in the intervention, but did not deliver the intervention. Weight loss outcomes after 24 months was -1.53 kg in the intervention arm and -0.5kg in the usual care arm. Additionally, the intervention arm participants had significant improvements in blood pressure.

These studies collectively demonstrate promise in obesity treatment clinical models that include counseling by allied health care professionals, community workers, remote support through phone calls or Internet, and health care provider support of weight loss efforts. While significant resources and staff training may be needed to successfully implement obesity treatment in clinical settings, it appears that treatment within these settings can result in clinically significant weight loss.

OBESITY TREATMENT FOR DIABETES PREVENTION IN THE REAL WORLD

Health Care Settings

A critical outcome of obesity treatment is the prevention of chronic disease such as diabetes. Concomitant with rising obesity rates are rising rates of diabetes worldwide. Landmark studies in diabetes prevention [14-17] have demonstrated the significant impact that lifestyle intervention has in reducing diabetes incidence among overweight and obese patients with risk factors for developing diabetes. The U.S. Diabetes Prevention Program reported a 58% reduction in diabetes incidence among participants at high risk of developing diabetes who received an intensive lifestyle intervention [18]. This reduction in diabetes risk was in part attributed to increases in physical activity and weight loss in the range of 5-7%. A medication that could provide a 7% weight loss and more than a 50% reduction in diabetes risk with no side effects would arguably be one of the most profitable medications in history.

The success of these lifestyle interventions, conducted in highly controlled clinical trial environments, have spurned an era of lifestyle intervention research focusing on how to achieve these outcomes in less controlled, more realistic day to day settings. In general, the magnitude of reduction in diabetes incidence has been lower in lifestyle interventions conducted in real world settings. However, the impact of modest weight reductions disseminated at the population level can contribute to significant population level improvements. These real world lifestyle interventions have been studied in health care systems, community centers, and churches.

In Finland, the national diabetes prevention program has implemented diabetes prevention in health care settings through changes in screening and health care delivery at primary care sites. The National Program for the Prevention of Type 2 Diabetes in Finland was implemented in five hospital districts throughout Finland using three strategies [19]. A population strategy raised awareness of diabetes and its risk factors in the general population, an early-treatment strategy provided diabetes treatment to those who were diagnosed during population based screening, and a high-risk strategy screened and identified patients who were at high risk for developing diabetes. Screening was done using the Finnish Diabetes Risk Score (FINDRISC), an 8-item questionnaire, where the total score provides a probability for developing type 2 diabetes. High score of 15 or greater represented high risk of developing type 2 diabetes. Screenings were done *via* the Internet, in primary and occupational health care settings, pharmacies, and at public health campaigns and health fairs. High-risk individuals were referred to health centers for additional testing and lifestyle intervention. Individual health centers were responsible for implementation of the lifestyle intervention. The default implementation strategy was a group intervention, and motivational interviewing approaches were used for lifestyle counseling [19]. In a one-year evaluation, over 10,149 participants were identified as being high risk based on the FINDRISC score [20]. Of these, 2,798 completed additional screening measures, received the lifestyle intervention and were followed for one year. Results of the one-year analysis demonstrated an average modest weight loss of 1.3 kg in women and 1.1 kg in men. 17.5% of participants lost more than 5% of their body weight, and in this group, diabetes risk reduction was 69%. Among those who lost 2.5-4.9% of their body weight, (16.8% of population) diabetes incidence was reduced by 29% [20]. Thus, while more modest in outcome, transforming health care settings to include lifestyle intervention as a standard of care succeeded in reducing diabetes risk among 34% of participants who received the lifestyle intervention.

Are there long-term benefits of lifestyle interventions conducted in primary health care settings? It is clear that the interventions conducted in primary care have had more modest risk reductions than those in clinical trials. In a national diabetes prevention program in Catalonia, Spain general practitioners conducted screening among participants in 18 health centers throughout Catalonia. The FINDRISC questionnaire identified patients at high risk for diabetes. High-risk individuals were assigned to receive either a lifestyle intervention (individual or group) or a standard intervention. The group intervention consisted of six hours of education divided into 2-4 group sessions. Telephone or text message contact was maintained with participants every 6-8 weeks to enhance motivation and adherence to lifestyle goals [21]. Of 2,049 individuals screened, 58% of them completed an OGTT, and 624 were found to be at high risk for developing diabetes. In a four-year evaluation, there was a 37% risk reduction in diabetes incidence among those receiving the intensive intervention delivered in a primary care setting [22]. It appears that there are long-term benefits of the modest weight reductions that are achievable in health care settings.

While primary health care settings have traditionally been thought of as the major resource for health information and interventions, delivery of lifestyle interventions in other community settings such as recreation centers have yielded encouraging outcomes.

Recreation Centers

The DEPLOY: Diabetes Education & Prevention with a Lifestyle Intervention Offered at the YMCA (Young Men's Christian Association) demonstrated the feasibility and success of lifestyle interventions implemented in community settings such as local YMCAs [23, 24]. The YMCA is a community organization that operates in 125 countries and 10,000 communities in the U.S and offers wellness resources to children and adults. In the DEPLOY study, YMCA personnel completed a 2.5 day training session to learn how to deliver the lifestyle group intervention [24, 25]. In a one year randomized trial, participants receiving the intervention lost significantly more weight than control group participants. These weight reductions were maintained at 28 months of follow-up [23].

Building on this data, the YMCA of the USA, the Centers for Disease Control, and United Health partnered together to create a low-cost group diabetes prevention program that can be disseminated nationally [26, 27]. The adapted lifestyle program is a one-year program that includes 16 core group sessions (weekly meetings) with a lifestyle coach, followed by 6 post-core sessions (monthly meetings). The program is focused on behavioral modification to improve diet and increase physical activity to 150 minutes a week. The YMCA has offered the lifestyle program in 68 YMCAs in 30 different states reaching about 6,000 participants [26]. While the success of these national partnerships and interventions will be evaluated in the future [27], these studies highlight the important role that recreation centers and trained lay non-medical staff can have in diabetes prevention.

Churches

The church in many communities can also be a resource for health care information and intervention. Churches provide a familiar setting for information and services for individuals who may feel alienated from the mainstream health care system because of differences in health beliefs, attitudes, or language, and thus often succeed where the health care system cannot [28, 29]. Churches also offer pre-existing social networks to facilitate the adoption and maintenance of health behaviors [30, 31]. This makes churches a valuable channel for delivery of evidence-based programs, with many advantages for undertaking behavior change programs targeting weight loss.

Studies conducted in churches have ranged from the promotion of preventive screenings and immunizations to weight loss and lifestyle modification. Regular church attendance has been linked to healthier lifestyle habits (*e.g.*, eating less fast food) as well as lower rates of cardiovascular disease [32, 33]. Beyond attending church, faith can also serve as a motivator to support behavior change. People who describe themselves as religious are more likely to engage in healthy behaviors as part of the commitment to their faith [34]. Engaging in prayer and meditation has also been shown to confer protective benefits on health and well being, resulting in lower rates of mortality [35, 36]. Studies conducted in church settings have included interventions focused on increasing fruit and vegetable intake [37-39], decreasing fat intake [40, 41], and weight loss [39, 41, 42]. Studies used group sessions, individual counseling (in-person or *via* telephone), self-help, and church wide programming to improve outcomes. In several church based interventions, the group based adapted diabetes prevention program curriculum was applied, resulting in significant weight reductions [42-45].

While, the vast majority of church based interventions have been conducted in African-American communities, it is likely that any community in which the church has a strong identity and influence can potentially benefit from church based lifestyle interventions.

Obesity Prevention in Schools

Among adults, one goal of obesity treatment is the prevention of chronic diseases. Children however are increasingly facing the diagnosis of chronic diseases at younger ages that are attributed to their weight. With increasing rates of childhood obesity, and a generation in the U.S. that is predicted to live shorter lives than their parents due to weight related comorbidities, it is clear that interventions targeting children are critical in combating this epidemic. Many of these interventions are focused on creating healthier lifestyles in the hopes of preventing obesity and its related comorbidities among children. Interventions have been conducted in school settings at all age ranges from pre-school ages (3-5 years old) to high school ages (13-17 years old). Such interventions have included changing the food environment in schools [46, 47], sending BMI report cards home to parents [48, 49], and increasing physical activity during the school day [50, 51]. Several meta-analyses have been done to evaluate the impact of these school-based interventions. These meta-analyses have concluded that interventions with combined classroom nutrition curriculum and physical activity were effective in reducing the prevalence of overweight and obesity [52], and interventions combining nutrition with physical activity and parental involvement resulted in significant reductions in BMI [53].

Information gained from long-term school intervention studies can be instrumental in informing future school based policies. The Kiel Obesity Prevention Study conducted in Germany, enrolled children beginning in 1996 and followed them for 8 years [54]. In this study, schools were randomized to intervention or non-intervention. In the intervention schools, first graders were taught 6 nutrition classes over a 2-3 week period during the first school year. The nutrition education focused on eating fruits and vegetables daily, reduction of high fat foods, physical activity of at least one hour each day, and reducing TV to less than one hour each day. After each class, physical activity was done for 20 minutes. A total of 780 first graders received the intervention. In an 8-year follow-up evaluation, 240 students who received the intervention were studied and compared to students who did not receive the intervention. Follow-up data demonstrated that the intervention showed improvement in BMI among children receiving the intervention, but the changes were statistically significant only among students with high socioeconomic status.

In the Cretan Health and Nutrition Education Program, intervention students received a 6-year health education curriculum from grades 1-6. The intervention included 13-17 hours of nutrition education each year, two 45-minute physical education sessions weekly, a student handbook about nutrition, and parental seminars [55]. An evaluation conducted 10 years after the intervention, demonstrated a significantly lower BMI z-score in the intervention arm, while the control group had an increase in BMI z-score. Additionally, this study showed beneficial effects on blood pressure, as intervention groups had significantly lower systolic and diastolic blood pressure at 10 years [56].

Findings from school based interventions highlight the importance of schools and the school environment in fighting obesity. Interventions that target combinations of nutrition and physical activity and involve familial support show great promise in reducing obesity in children.

MULTI-COMPONENT INTERVENTIONS

Each of the community environments discussed in this chapter: health care, recreation centers, schools, and churches may yield limited outcomes given the larger obesogenic environments in which they exist. To truly combat this epidemic, multi-level interventions that impact different aspects of the obesogenic environment simultaneously will likely be needed. Shape Up Somerville offers an insight into what such multilevel interventions may entail and what outcomes may be achievable.

Shape Up Somerville (SUS) is a model of community based participatory research that engaged researchers, community stakeholders, and policy makers in a collaborative effort to reduce childhood obesity [57]. The initial research project was conducted from 2002-2005 and included multiple interventions to impact the before school, during school, and after school environments. Examples of interventions included changing the food environment for school breakfasts and lunch to increase fresh fruits, low-fat milk, and whole grains, having monthly taste tests and introducing vegetarian recipes and healthy snacks. During school, a curriculum that included 30-minute nutrition and physical activity lessons, were delivered once a week and students had enhanced recess. After school programming included increased physical activity, cooking lessons, and walks from school campaigns. The home environment was impacted through parent newsletters, parent education, family events and an annual child health report card. The health care environment was impacted through training of local health care professionals on childhood obesity guidelines and screening practices. Additional community changes included changing food options in restaurants and expanded pedestrian safety policies.

To evaluate the impact of this multi-component intervention, children in the Somerville community were compared to 2 control cities that were sociodemographically similar to Somerville. Following an eight-month intervention, a significant reduction in BMI z-score was observed among students in the Somerville community [57]. While SUS began as a research study, the community subsequently obtained funding to continue a citywide campaign to increase physical activity and healthy eating.

CONCLUSION

Fundamentally, the solutions to addressing obesity seem simple; healthy eating and increased physical activity. However within the obesogenic, increasingly industrialized environments in which many live, the default behavior leads toward unhealthy diets and minimal physical activity. It is important to recognize that obesity is not simply a result of individual choice. For many, achieving healthy diets and increased physical activity requires significant effort. Thus multi-level interventions and policies that facilitate healthy behaviors are needed. Such policies may include environmental changes that lead to increased walkability of city streets, increased availability and affordability of fresh produce, reducing portion sizes in restaurants, and healthcare models that focus on prevention of chronic disease rather than treatment. Policies incorporating these strategies have been implemented in some settings or are currently being tested. It is clear that one single policy or intervention is not going to be the solution. Rather, changes in many sectors will need to occur to achieve population reductions in the prevalence of overweight and obesity. It is encouraging that in some areas of the United States; the population prevalence has not significantly increased in the past few years. With continued focus at both the individual and community level, the hope is that we will begin to see declines in the prevalence of overweight and obesity.

ACKNOWLEDGEMENTS

Declared none.

CONFLICT OF INTEREST

The authors confirm that this chapter contents have no conflict of interest.

REFERENCES

[1] World Health Organization. 10 Facts on Obesity. [Cited March, 2013]. Available from http://www.who.int/features/factfiles/obesity/en/index.html]

[2. Wang Y, Beydoun MA, Liang L, Caballero B, Kumanyika SK. Will all Americans become overweight or obese? estimating the progression and cost of the US obesity epidemic. Obesity (Silver Spring) 2008; 16:2323-2330.

[3] Institute of Medicine: Accelerating Progress in Obesity Prevention. Solving the Weight of the Nation. Washington, DC; 2012.

[4] Galuska DA, Will JC, Serdula MK, Ford ES. Are health care professionals advising obese patients to lose weight? JAMA 1999; 282:1576-1578.

[5] Davis NJ, Emerenini A, Wylie-Rosett J. Obesity management: physician practice patterns and patient preference. Diabetes Educ 2006; 32:557-561.

[6] Foster GD, Wadden TA, Makris AP, *et al.* Primary care physicians' attitudes about obesity and its treatment. Obes Res 2003; 11:1168-1177.

[7] McQuigg M, Brown J, Broom J, *et al.* Empowering primary care to tackle the obesity epidemic: the Counterweight Programme. European Journal of Clinical Nutrition 2005; 59:S93-S100.

[8] Counterweight Project T: Evaluation of the Counterweight Programme for obesity management in primary care: a starting point for continuous improvement. Br J Gen Pract 2008; 58:548-554.

[9] Trueman P, Haynes SM, Felicity Lyons G, *et al.* Long-term cost-effectiveness of weight management in primary care. Int J Clin Pract 2010; 64:775-783.
[10] The implementation of the Counterweight Programme in Scotland, UK. Fam Pract 2012; 29 Suppl 1:i139-i144.
[11] Appel LJ, Clark JM, Yeh HC, *et al.* Comparative effectiveness of weight-loss interventions in clinical practice. N Engl J Med 2011; 365:1959-1968.
[12] Wadden TA, Volger S, Sarwer DB, *et al.* A two-year randomized trial of obesity treatment in primary care practice. N Engl J Med 2011; 365:1969-1979.
[13] Bennett GG, Warner ET, Glasgow RE, *et al.* Obesity Treatment for Socioeconomically Disadvantaged Patients in Primary Care Practice. Arch Intern Med 2012.
[14] Lindstrom J, Louheranta A, Mannelin M, *et al.* Finnish Diabetes Prevention Study G. The Finnish Diabetes Prevention Study (DPS): Lifestyle intervention and 3-year results on diet and physical activity. Diabetes Care 2003; 26:3230-3236.
[15] Knowler WC, Barrett-Connor E, Fowler SE, *et al.* Reduction in the incidence of type 2 diabetes with lifestyle intervention or metformin. New Engl J Med 2002; 346:393-403.
[16] Knowler WC, Fowler SE, Hamman RF, *et al.* 10-year follow-up of diabetes incidence and weight loss in the Diabetes Prevention Program Outcomes Study. Lancet 2009; 374:1677-1686.
[17] Li G, Zhang P, Wang J, *et al.* The long-term effect of lifestyle interventions to prevent diabetes in the China Da Qing Diabetes Prevention Study: a 20-year follow-up study. Lancet 2008; 371:1783-1789.
[18] Knowler WC, Barrett-Connor E, Fowler S, *et al.* Reduction in the incidence of type 2 diabetes with lifestyle intervention or metformin. N Engl J Med 2002; 346:393-403.
[19] Saaristo T, Peltonen M, Keinanen-Kiukaanniemi S, *et al.* National type 2 diabetes prevention programme in Finland: FIN-D2D. Int J Circumpolar Health 2007; 66:101-112.
[20] Saaristo T, Moilanen L, Korpi-Hyovalti E, *et al.* Lifestyle intervention for prevention of type 2 diabetes in primary health care: one-year follow-up of the Finnish National Diabetes Prevention Program (FIN-D2D). Diabetes Care 2010; 33:2146-2151.
[21] Costa B, Cabre JJ, Sagarra R, *et al.* Rationale and design of the PREDICE project: cost-effectiveness of type 2 diabetes prevention among high-risk Spanish individuals following lifestyle intervention in real-life primary care setting. BMC Public Health 2011; 11:623.
[22] Costa B, Barrio F, Cabre JJ, *et al.* Delaying progression to type 2 diabetes among high-risk Spanish individuals is feasible in real-life primary healthcare settings using intensive lifestyle intervention. Diabetologia 2012; 55:1319-1328.
[23] Ackermann RT, Finch EA, Brizendine E, Zhou H, Marrero DG. Translating the Diabetes Prevention Program into the community. The DEPLOY Pilot Study. Am J Prev Med 2008; 35:357-363.
[24] Ackermann RT, Marrero DG: Adapting the Diabetes Prevention Program lifestyle intervention for delivery in the community: the YMCA model. Diabetes Educ 2007; 33:69, 74-65, 77-68.
[25] Finch EA, Kelly MS, Marrero DG, Ackermann RT. Training YMCA wellness instructors to deliver an adapted version of the Diabetes Prevention Program lifestyle intervention. Diabetes Educ 2009; 35:224-228, 232.
[26] Centers for Disease Control and Prevention. National Diabetes Prevention Program. [cited October 5th, 2012]. Available from http://www.cdc.gov/diabetes/prevention/about.htm
[27] Ackermann RT, Holmes AM, Saha C. Designing a natural experiment to evaluate a national health care-community partnership to prevent type 2 diabetes. Prev Chronic Dis 2013; 10:E12.
[28] Churches as an Avenue to High Blood Pressure Control. pp. xii, 97 p. [Bethesda, Md.]. U.S. Dept. of Health and Human Services, Public Health Service, National Institutes of Health, National Heart, Lung, and Blood Institute, National High Blood Pressure Education Program; 1987:xii, 97 p.
[29] Saunders E, Kong BW. A role for churches in hypertension management. Urban Health 1983; 12:49-51, 55.
[30] Campbell MK, Hudson MA, Resnicow K, Blakeney N, Paxton A, Baskin M. Church-based health promotion interventions. Evidence and lessons learned. In Annu Rev Public Health. Volume 28; 2007: 213-234: Annual Review of Public Health].
[31] Lasater TM, Wells BL, Carleton RA, Elder JP. The role of churches in disease prevention research studies. Public Health Rep 1986; 101:125-131.
[32] Dodor B: The impact of religiosity on health behaviors and obesity among African Americans. Journal of Human Behavior in the Social Environment 2005; 22:451-462.

[33] Holt-Lunstad J, Steffen PR, Sandberg J, Jensen B. Understanding the connection between spiritual well-being and physical health: an examination of ambulatory blood pressure, inflammation, blood lipids and fasting glucose. J Behav Med 2011; 34:477-488.
[34] Holt CL, Lewellyn LA, Rathweg MJ. Exploring religion-health mediators among African American parishioners. J Health Psychol 2005; 10:511-527.
[35] Chida Y, Steptoe A, Powell LH. Religiosity/spirituality and mortality. A systematic quantitative review. Psychother Psychosom 2009; 78:81-90.
[36] Helm HM, Hays JC, Flint EP, Koenig HG, Blazer DG. Does private religious activity prolong survival? A six-year follow-up study of 3,851 older adults. J Gerontol A Biol Sci Med Sci 2000; 55:M400-405.
[37] Campbell MK, Demark-Wahnefried W, Symons M, *et al*. Fruit and vegetable consumption and prevention of cancer: The Black Churches United for Better Health Project. American Journal of Public Health 1999; 89:1390-1396.
[38] Resnicow K, Jackson A, Wang T, De AK, McCarty F, Dudley WN, Baranowski T. A motivational interviewing intervention to increase fruit and vegetable intake through Black churches: results of the Eat for Life trial. Am J Public Health 2001; 91:1686-1693.
[39] Wilcox S, Laken M, Bopp M, *et al*. Increasing physical activity among church members - Community-based participatory research. American Journal of Preventive Medicine 2007; 32:131-138.
[40] Bopp M, Wilcox S, Laken M, *et al*. 8 Steps to Fitness: a faith-based, behavior change physical activity intervention for African Americans. J Phys Act Health 2009; 6:568-577.
[41] Djuric Z, Mirasolo J, Kimbrough L, *et al*. A pilot trial of spirituality counseling for weight loss maintenance in African American breast cancer survivors. J Natl Med Assoc 2009; 101:552-564.
[42] Boltri JM, Davis-Smith YM, Seale JP, Shellenberger S, Okosun IS, Cornelius ME. Diabetes prevention in a faith-based setting: results of translational research. J Public Health Manag Pract 2008; 14:29-32.
[43] Dodani S, Fields JZ: Implementation of the fit body and soul, a church-based life style program for diabetes prevention in high-risk African Americans: a feasibility study. Diabetes Educ 2010; 36:465-472.
[44] Yeary KH, Cornell CE, Turner J, Moore P, Bursac Z, Prewitt TE, West DS. Feasibility of an evidence-based weight loss intervention for a faith-based, rural, African American population. Prev Chronic Dis 2011; 8:A146.
[45] Boltri JM, Davis-Smith M, Okosun IS, Seale JP, Foster B. Translation of the National Institutes of Health Diabetes Prevention Program in African American churches. J Natl Med Assoc 2011; 103:194-202.
[46] Slusser WM, Cumberland WG, Browdy BL, Lange L, Neumann C. A school salad bar increases frequency of fruit and vegetable consumption among children living in low-income households. Public Health Nutr 2007; 10:1490-1496.
[47] French SA, Stables G. Environmental interventions to promote vegetable and fruit consumption among youth in school settings. Prev Med 2003; 37:593-610.
[48] Chomitz VR, Collins J, Kim J, Kramer E, McGowan R. Promoting healthy weight among elementary school children *via* a health report card approach. Arch Pediatr Adolesc Med 2003; 157:765-772.
[49] Evans EW, Sonneville KR: BMI report cards. Will they pass or fail in the fight against pediatric obesity? Curr Opin Pediatr 2009; 21:431-436.
[50] Harris KC, Kuramoto LK, Schulzer M, Retallack JE. Effect of school-based physical activity interventions on body mass index in children: a meta-analysis. CMAJ 2009; 180:719-726.
[51] Dobbins M, Husson H, DeCorby K, LaRocca RL. School-based physical activity programs for promoting physical activity and fitness in children and adolescents aged 6 to 18. Cochrane Database Syst Rev 2013; 2:CD007651.
[52] Gonzalez-Suarez C, Worley A, Grimmer-Somers K, Dones V. School-based interventions on childhood obesity: a meta-analysis. Am J Prev Med 2009; 37:418-427.
[53] Katz DL, O'Connell M, Njike VY, Yeh MC, Nawaz H. Strategies for the prevention and control of obesity in the school setting: systematic review and meta-analysis. Int J Obes (Lond) 2008; 32:1780-1789.

[54] Plachta-Danielzik S, Landsberg B, Lange D, Seiberl J, Muller MJ. Eight-year follow-up of school-based intervention on childhood overweight--the Kiel Obesity Prevention Study. Obes Facts 2011; 4:35-43.

[55] Manios Y, Moschandreas J, Hatzis C, Kafatos A. Evaluation of a health and nutrition education program in primary school children of Crete over a three-year period. Prev Med 1999; 28:149-159.

[56] Kafatos I, Manios Y, Moschandreas J, Kafatos A. Health and nutrition education program in primary schools of Crete: changes in blood pressure over 10 years. Eur J Clin Nutr 2007; 61:837-845.

[57] Economos CD, Hyatt RR, Goldberg JP, Must A, Naumova EN, Collins JJ, Nelson ME. A community intervention reduces BMI z-score in children: Shape Up Somerville first year results. Obesity (Silver Spring) 2007; 15:1325-1336.

CHAPTER 19

Life-Course Approach to Obesity Management: The Role of Family and Environment

Denise C. Tahara*

[1]*Department of Health Policy & Management, New York Medical College School of Health Sciences and Practice, Valhalla, NY 10530, USA*

Abstract: Pediatric obesity is a significant public health concern. It is also, to some degree, designed into lifestyles that encourage sedentary behaviors and convenience. Our children move their fingers and their ideas across networks connected by electronic webs. Their social meet ups are often online and their friends are on Facebook rather than waiting on the field. E-culture is here and so are its consequences for children's well-being. The design of our healthcare system will need to adapt to the changing conditions of our world and help children re-design their behaviors to encourage healthy choices. Communities need to be engaged in developing environments to reinforce well-being. To address this significant public health issue, a systems approach to analysis and improvement is required. The first step is to understand the existing delivery system by documenting the patient's experience, identifying environmental, social, and economic barriers and challenges to engaging them in their care and well-being. This should also include identifying lifestyle and infrastructure failures and leveraging opportunities to reinforce healthy choices and coordinated care. Every patient interaction should be viewed as an opportunity to improve health and well-being. New models of care will require that physicians take a proactive approach to managing patients' health and wellness, collaboratively. Values, preferences, and beliefs should be considered in designing strategic health treatment plans that will engage and empower patients and their families; taking a life-course approach to care.

Keywords: Coordinated and collaborative care, e-culture, global health, life-course approach, nutrition, obesity, overweight, patient accountability, patient centeredness, patient engagement, public health, risk, strategic design, systems thinking, wellness.

INTRODUCTION

Pediatric obesity is a significant public health concern. It is also, to some degree, designed into lifestyles that encourage sedentary behaviors and convenience. Our

***Corresponding author Denise C. Tahara:** Department of Health Policy & Management, New York Medical College School of Health Sciences and Practice, Valhalla, NY 10530, USA; Tel: (914) 594-4250; Fax: (914) 594-4292; E-mail: denise_tahara@nymc.edu

Judith Wylie-Rosett & Sunil S. Jhangiani (Eds)

children move their fingers and their ideas across networks connected by electronic webs. Their social meet ups are often online and their friends are on Facebook rather than waiting on the field. E-culture is here and so are its consequences for children's well-being.

The design of everyday life will continue to emphasize easy connectedness without real physical movement and fast food fed young bodies filled with calorie-dense foods. Urban green space is being replaced with modern high-rise buildings. In the suburbs, children are driven to school and their leisure activities and as a result, walk less. In urban areas walking is a safety concern in many lower income neighborhoods due to high traffic and violence. The design of our healthcare system will need to adapt to the changing conditions of our world and help children re-design their behaviors to encourage healthy choices. This chapter focuses on the role of community systems in preventing and managing obesity. The challenges associated with increased use of technologies can be turned into opportunities to address obesity.

ADDRESSING THE CHALLENGE

Healthcare needs to become part of community systems to develop a collaborative approach to obesity prevention and management. The Institute of Medicine (IOM) groundbreaking report [1] Crossing the Quality Chasm, suggested that quality healthcare should achieve (at a minimum), six aims:

- Care should be safe;
- Care should be effective;
- Care should be patient-centered;
- Care should be timely;
- Care should be efficient; and
- Care should be equitable.

Based on these aims, our healthcare delivery system is failing to meet the requisite needs of our population. Of the 32 million Americans [2] who are newly covered by the Patient Protection and Affordable Care Act (ACA), many may have never utilized the healthcare system. For others, their only encounters may have been episodic care delivered in hospital emergency departments (EDs). The Commonwealth Fund [3] ranks the United States (US) last of 16 industrial countries with regard to mortality amenable to medical care in their Third National Health Care Scorecard. In 2008, 44% of adults reported that they did not have accessible primary care providers and only half received the recommended preventive care. Minorities were less likely to receive preventive care or have an accessible source of primary care. Further, respondents discussed delays in care and experienced poorly coordinated care, uncontrolled chronic diseases, untreated dental caries, and generally worse outcomes [4]. Racial and socioeconomic disparities continue to exist, particularly in urban and low income areas. "As the degree of urbanization and national income increase, so too does the prevalence of diabetes, heart disease, obesity, mental health problems, alcohol and drug abuse, and violence" [5]. For example, several developing countries experiencing rapid socioeconomic development such as Brazil, Chile, and urban regions of China, reported an increased prevalence of obesity [6].

According to the Centers for Disease Control and Prevention (CDC) [7], in 2009-2010, 16.9% of children two to nineteen years old were classified as obese and 31.7% were classified as overweight or obese. In England, recent surveys of obesity prevalence indicated that 17% of children two to ten years old and 21% of children eleven to fifteen years old were obese. Portugal and Italy also reported similar trends: 11% of children seven to nine years old and 21% of children six to eleven years old, respectively [8]. In the immediate term, these children are at high risk for cardiovascular diseases, diabetes, bone and joint problems, as well as psychosocial problems. In the long term, they are likely to be obese as adults and more at risk for heart disease, stroke, and type 2 diabetes [9]. Further, in the US, prevalence of obesity among Hispanic boys (28.9%) and non-Hispanic black girls (24.8%) were disproportionately higher [10].

"Obesity has become increasingly more prevalent among socially disadvantaged groups" [11], and frequently in these same populations, we see high rates of underweight and malnutrition. Approximately 23.5 million people in urban and rural areas in the United States live in food deserts as reported by the Department of Agriculture [12]. Food deserts are areas, neighborhoods, or communities that lack access to foods that are essential to a healthy diet such as fresh vegetables, low fat milk, and whole grains [13]. Although the number of people who suffer from malnutrition and hunger continues to fall worldwide, in 2010 approximately 925 million people suffered from chronic hunger. Further, although the proportion of underweight children under five in developing regions declined from 31% in

1990 to 26% in 2008, it is not likely that United Nations Millennium Development Goal #1 (Eradicate Extreme Poverty and Hunger target: reduce the proportion of people who suffer from hunger by half), will be met [14]. Addressing pediatric obesity is critical to reducing the risk of chronic diseases such as diabetes, asthma, hypertension, hyperlipidemia, and cardiovascular diseases. These co-morbidities can require a lifetime of chronic disease management and limited quality of life. Direct healthcare costs for childhood obesity are about $14 billion per year [15].

Of equal concern is the high rate of dental caries, the most prevalent chronic disease in children and adolescents in the United States [16]. Worldwide, 60-90% of school children have dental cavities [17]. Racial, ethnic, and socioeconomic disparities continue to exist as well. In the United States from 1999 to 2004, the rate of primary dentition caries among children aged two to eleven years old was 55% for Hispanic children, 43% for black children, and 39% for white children [18]. Further, higher rates were reported among children living in households at or below the federal poverty level [19].

Modifiable lifestyle risk factors including dietary choices, access to calorie-dense foods, high costs of nutrient-rich foods, parental role modeling, oral hygiene, and use of tobacco [20] contribute to poor oral health as well as pediatric obesity. Socioeconomic factors play a role in accessing oral healthcare. In the US, State Children's Health Insurance Programs (SCHIP) have improved access to dental coverage, however, a preponderance of dental care needs of low-income children remain unmet. Data from the 2008 National Health Interview Survey indicate that 7% of all children aged two to seventeen years old had unmet dental needs because their families could not afford dental care. This is in comparison with 2.8% who had unmet medical care for the same reason [21]. Integrating oral healthcare with chronic disease prevention requires a patient-centered approach to improving health and well-being.

To address this significant public health issue, a systems approach to analysis and improvement is required. The first step is to understand the existing delivery system by documenting the patient's experience, identifying barriers and obstacles to engaging them in their care and well-being, including lifestyle and infrastructure failures, and leveraging opportunities to reinforce healthy choices and coordinated care. A systems approach requires both provider-based and patient-based care which engages the whole patient/family constellation and reorients care from episodic treatment to ongoing health management and well-being; supporting changes in the ecology of place and lifestyle behaviors [22]. This approach also considers the need for physicians to become engaged as champions who can help co-design collaboration and integration efforts, encourage agency in patients and their families, and support parents to advocate as role models and change agents.

FINDING SOLUTIONS

Patient-Centered Health Care at the Core

From the start, medical school education is organized into modules starting with the sciences, anatomy, and then functional systems. Clinical clerkships then follow the same format, where students spend their rotations in specific functional departments, *i.e.*, surgery, pediatrics, radiology, a sub-specialty, *etc.* Students study the science of diagnosing and treating individual diseases, even though the concept of patient-centered medicine has been around for a long time. This format reinforces the individual disease focus of the curriculum and approach to care.

Balint [23] first introduced the idea of patient-centered medicine as an approach for physicians to be able to treat their patients by understanding the individual patients, their beliefs and values, and by engaging them in their care. The intent was for physicians to gain an understanding of the patient and their disease so that they could provide the appropriate care [24]. Care and treatment decisions should be informed by patient values and preferences [25]. The goal is to then identify social, cultural, behavioral, environmental, and socioeconomic factors that affect the knowledge and decision making of patients and their families; to take a life-course approach.

In another international study by the Commonwealth Fund [26], they determined that patients with complex care needs who received healthcare through a coordinated care model had better health outcomes than those who navigated the systems themselves. There was better communication among providers, sharing of patient data, and costs were less. Patients with medical homes (in all eleven countries studied) reported better care experiences than those without medical homes. Further, patients reported fewer coordination failures with their care, including medical errors and duplicate testing [27]. Much of this is attributed to the strong relationships developed with the primary care physicians, a hallmark of the Patient Centered Medical Home (PCMH) model of care. The survey concluded that coordinating care for all patients is needed.

According to the IOM, patient-centeredness refers to healthcare that establishes a partnership among practitioners, patients and their families to ensure that decisions respect patients' wants, needs, values, and preferences, and that patients have the education and support they require to make decisions and participate in their own care [28]. The Agency for Healthcare Research and Quality (AHRQ) identified five primary functions and attributes of Patient Centered Medical Homes:

- **Patient Centered**-The primary care medical home provides primary care that is relationship-based with an orientation toward the whole person.
- **Comprehensive Care**-The PCMH is accountable for meeting the large majority of each patient's physical and mental health care needs, including prevention and wellness, acute, and chronic care.
- **Coordinated Care**-The PCMH coordinates care across all elements of the broader healthcare system including specialty care, hospitals, home healthcare, and community services and support.
- **Superb Access to Care**-The PCMH delivers accessible services with shorter waiting times for urgent needs, enhanced in-person hours, round-the-clock telephone or electronic access to a member of the care team, and alternative methods of communication such as patient web portals, email, and telephone care.
- **Systems-based Approach to Quality and Safety**-The PCMH demonstrates a commitment to quality and quality improvement through ongoing engagement in performance improvement activities [29].

The promise of PCMHs is comprehensive care coordination where there is centralization and communication of patient data to improve quality, appropriateness, efficiency, and overall health of the patient. The PCMH model was developed to address socioeconomic barriers to care by providing patients with a usual source of care including preventive and wellness care. Increased utilization of primary care services results in decreased hospitalizations and ED use. This approach enables providers to focus on whole patient care, by planning and coordinating services and activities within and outside the healthcare setting, aimed at addressing lifestyle behaviors and practices to improve health and wellness across the life span. To optimize the benefits including improved outcomes from patient-centered care, communication and coordination across settings should facilitate information exchange between clinicians and their patients, and increase accountability. In other words, creating a functioning medical neighborhood [30].

Role of Physicians

New models of care will require that physicians take a proactive approach to managing patients' health and wellness, collaboratively. Physicians will need to coordinate services and deliver care where they will have a different role, responsibilities, and accountability; teams will not be organized vertically around the physician, but rather horizontally around the patient's needs [31]. Physician training will need to include these new communication and leadership skills to better manage the whole patient, in some cases with multiple diseases. Further, medical school education will need to include more training in oral health, particularly for those pursuing family medicine or pediatrics. Continuing medical education activities in oral health aimed at these providers will improve their ability to address oral health concerns which can lead to other chronic comorbidities. However, assigning physicians these new roles without the requisite training is no different from giving patients a prescription for diet and lifestyle changes without the training and knowledge to adopt those activities and make choices at home and in the community. Further, care will need to be responsive and accessible to patient preferences, needs, and values so that they can actively participate in their treatment decision making and care [32].

The Process

Systems analysis is the first step toward redesigning care that achieves the desired outcomes of improved health, improved care and reduced cost, the triple aim of our system as defined by Berwick [33]. If we are to reduce the prevalence of pediatric obesity, then a systems approach is required. To achieve this objective we need to first examine all the components of the operating environment in which our children live. According to Katz and Kahn [34] in every open system there is an exchange of inputs and outputs with the operating environment. The structure, relationships, and supporting environment affect all outcomes of the system. Systems are optimized when the benefits are maximized to all participants. Stakeholders, their expectations, and their role in achieving improved outcomes should be defined. Inputs can be filtered into the system through standards, criteria, and reimbursements which have been instituted through policy and legislation. The design of processes and interactions should address the challenges, reduce the barriers, and facilitate behaviors that are sustainable in the community. There must be a commitment to wellness and well-being (Fig. **1**).

The current design of our healthcare system encourages fragmentation and results in sub-optimal efficiencies and effectiveness of care delivery. The first step in every change initiative is to identify opportunities for improvement by performing a process analysis. This starts with documenting the current system including all patient touch points and resulting patient interactions. This analysis should focus on the patient's experience navigating the system; evaluating the system from the patient's perspective. Current flows, redundancies, gaps in service, bottlenecks, capacity limiters, and non-value added services should be identified; inventories of system competencies, capabilities, and capacity should be included.

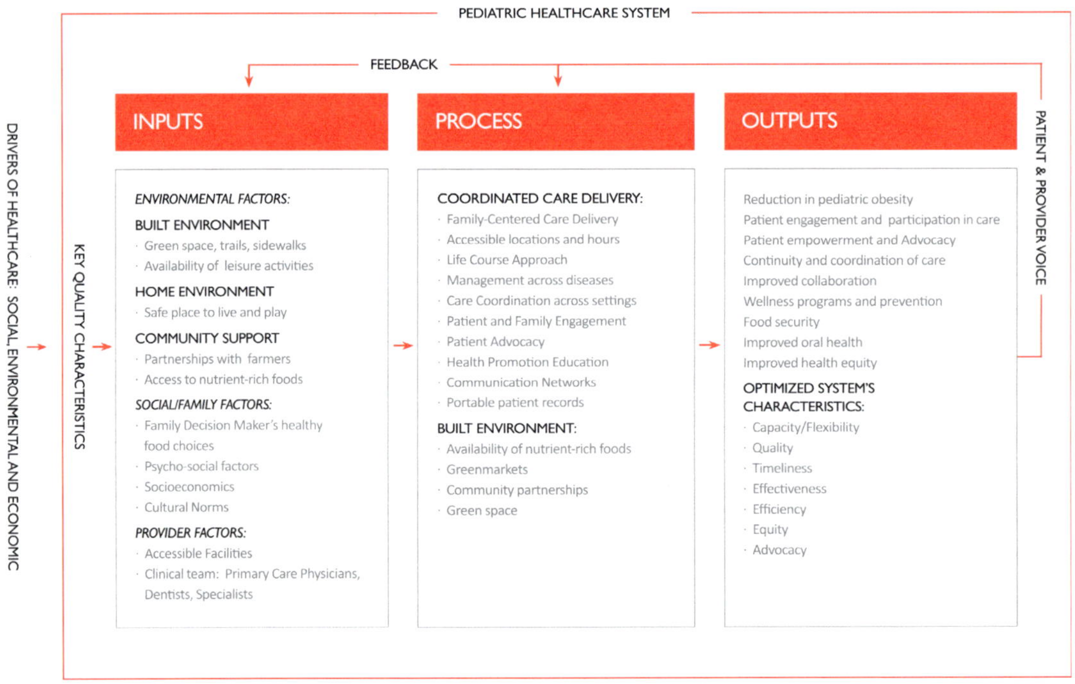

Fig. (1). Pediatric healthcare system.

After the internal analysis is performed, next steps focus on interactions with the environment that affect timely provision of healthcare. Through these interactions, barriers to access and health equity can be addressed to facilitate utilization and sustainability. Further, lifestyle behavioral risk factors should also be identified so that community-based supported interventions can be designed. "Health must be incorporated into every aspect of society and daily life" [35].

To evaluate the capabilities of the providers and capabilities of the users to engage in lifestyle and behavior changes as well as support healthy choice solutions to infrastructure and socio-economic barriers, the healthcare service delivery process should be analyzed. Documenting the process is the first step towards designing a system that engages patients in their care.

Inputs to care (and treatment) should be identified to determine whether there are sufficient resources to provide the needed care to achieve the desired outcomes of health and well-being, including access to primary care providers to champion strategic health planning. Medical schools do not routinely promote the provision of primary care in urban settings or promote the importance of rural healthcare. Consider that in the US there has been a 51% decline in medical students entering family practice residencies [36]. This trend is seen in the dental workforce as well where the dentist-to-population ratio is declining while rural and underserved communities suffer the most [37].

While the diversity of our population has increased, the diversity of the workforce servicing these at-risk communities in particular has not [38]. For example, although Hispanics comprised approximately 16% of the US population in 2008, they comprised less than 6% of all physicians [39]. Of equal concern is that African Americans comprised only a little over 6% of all physicians [40]. Studies have shown that diversity in the physician workforce ensures the responsiveness to population healthcare needs, improving access, patient satisfaction, and culturally competent providers [41]. Redistributing clinicians to at-risk and medically disenfranchised populations will be necessary and will need to be designed into the medical school experience. Programs to incentivize particular residencies and specific practice specialties should be designed and developed. Training programs to support physician assistants, nurses, and nurse practitioners should be designed and expanded to supplement clinical supply [42].

To evaluate the patient's service experience *i.e.*, navigating the system, a process flow chart should be created to document how they move through the system; the challenges and barriers they face as they navigate the system. The process flow chart is an important tool as it helps to identify interactions between the patient and the system. The benefits include:

- It is a visual depiction of the system;
- Documents the patient's experience;

- Identifies failure points; and
- Identifies value-added services.

Process structure and design must be appropriate for the service and also for the end user; the patient and his/her family. As such, we need to design a healthcare delivery process that considers points of entry into the system, facilitates communication, collaboration and coordination, continuity and transitions of services across multiple settings and into the community, including patient hand-offs, and reinforces patient agency. Poorly coordinated transitions *i.e.*, patients unable to follow treatment recommendations, specific care instructions or are not ready to move to a new setting, are the primary cause of hospital readmission [43].

From this preliminary analysis we can develop both short-term and long-term solutions to improve patient engagement, compliance and well-being. Process flow charts help identify system failures such as:

- Patient interactions, where their input is not supported by the service concept; *i.e.*, where the system does not support required decisions by the family. Examples include initial access to primary care providers and, once identified, long lead time from when a patient calls to schedule an appointment to when they are seen by a provider for both emergent and routine care.
- Inadequate integration between patient involvement and the system-where the provider cannot deliver. For example, are translators or translating services available in the patient's native language?
- Operations infrastructure is poorly designed (*i.e.*, support services and other ancillary services). Process structure or design must be appropriate for the service and community.
    - Are there evening and weekend appointments for working parents or dual income-parents, who do not have regular caregivers? Is there after hour availability and access?
    - At institution-based and large pediatric practice groups, is there a case manager to enroll the patient in Medicaid (SCHIP) or other insurance which they are eligible? Will coverage begin when the patient seeks care

or will they need to wait to see the provider? Once the provider is established as the patient's usual source of care, will the case manager monitor coverage and alert families when they need to re-enroll so the coverage does not lapse?

- o Are follow-up appointments for diagnostic services and specialty providers (on-site and off-site) initiated and coordinated by the provider *before* the patient leaves? Does the front desk staff make these appointments for the patient before they check out? Does the patient know where to go for these services and what information s/he needs to provide *i.e.*, insurance card, medication list (or the bottles themselves)?
- o Are oral health providers available at the practice or nearby?
- o Will the specialty care be coordinated by the primary care provider?
- o Is the patient's health information portable or available to the specialty providers?
- o Are test results communicated and available to physicians so that care can be coordinated, duplicate testing avoided, transitions facilitated, and hand-offs complete?

Once these system failures have been identified, cross-functional teams from within the organization should work together to redesign the service experience and the delivery process identifying innovative ways to perform tasks and deliver care. To improve the efficiency and effectiveness of the delivery process, these teams should focus improvement initiatives on:

- Where steps are unclear;
- Where there are redundant steps;
- Where steps are misplaced (perhaps need to re-sequence);
- Where steps do not serve a purpose or add value;
- Where it is resource intensive and costs a lot;
- Where there are inefficiencies in equipment, supplies, and task assignments;

- Where the process affects other processes; and
- Replicating steps that add value and engage patients.

In 2008, the World Health Organization Commission on Social Determinants of Health (CSDH) reported that "communities and cities that ensure access to basic goods, that are socially cohesive, that are designed to promote good physical and psychological well-being, and that are protective of the natural environment are essential for health equity" [44].

Designing a system for improved health and wellness can be organized to address three areas of opportunity: environmental, social, and economic. The barriers and challenges faced by patients as they navigate care and follow up with prescribed health plans, that result from contributing factors in these three areas are described in Fig. (**2**).

By defining the current challenges in the operating environment we can then focus on coordinating wellness care and the management of pediatric obesity, oral health, as well as those with co-morbidities. Every patient interaction should be viewed as an opportunity to improve health and well-being. The focus cannot be only on the chief complaint, but on the whole patient; understanding the needs of the patient *vs* focusing on the disease [45]. To address these challenges, communities need to be engaged in developing environments to reinforce healthy choices. The solutions are greater than the household environments and behaviors need to be supported in the community, schools, and by caregivers in addition to parents-all must make healthy choices.

- Workplaces, schools and faith-based organizations (also see CHAPTER 18: Obesity: Integration with Community-Based Systems) should model healthy behaviors by serving nutrient-rich *vs* calorie-dense foods at gatherings and functions.
- School cafeterias should create partnerships for farmer-to-school programs. Vending machines should stock less sugar and calorie-dense foods, and instead provide foods that meet dietary guidelines. Community gardens should be created in the schools and the community.
- Smartphone applications and social media applications should be used to facilitate patient management of follow-up instructions such as monitoring

ENVIRONMENTAL

HOME ENVIRONMENT:

· Limited access to (healthy) food – nutrient-rich vs. calorie-dense foods and sugary beverages
· Supersized food portions/ Inadequate food portions
· Safe places to play
· High levels of screen-time
· Direct marketing on television of food to children
· Access to fluoride programs

BUILT ENVIRONMENT:

· Availability and distribution of pediatric clinicians, dental providers, and community-based developmental services
· Lack of access to: sidewalks, bike lanes, parks, playgrounds and other recreational facilities, after-school programs and day care that includes physical activity
· Food Insecurity
· Food Deserts and Food Swamps
· Disruption and depletion of natural resources in our ecosystem
· Availability of calorie-dense foods and sugary beverages at school cafeterias
· Insufficient meal time
· Availability of calorie-dense foods at fast-food restaurants, local bodegas and grocery stores with convenient packaging
· Lack of farmers' markets or fresh produce in neighborhood stores
· High physician-to-population ratios particularly dental health providers
· Needed training for practicing pediatricians in oral health

SOCIAL:

· Health literacy
· Parental level of education
· Food choice purchase decisions out of control of children; made by parents
· Limited development of food palates
· Lack of knowledge of how to prepare nutrient-rich foods
· Peer pressure
· Marketing of fast-food and calorie-dense foods to children and adolescents
· Poor food choices reinforced at social events and other leisure time activities
. Body image, self-esteem and psycho-social stigmas

ECONOMIC:

· Socio-economic level
· Difficulty paying for health supplies to comply with treatment recommendations
· Lack of access to affordable nutritious foods such as vegetables and fruits
· Promotional pricing and placement to encourage purchase of calorie-dense foods
· Inadequate reimbursements for medical and dental health practitioners

Fig. (2). Barriers and challenges to care.

and tracking food consumption (nutrition and calories), and physical activity, as well as maintaining food diaries and access to easy nutrient-rich recipes. (also see CHAPTER 20: From Intervention to Innovation: Health Information Technology.)

- The service design of healthcare systems will need to include school-based health centers, oral health campaigns, immunization and vaccine awareness, tobacco cessation and anti-obesity programs to create a population of more educated service users.

- Designing medical neighborhoods to improve coordination and continuity of services by primary care providers and specialty providers to overcome the challenge represented by the management of patient care and medications.

- Healthcare encounters should be leveraged as opportunities to educate and reinforce wellness and well-being and empower patients and their families. For example, patient data collection forms (questionnaires) should include questions about the patient's home and built environments such as: access to fresh air (do the windows open?), number of smokers in the home, screen time, after school care, typical breakfast, lunch and dinner, access and use of playgrounds and what activities they participate in. This information can guide recommendations for management of the chronic illness and wellness planning.

Healthcare Encounters: Leveraging Wellness Visits to Empower Parents and Reduce Obesity

Educating patients on how to use the healthcare system must begin at the front end. In the case of new participants, health literacy plays a large role. A service experience designed for this kind of participant must begin before they officially enter the facility. It must educate them on the basics of well-being and illustrate the behaviors that will support a healthy lifestyle. All experience design must be tailored to increase participant awareness, interest and desire to act. In the design of the healthcare experience, particularly in utilizing preventive and wellness services and establishing a usual source for care, we cannot assume that new participants are either aware or clear about the actions to take to secure well-being. If we want them to succeed and if we want to be able to predict and control outcomes, we must design to guide their experience through awareness to action.

Then, and only then, can we succeed in designing actions and encouraging behaviors related to effective use of the system [46].

Although there will be increased numbers of children accessing and utilizing the healthcare system as a result of the passage of the ACA, there will not be a corresponding increase in providers, particularly pediatricians and oral health providers. There is also a maldistribution of providers in urban and rural disenfranchised communities. Providers will be more time constrained and therefore will need to develop innovative solutions to deliver care in a more cost-effective way. Through systems analysis they can evaluate how they provide the requisite services during each encounter, leveraging skills and competencies of all members of the healthcare delivery team to achieve the triple aim of improved health, improved care and reduced costs. The structure and content of each visit should be reviewed to optimize care management and agency of the patient and their families.

To maximize the effectiveness of each wellness visit we must first consider the desired outcome from the encounter. Then physicians can set goals for each visit to better manage the child's overall health over their life span, reduce duplication of services and increase surveillance of developmental milestones, while improving continuity of care. Taking a life-course approach considers social determinants of health and can help physicians better understand the environment in which the patient lives, learns, plays, and prays, and the values that influence their lifestyle choices. Content, format, and communication modalities should be evaluated for clear messaging so that it is retained by the patient and prescribed treatments followed up in the community. Many patients and their families do not understand their instructions or are unable to follow treatment plans due to socioeconomic and environmental barriers as well as health literacy. This includes knowledge and access to requisite community-based services and services by specialty providers.

Designing improved coordination and continuity of services by primary care providers and specialty providers can help to overcome the challenge represented by the management of complex patient care and medications, and can improve patient empowerment. For example, patients in underserved communities tend to have chronic diseases and co-morbidities that put them more at risk, and more importantly, require a more integrated management of their diseases and lifestyle behaviors. A recent study in Nigeria reported a higher incidence of chronic childhood malnutrition among urban poor compared to those living in rural areas

[47]. Many of the risk factors for these diseases are modifiable. Systems must be designed for these conditions including early detection and prevention of chronic diseases [48] engaging patients and their families in their care and treatment.

Wellness visits provide opportunities to educate and engage. Barriers to managing information exchange affect both providers and patients. Time constraints, high administrative costs, and reimbursements that focus on treatment *vs* prevention, present challenges to primary care providers. Value-based design insurance plans are a successful approach to reducing healthcare costs. Patients, particularly those with chronic conditions are "rewarded" for following recommended health management strategies. As adherence increases, the patient's out-of-pocket costs decrease. This includes expenditures for health supplies as well as co-pays for visits. Further, it is believed that indirect medical expenses such as worker productivity improve as a result of this adherence [49].

Oral Health

A policy approach to health and wellness that is proving effective is the requirement for screenings and examinations of oral health for school-aged children. Disappointingly, only about a quarter of the states in the US have any type of policy in place for routine screenings and examinations.

Access to oral health exams and screenings remain a challenge. Low reimbursements to providers are a disincentive for oral health practitioners to provide services in at-risk communities. Lack of education of parents also affects the frequency of oral health screenings and examinations. Utilization of preventive dental care varies by age, health insurance status, and race and ethnicity. In a 2007 study of children aged six to eleven years old, 89.5% received preventive dental care in the past year, as did 87.8% of those aged 12 to 17 years old, compared to 53.5% of children aged one to five years [50]. Mobile dental vans have been a solution to the geographic challenges of oral health care. However, these vans and the equipment are expensive to maintain. More cost-effective solutions include primary or secondary schools partnering with providers to bring the preventive services on site at the schools or at the beginning of each school year.

Resources for pediatricians for CME training in oral health and examples of successful partnerships include:

In North Carolina, Into the Mouths of Babes

http://www.ncdhhs.gov/dph/oralhealth/partners/IMB.htm

In California, First Smiles

http://www.first5oralhealth.org/

American Academy of Pediatricians toolkit

http://www2.aap.org/oralhealth/EducationAndTraining.html

American Dental Association, MouthHealthy Initiative:

http://www.mouthhealthy.org/

Immunizations

Well visits required for school-age children afford an opportunity to reinforce health promotion and disease prevention through immunizations and psychosocial screenings, including BMI and oral health assessments. The federal government requires state Medicaid programs to establish their own schedules for screenings. States generally follow the American Academy of Pediatricians' immunization recommendations and can be found at: http://www2.aap.org/immunization/IZSchedule.html

Immunizations have proven to be one of the most effective tools to prevent epidemics of infectious and preventable diseases. Childhood immunization programs provide a high return on investment, by reducing direct and indirect healthcare costs [51]. Data from the 2007 National Immunization Survey indicate that only 77.4% of toddlers 19 to 35 months of age had completed the combined immunization series (Dtap, Td, Hib, Hep B, MMR, Polio, and Varicella). Immunization rates for adolescents also remain below Healthy People 2020 objectives. Improvements in infant and child mortality rates are largely associated with infectious disease immunization programs, even though racial and ethnic disparities exist. Even so, there is a lot of misinformation available, particularly on the internet and social media with unsupported claims of serious side effects of immunizations, links to autism and death, reinforcing existing cultural fears of immunizations. Many parents avoid or delay pre-school age immunizations until they are mandated for school attendance. Even then, parents opt out based on available exclusions.

Communication

Activities that coordinate care and wellness are generally not reimbursed. Many pediatricians lack the needed training in child development and oral health that would aid in psychosocial, behavioral, developmental, and oral health risk assessment. There is variation in the quality of care, particularly that experienced by minority patients [52]. Patients and their families frequently do not get the guidance they seek regarding raising their children. This includes discussions about the advantages of breast feeding, introduction and reintroduction of healthy foods even if initially rejected, appropriate sleep habits, levels of physical activity, risk of injury of night walking, oral health, dietary choices including portion sizes, and how to promote a safe environment at home.

These barriers and challenges can be addressed by more innovative and cooperative approaches to care, to ensure the exchange of health information. For example, patient screenings and updates in health should be collected prior to the patient meeting with the physician. These should be reviewed and maintained by the healthcare team at each visit. Patient medical records including immunization records should be up-to-date and information centralized to maintain continuity of care as patients transition across healthcare settings. Knowledge of patient histories, values and preferences can improve coordinated care and management of chronic diseases in particular. Appropriate screenings and monitoring of chronic conditions should be performed at these wellness visits including BMI and oral health.

Time before and after the interaction with the physician should be maximized to exchange health information. For example, setting up follow-up appointments to keep patients on the recommended immunization schedule, discussions with nurse practitioners, registered dieticians, or health educators regarding follow-up health treatment instructions, short-term and long-term care plans that include lifestyle activities, and healthy food choices should be included in each healthcare encounter and aligned with community resources. Contact information should be verified so that reminders and other information can be communicated in a timely manner. Barriers to access should be discussed and the clinicians should connect patients with community-based resources that will support new behaviors. These include social services (to facilitate enrollment in programs such as WIC, AFDC, and SCHIP) that support improved health and well-being.

CONCLUSION

Healthcare delivery must be seen for what it is-a service experience. That service experience must be designed to improve the health and wellness of the population by engaging patients and their families in behaviors that can be maintained and can sustain well-being outside the system of service delivery [53]. As we move toward family-centered care, physicians will have new roles and leadership responsibilities. Environmental, social and economic barriers must be addressed so that patients can take ownership of their health and well-being. Communities must support these efforts.

Resources - Systems Analysis Templates

Pediatric Healthcare Systems Approach Template

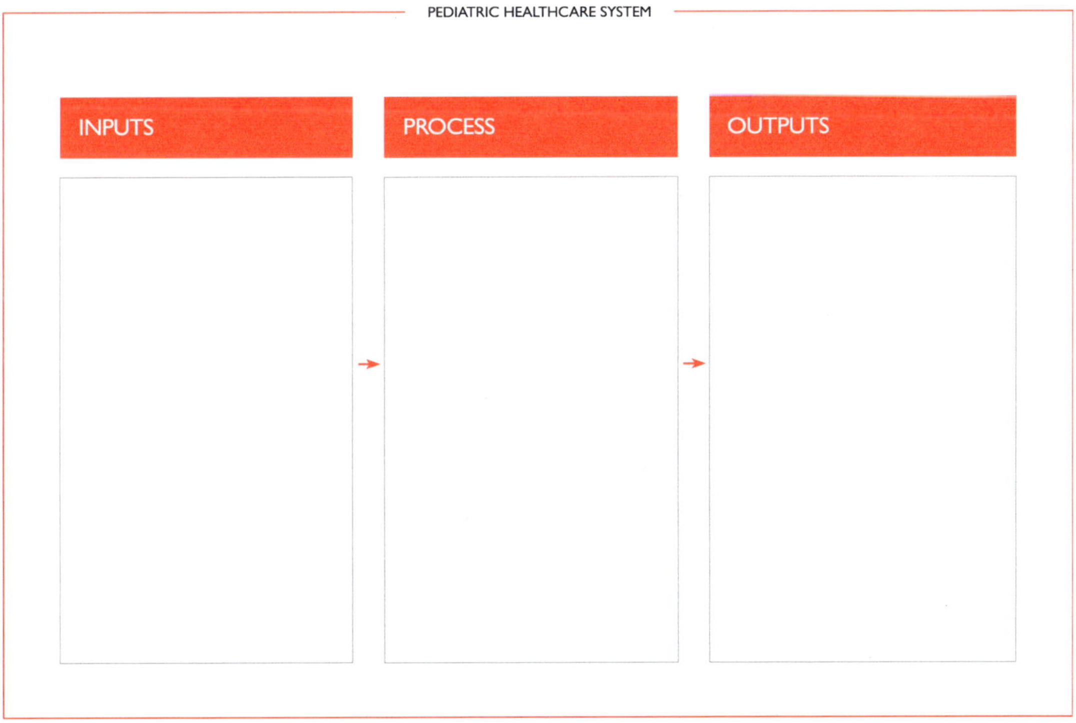

Pediatric Obesity Root Cause Analysis Template

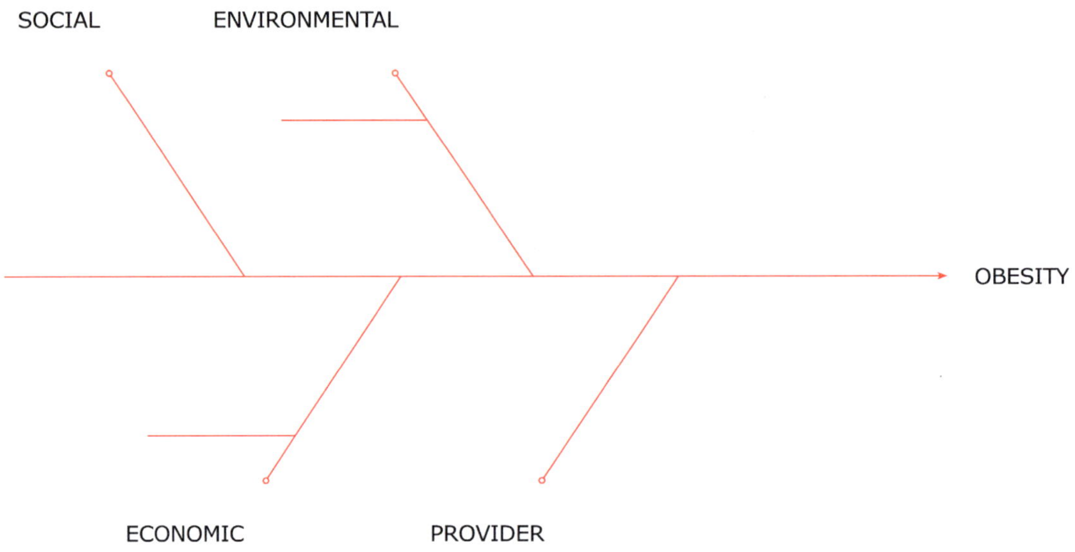

Additional Resources & Links

Healthy People 2020:

http://www.healthypeople.gov/2020/topicsobjectives2020/ebr.aspx?topicId=32

Agency for Healthcare Research and Quality:

http://www.pcmh.ahrq.gov/page/patient-centered-care

American Academy of Pediatrics:

http://www2.aap.org/immunization/IZSchedule.html

http://pedialink.aap.org/visitor

Bright Futures:

http://brightfutures.aap.org/

CDC's Community Preventive Services Task Force:

http://www.thecommunityguide.org/index.html

CDC's Healthy Communities Programs: Pioneering Healthier Communities:

http://www.cdc.gov/healthycommunitiesprogram/communities/phc/index.htm

CDC's Racial and Ethnic Approaches to Community Health (REACH) at:

http://www.cdc.gov/reach/

CDC's School Health Guidelines to Promote Healthy Eating and Physical Activity:

http://www.cdc.gov/healthyyouth/npao/strategies.htm

CDC's Vaccine Safety Datalink:

http://www.cdc.gov/vaccinesafety/Activities/VSD.html

Communities Creating Healthy Environments:

http://ccheonline.org/

The Convergence Partnership:

http://www.convergencepartnership.org/site/c.fhLOK6PELmF/b.3917533/k.F45E/Whats_New.htm

Departments of Health and Human Services and Agriculture:

http://health.gov/dietaryguidelines/

Food and Drug Administration:

http://www.iom.edu/~/media/Files/Report%20Files/2010/Enhancing-Food-Safety-The-Role-of-the-Food-and-Drug-Administration/Enhancing%20Food%20Safety%202010%20Report%20Brief.pdf

Fresh Food Financing Initiative:

http://www.thefoodtrust.org/php/programs/fffi.php

Global Research Network on Urban Health Equity (GRNUHE):

http://www.ucl.ac.uk/gheg/GRNUHE

Healthy Food Financing Initiative:

http://www.acf.hhs.gov/programs/ocs/resource/healthy-food-financing-initiative-0

Healthy Steps:

http://www.healthysteps.org/

Healthy Weight Collaborative through HRSA:

http://www.collaborateforhealthyweight.org/

Institute of Medicine:

http://www.iom.edu/~/media/Files/Report%20Files/2013/Childhood-Immunization-Schedule/ChildhoodImmunizationScheduleandSafety_RB.pdf

International Pediatric Association:

http://www.ipa-world.org/page.php?id=141

Kids Safe and Healthful Foods Project:

http://www.healthyschoolfoodsnow.org/

Let's Go!:

http://www.letsgo.org/

Let's Move!:

http://www.letsmove.gov/

National Conference of State Legislators:

http://www.ncsl.org/research/health/childhood-obesity-legislation-2013.aspx

National Prevention Council:

http://www.cdc.gov/features/preventioncouncil/

Office of Minority Health at the US Department of Health and Human Services:

http://minorityhealth.hhs.gov/

The Policy Link:

http://www.policylink.org

Robert Wood Johnson Foundation:

http://www.rwjf.org/en/our-topics.html

United Nations Millennium Development Goals:

http://www.un.org/millenniumgoals/

United Nations Population Fund:

http://www.unfpa.org/public/home/sitemap/7Billion

United Nations Seven Billion Actions:

https://www.youtube.com/watch?v=mdu71FSKJvI

WHO Global Strategy on Diet, Physical Activity and Health:

http://www.who.int/dietphysicalactivity/implementation/toolbox/en/index.html

WHO World Health Statistics 2012:

http://www.who.int/gho/publications/world_health_statistics/2012/en/index.html

ACKNOWLEDGEMENTS

Declared none.

CONFLICT OF INTEREST

The authors confirm that this chapter contents have no conflict of interest.

REFERENCES

[1] Committee on Quality of Health Care in America, Institute of Medicine. "Front Matter." Crossing the quality chasm: A new health system for the 21st century. Washington, DC: The National Academies Press: 2001.
[2] Congressional Budget Office Testimony. CBO's analysis of the major health care legislation enacted in March 2010. [Updated 2011 Mar 30; cited 2013 Sept 3]. Available from: http://cbo.gov/sites/default/files/cbofiles/ftpdocs/121xx/doc12119/03-30-healthcarelegislation.pdf
[3] The Commonwealth Fund. Why not the best? Results from the national scorecard on US health system performance. c2011. [Updated 2011 October 18; cited 2013 Sept 3]. Available from: http://www.commonwealthfund.org/Publications/Fund-Reports/2011/Oct/Why-Not-the-Best-2011.aspx
[4] The Commonwealth Fund. Why not the best? Results from the national scorecard on US health system performance. c2011. [Updated 2011 October 18; cited 2013 Sept 3]. Available from: http://www.commonwealthfund.org/Publications/Fund-Reports/2011/Oct/Why-Not-the-Best-2011.aspx
[5] Friel S, Akerman M, Hancock T, *et al*. Addressing the social and environmental determinants of urban health equity: Evidence for action and a research agenda. J Urban Health.2011; 88(5): 862.
[6] Hughes AR, Reilly JJ. Disease management programs targeting obesity in children: Setting the scene for wellness in the future. Dis Manage Health Outcomes 2008; 16(4): 255-266.
[7] Ogden CL, Carroll MD, Kit BK, Flegal KM. Prevalence of obesity and trends in body mass index among US children and adolescents, 1999-2010. JAMA 2012; 307(5): 483-490.
[8] Hughes AR, Reilly JJ. Disease management programs targeting obesity in children: Setting the scene for wellness in the future. Dis Manage Health Outcomes 2008; 16(4): 255-266.
[9] The Centers for Disease Control and Prevention: CDC grand rounds: Childhood obesity in the United States. JAMA 2011; 305(10): 988-991.
[10] Ogden CL, Carroll MD, Kit BK, Flegal KM. Prevalence of obesity and trends in body mass index among US children and adolescents, 1999-2010. JAMA 2012; 307(5): 483-490.
[11] Friel S, Akerman M, Hancock T, *et al*. Addressing the social and environmental determinants of urban health equity: Evidence for action and a research agenda. J of Urban Health 2011; 88(5): 863.
[12] The Centers for Disease Control and Prevention: CDC grand rounds: Childhood obesity in the United States. JAMA.2011; 305(10): 988-991.
[13] Centers for Disease Control and Prevention. A look inside food deserts. [Updated 2012; cited 2014 Feb 18]. Available from: http://www.cdc.gov/features/fooddeserts/
[14] United Nations Department of Public Information. UNMDG #1: Eradicate poverty and hunger Fact Sheet DPI/2650 A/Rev.1. c 2010. [Cited 30 Sept 2013]. Available from: http://www.un.org/millenniumgoals/pdf/MDG_FS_1_EN.pdf
[15] Robert Wood Johnson Foundation. Which approaches encourage patients to become more engaged in their own health care? Health Policy Snapshot Issue Brief. c2012. [Cited 2013 October 15]. Available from: http://www.rwjf.org/content/dam/farm/reports/issue_briefs/2012/rwjf72086
[16] US Department of Health and Human Services. Oral health in America: A report of the Surgeon General. Rockville, Md: US Department of Health and Human Services, National Institutes of Health, National Institute of Dental and Craniofacial Research, 2000. NIH Publication 00-4713.
[17] World Health Organization. Fact Sheet No 318 Oral Health. c 2012. [Cited 2013 October 15]. Available from: http://www.who.int/mediacentre/factsheets/fs318/en/
[18] Guarnizo-Herreño CC, Wehby, GL. Explaining racial/ethnic disparities in children's dental health: a decomposition analysis. Am J of Public Health 2012; 102(5): 859-866.
[19] Dye BA, Tan S, Smith V. *et al*. Trends in oral health status: United States, 1988-1994 and 1999-2004. Vital Health Stat 2007; 11: 1-92 as presented in Mobley C, Marshall TA, Milgrom P, Coldwell SE.

The contribution of dietary factors in dental caries and disparities in caries. Acad Pediatr 2009; 9(6): 410-414.
[20] Petersen PE. World Health Organization global policy for improvement of oral health-World Health Assembly 2007. International Dental Journal 2008; 58(3).
[21] Centers for Disease Control and Prevention. Vital and health statistics. Series 10, No. 244. c2009. [Cited 2013 October 15]. Available from: http://www.cdc.gov/nchs/data/series/sr_10/sr10_244.pdf
[22] Tahara D, McBride M. Chronic diseases and the strategic design of patient care (not published) 2013.
[23] Balint E. The possibilities of patient-centered medicine. Br J Gen Pract 1969; 17(82): 269-276.
[24] Saha, S, Beach MC, Cooper LA. Patient centeredness, cultural competence and healthcare quality. J Nat Med Assoc 2008; 100(11): 1275-1285.
[25] Committee on Quality of Health Care in America, Institute of Medicine. "Front matter." Crossing the quality chasm: A new health system for the 21st century. Washington, DC: The National Academies Press 2001.
[26] Schoen C, Osborn R, Squires D, Doty M, Pierson R, Applebaum A. New 2011 survey of patients with complex care needs in eleven countries finds that care is often poorly coordinated. Health Aff 2011; 30(12). [Cited 2013 Sept 3]. Available from: http://www.commonwealthfund.org/Publications/In-the-Literature/2011/Nov/2011-International-Survey-Of-Patients.aspx
[27] Schoen C, Osborn R, Squires, D, Doty M, Pierson R, Applebaum, A. New 2011 survey of patients with complex care needs in eleven countries finds that care is often poorly coordinated. Health Aff.2011; 30(12). [Cited 2013 Sept 3]. Available from: http://www.commonwealthfund.org/Publications/In-the-Literature/2011/Nov/2011-International-Survey-Of-Patients.aspx
[28] Committee on Quality of Health Care in America, Institute of Medicine. "Front matter." Crossing the quality chasm: A new health system for the 21st century. Washington, DC: The National Academies Press 2001.
[29] Agency for Healthcare Research and Quality (n.d.)). [Cited 2013 Sept 3]. Available from: http://www.pcmh.ahrq.gov/portal/server.pt/community/pcmh home/1483
[30] U.S. Department of Health and Human Services. HHS action plan to reduce racial and ethnic disparities: A nation free of disparities in health and health care. Washington, D.C.: U.S. Department of Health and Human Services 2011). [Cited 2013 Sept 3]. Available from: http://www.minorityhealth.hhs.gov/npa/templates/content.aspx?lvl=1&lvlid=33&ID=285
[31] Tahara D, Green R. Strategic re-design of team-based patient-focused healthcare services. Advances in Healthcare Management: Population Health Management in Health Care Organizations 2014; 16: 3-22.
[32] Ogden CL, Carroll MD, Kit, BK., Flegal, KM. Prevalence of obesity and trends in body mass index among US children and adolescents, 1999-2010. JAMA.2012; 307(5): 483-490.
[33] Berwick DM, Nolan TW, Whittington J. The triple aim: Care, health and cost. Health Aff 2008; 27(3) 750-769.
[34] Katz D, Kahn RW. The social psychology of organizations. Hoboken, NJ: John Wiley & Sons, Inc 1966.
[35] Williams DR, McClellan MB, Rivlin AM. Beyond the Affordable Care Act: Achieving real improvements in Americans' health. Health Aff 2010; 29(8): 1481.
[36] Woo B. Primary care-the best job in medicine? N Engl J Med 2006; 355(9): 864-866.
[37] Mertz E, Mouradian WE. Addressing children's oral health in the millennium: Trends in the dental workforce. Acad Pediatr 2009; 9(6): 433-439.
[38] Mertz E, Mouradian WE. Addressing children's oral health in the millennium: Trends in the dental workforce. Acad Pediatr 2009; 9(6): 433-439.
[39] Association of American Medical Colleges. Diversity in the physician workforce: Facts & figures 2010. Washington, DC: c2010. US Census Bureau 2008 Population Reports.
[40] Association of American Medical Colleges. Diversity in the physician workforce: Facts & figures 2010. Washington, DC: c2010. US Census Bureau 2008 Population Reports.
[41] Association of American Medical Colleges. America needs a more diverse physician workforce. [Cited 2013 Oct 15]. Available from: https: //www.aamc.org/download/87306/data/
[42] Tahara D, McBride M. Beyond patient management: Healthcare by design. The Int J Constr Environ 2013; (4): 51-61.

[43] Robert Wood Johnson Foundation. Which approaches encourage patients to become more engaged in their own health care? Health Policy Snapshot Issue Brief. c2012. [Cited 2013 Oct 15]. Available from: http://www.rwjf.org/content/dam/farm/reports/issue_briefs/2012/rwjf72086
[44] Friel S, Akerman M, Hancock T, *et al*. Addressing the social and environmental determinants of urban health equity: Evidence for action and a research agenda. J Urban Health 2012; 88(5): 863.
[45] Saha S, Beach MC, Cooper LA. Patient centeredness, cultural competence and healthcare quality. J Nat Med Assoc 2008; 100(11): 1275-1285.
[46] Tahara, D, McBride M. Beyond patient management: Healthcare by design. Int J Constr Environ 2013; 2(4): 51-61.
[47] Friel S, Akerman M, Hancock T, *et al*. Addressing the social and environmental determinants of urban health equity: Evidence for action and a research agenda. J Urban Health 2012; 88(5): 863.
[48] Tahara D, McBride M. Beyond patient management: Healthcare by design. Int J Constr Environ 2013; 2(4): 51-61.
[49] Choudhry NK, Rosenthal MD, Milstein A. Assessing the evidence for value-based insurance design. Health Aff 2010; 29 (22): 1988-1994.
[50] US Department of Health and Human Services, Health Resources and Services Administration, Maternal and Child Health Bureau. The national survey of children's health 2007. Rockville, Md: US Department of Health and Human Services. c2009. [Cited 2013 Oct 15]. Available from: http://mchb.hrsa.gov/nsch/07main/national/1child/2healthcare/pages/05pdc.html
[51] US Department of Health and Human Services. Healthy People 2020 Objectives. c2010. [Cited 2013 Oct 15]. Available from: http://healthypeople.gov/2020/topicsobjectives2020/overview.aspx?topicid=23
[52] Schor EL. Rethinking well-child care. Pediatr 2004; 114: 210-216.
[53] Tahara D, McBride M. Beyond patient management: Healthcare by design. Int J Constr Environ 2013; 2(4): 51-61.

CHAPTER 20

From Intervention to Innovation: Health Information Technology

Denise C. Tahara[*,1] **and Guy Laufer**[2]

[1]*Department of Health Policy & Management, New York Medical College School of Health Sciences and Practice, Valhalla, NY 10530, USA;* [2]*Global Digital Learning, McCann Worldgroup, USA*

Abstract: Health information technology is changing the way we deliver quality care, and improves our ability to access and treat patients, particularly those in remote or health resource-poor communities and those most at-risk. As healthcare providers, we find ourselves competing with businesses, friends and family members for the patient's attention and time. To develop effective interventions, a systems approach to analysis and improvement is required that considers cultural, human and environmental factors. New models of care will require that physicians take a proactive approach to managing patients' health and wellness, collaboratively. Our patients are constantly assaulted by stimuli, some of them traditional, others products of technology. To enable behavior change, we must devise effective methods of engaging our patients. We propose that healthcare innovations should be developed to focus on the patient's experience and portability. The design of these innovations should promote competence and confidence and provide the requisite level of functionality required by the user. Effective innovations must begin with the patient. As appropriate, designing in certain elements, Gamification, Phygital™, and Social Engagement are essential to engage patients. Integrating these innovations into healthcare delivery can bring about definitive public health benefits.

Keywords: Behavior, design thinking, digital, eHealth, EMRs, gamification, global health, health information technology, innovation, lifestyle diseases, mHealth, mobile, obesity, overweight, patient engagement, patient experience, risk, telehealth, wellness.

INTRODUCTION

Technology has changed the way we communicate and interact as well as our day-to-day experience. As healthcare providers, we find ourselves competing with

***Corresponding author Denise C. Tahara:** Department of Health Policy & Management, New York Medical College School of Health Sciences and Practice, Valhalla, NY 10530, USA; Tel: (914) 594-4250; Fax: (914) 594-4292; E-mail: denise_tahara@nymc.edu

Judith Wylie-Rosett & Sunil S. Jhangiani (Eds)

businesses, friends, and family members for the patient's attention. Advertisers use flashy, moving gimmicks, anything to grab attention. Regardless, as healthcare providers it is incumbent upon us to create an authentic approach, informed by accurate content that will establish a meaningful, long-term relationship with our patients. Our patients are constantly assaulted by stimuli, some of them traditional, others products of technology. This chapter focuses on how to enable behavior change with effective methods of engaging patients. Healthcare innovations that focus on the patient's experience and portability are considered. This chapter discusses why the design of these innovations needs to promote not just competence and confidence, but also provide the requisite level of functionality required by the user.

LET'S GO DIGITAL!

In this digital age, kids are active on social media sites and online games; expanding their community. They seek approval, praise, support, and sometimes just want to share. It is a media they are familiar with and therefore healthcare plans, other interventions, and guidelines should be delivered through this channel. According to a recent survey, 93% teens share a computer or have access to one and 74% of older teens are "mobile internet users" meaning that they access the internet through their mobile devices. Furthermore, 95% of teens use the internet and 82% are on social networking sites. Children, adolescents, and teens spend more time with media, than they do in school [1]. Racial differences persist as 81% of white teens *versus* 64% of black teens own a computer [2].

Health communication and care plans should be designed to engage patients as well as maximize participation and adherence. We propose that healthcare innovations should be designed for the user experience and portability. Unlike traditional product design, the digital product/service constantly needs to be updated to fit the needs and requirements of the user, which simultaneously change over time as well. In this agile process, once the innovation has been launched, the tracking begins to measure patient behavior and feedback on an ongoing basis. After analyzing what can be improved, providers should address these issues, adjust them accordingly, and send the improved version back to the patient. This is an unending feedback/refinement cycle, or Plan-Do-Study-Act, frequently referred to as the Deming Cycle for performance improvement. For example in July 2013, Facebook's Graph Search was launched. Graph Search is an inner search engine within Facebook that helps the user to easily search on Facebook. Sample users tested this product for nearly six months before reaching the mass audience. Facebook continually refined the service in response to user feedback. For more information click here.

User-centered thinking and design encompasses the following elements: Gamification, Phygital™, and Social Engagement and is illustrated in Fig. (**1**). These elements provide a holistic blend, combined with the ongoing experience of our patients. At the center of the design of the healthcare innovation is the patient. The core factors: design, purpose, utility, engagement, personalization and friendliness are common to all three spheres of Gamification, Phygital™, and Social Engagement, and are essential to the patient.

Gamification is the usage of game thinking and design in a non-game environment/context. It adds a layer of game-thinking to create a sense of competition among other patients, or among themselves; it imparts to the user a story line, which creates a rich experience. Phygital™ (the blending of two words, physical and digital) adds a digital layer to our physical environment, which provides additional information, as well as a new way of engaging with one's surroundings. These three elements are not stand-alone, but their interactive combination, coupled with the patient at the center, creates a meaningful and long-lasting engagement. In the patient's experience, he/she should be exposed to these elements in a coherent, clear-cut manner. Our target population continuously Tweets, Shares, and Likes all of this being done on social networks. This branch in the digital sphere is a major element, and should be a pivotal part of our healthcare innovations.

Gamification

Gamification motivates the user to perform mundane tasks or services by providing a dimension of fun. Adding a layer of gamification encourages and stimulates the patient to engage.

The foundation of gamification is built on a perception of human nature; people enjoy competition in a variety of forms, particularly children. People have an inherent desire for self-expression and the achievement of status. Rewards in this competitive process could be points, badges, levels, or any category that provides a sense of pride and accomplishment.

Gamification contributes a layer of enjoyment to tasks that could otherwise be considered burdensome or downright dull. It motivates actions, gives feedback,

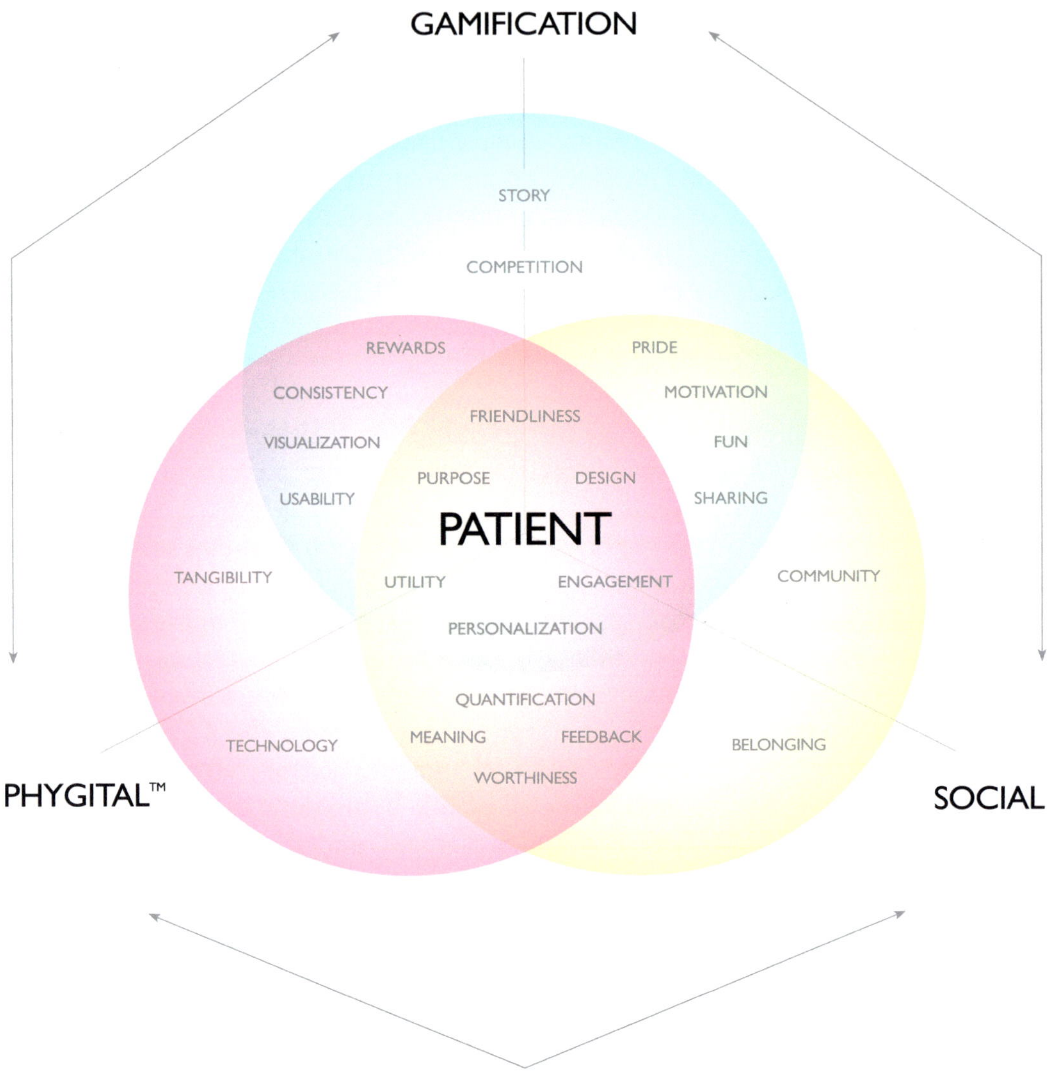

Fig. (1). From intervention to innovation framework, ©2013, Tahara & Laufer.

and reinforces the user's involvement with sundry rewards. The user is engaged and motivated to continue to participate. This is a key factor for protocol adherence for children. Feedback highlights a sense of identity and expectation; the urge to improve is a highly desirable psychological and intellectual value. Gamification gives a clear path-in the form of a story line-to ascertain and evaluate outcomes. Status and feedback are essential in prompting the user to continue his/her engagement. Moreover, this story line gives the user a sense of measurable progress *vs* monitoring and reporting. It promotes the belief that with more time, effort, and dedication, higher levels of achievement, along with a process of discovery, can be realized; there is an incentive to follow protocols and adhere to care and treatment plans.

Not knowing how the story will turn out strengthens one's sense of curiosity, and moves the patient to want to know more, to continue to participate. This kind of competition also creates a sense of ongoing social interaction. In sum, gamification-a sense of play-has always been a highly valued motivational strategy. Resources include:

http://www.hopelab.org/

http://www.forbes.com/sites/gartnergroup/2013/01/21/the-gamification-of-business/

http://mashable.com/category/gamification/

http://www.gamification.co/

http://www.brandingmagazine.com/2012/04/06/the-principles-of-gamification/

Phygital™

Phygital™ is a blending of two words-physical and digital-that are often brought to bear in the world of technology, and specifically in the field of marketing and is trademarked by Momentum Advertising Agency. Initial entries into this sphere include exergames such as those developed by Nintendo (Wii), Microsoft (Xbox 360 Kinect), and Sony (PlayStation). For example, the aim of Kinect Training by Nike is to utilize technology to narrow the gap between the physical and digital worlds. Today, the number of smartphone users worldwide is estimated at 1.4 billion, representing nearly one in three mobile phone users, or about one-fifth of the global population. It is estimated that by 2017 more than one third of the human population will use a smartphone [3] placing the digital sphere at everyone's fingertips, thus connecting the two worlds. Some of the best examples of this process are QR codes, Augmented Reality, Nike+ FuelBand, and Google Glass. These innovations provide the user with the benefits of both worlds. Similar to gamification, to maintain an ongoing engagement with the user, a Phygital™ product or service should always provide feedback. Feedback is an essential component of systems thinking and design. It provides important information about the user's experience with both content and delivery. Feedback can be either a single summary or a more sustainable mechanism in the form of a dashboard, which enables the user to track his or her results, narrowing the gap between the physical world and the digital sphere. Resources include: http://phygitalien.com/what-is-phygital/ and http://www.thedrum.com/knowledge-bank/2011/12/19/creating-phygital-ecosystem-between-brands-and-consumers

SOCIAL ENGAGEMENT

Social Engagement is the interaction between users in virtual communities. It might be expressed in the form of sharing ideas, information, or any other kind of content. User-generated content such as messages, images, and ratings, connects people from around the globe without a middleman. The participants in this process may be followers, friends, and contacts. Each community possesses its own set of ground rules and modes of communication. This, in brief, is the way that the "game" is played. For example, a posting by a mother of a child with diabetes on www.spoonful.com, resulted in collaboration between Eli Lilly and Disney Publishing and the development of Fantasy Diabetes, which is modeled after Fantasy Football [4]. Instead of focusing on NFL scores, children guess the blood sugar level of the child with diabetes. As in Fantasy Football, points are awarded for the best guess.

People spend more time on social networks than on any other category of sites [5]. It is human nature to seek engagement and to belong to a community. Moreover, younger generations feel this need even more urgently and they constantly look for feedback. They value the opinions of their peers. Group identity offers a support system, and it reinforces motivation. According to an eMarketer report [6] nearly one in three people worldwide will use social networks in 2014. We are living in a constantly changing world in which technology is always evolving; however, the need and desire for a sense of community remains intact. http://www.forbes.com/sites/piyankajain/2013/06/25/6-social-media-insights-bound-to-change-your-customer-support/

INTEGRATING INFORMATION TECHNOLOGY INTO HEALTHCARE

Getting Started

When integrating information technology into healthcare, there are two elements that need to be synchronized: content and delivery. Questions to consider in the design process include: What do we mean by content? Is it relevant to our patients? Is it personalized to fit his/her needs? At the same time, how do we deliver the actual content? Is it accessible? What is its format? Is it mindful of the patient's personal habits, health literacy and cultural traditions?

Optimally, in the design of healthcare innovations, our team should consist of analytical "brains" and "design thinkers". Healthcare providers, the "brains" focus on content *versus* messaging. During interactions, communications, and subsequent care, the provider concentrates on the patient's clinical needs; treatment plans are developed to manage the patient's health and wellness. This expertise is essential for every healthcare intervention. Designers tend to emphasize the affective dimension rather than the analytical, because they understand that customers frequently "go with their gut" in the selection of services and products more than upon considerations of utility and cost. Designers translate the product or service simply and intuitively in a user-friendly manner. However, while emotional appeal can initially engage potential users, analysis contributes legitimacy to the process of decision making. Such an approach creates "healthy tension", highlighting a blend of the advantages of both worlds, responding to the needs of the patient.

This process starts with four questions that must be addressed in order to create a complete patient-centered innovation.

Question #1: "What Is?"

Explain the project's intention. As providers, what do we need to learn? What is the outcome we want to achieve?

Question #2: "What If?"

After understanding both the provider's capabilities and the patient's needs, it is time to identify possibilities and opportunities. Brainstorming, gathering ideas from a cross-section of the team (including providers and designers) is the place to start. Successful brainstorming requires context and structure. Winnowing and combining ideas leads to the next question.

Question #3: "What Wows?"

Choose the best ideas. What best captures the user's attention and interest to effectively engage him/her? What are the provider's "in house" capabilities? In this stage you should consider the perspective of the patient in order to provide a different view of the service or capability, in other words picking the best of the ideas. This phase is equivalent to an editing room with production unit. It looks at what can be done in house and what should be outsourced.

Question #4: "What works?"

Now it is time to put the innovation into practice. Present the service or capability to a pilot group. Determine their experience and obtain their feedback. This will enable you to adjust to the specific needs and interests of the patient. This process has been employed by Facebook as previously described.

Mobile Technology

There is no doubt about the importance of mobile technology in the near future. Major companies are changing their business models after realizing that the web's future will be mobile. "We've transitioned, and are now a mobile company," says Mark Zuckerberg [7]. Many more businesses understand that their customers will utilize information through smartphones, tablets, and portable devices. Accordingly, healthcare providers must respond to this new reality by utilizing the mobile platform to communicate with and inform their patients.

For providers the question remains whether to build a mobile-optimized website or a stand-alone mobile app to communicate with their patients. How the patient interacts with healthcare services through the mobile device will determine the manner in which the actual content should be delivered. As recently as two years ago, users spent about 20 or more minutes per day on browser-based sites rather than on mobile apps. However, by last September mobile apps were outdistancing browser-based sites by more than 20 minutes a day [8]. How does this relate to health information technology? Currently only a quarter of all patients are accessing their medical records through websites or mobile devices, although, according to a recent survey, more than 52% are clearly interested in using electronic medical records (EMRs) [9]. This represents a dynamic opportunity for healthcare providers to accelerate implementation of EMR systems, and integrate health information technology into their practices. It also provides an incentive to providers to implement EMR systems with the requisite interoperability to facilitate connectivity to mobile communications. In Fig. (**2**), we compare the advantages and disadvantages of each approach.

MOBILE SITE	MOBILE APP
STATIC AND LIMITED USER INTERFACE	INTERACTIVE USER INTERFACE
ACCESSED THROUGH BROWSING	ACCESSED AFTER INSTALLED
REQUIRES CONNECTION	AVAILABLE OFFLINE
LIMITED FEATURES	CAN USE OTHER PHONE FEATURES SUCH AS GPS, CAMERA, ETC
FAST	FASTER
NO APPROVAL AND NO REGULATION	MOST APPS REQUIRE AN APPROVAL PROCESS, AND CAN BE FOUND IN THE APP STORE
USES AN EXISTING SITE AND ADJUSTS TO MULTIPLE SCREENS, INCLUDING MOBILE DEVICES AND TABLETS	EXPENSIVE
CONNECTIVITY TO PATIENT ELECTRONIC MEDICAL RECORDS (EMR)	LACK OF CONNECTIVITY TO PATIENT ELECTRONIC MEDICAL RECORDS (EMR)

Fig. (2). Mobile site *vs* mobile app.

In this chapter we created a framework to maximize patient engagement in their health and well-being. However, this framework will not ensure engagement if not effectively implemented using a systems approach to its design. We discussed the requisite components, being mindful of the patient's point of view-in effect, asking the question, "*What's in it for them?*" As we design healthcare interactions, this is the question we should continually ask. Possessing the components does not ensure success; however, in the digital sphere we always have the option to adjust and refine; we are never done.

A SYSTEMS APPROACH

To develop effective interventions, a systems approach to analysis and improvement is required. The first step is to understand the existing delivery system by documenting the patient's experience; identifying barriers and obstacles to engaging them in their care and well-being, including lifestyle and infrastructure failures, and leveraging opportunities to reinforce healthy choices and coordinated care. A systems approach requires both provider-based and patient-based care which engages the whole patient/family constellation and reorients care from episodic treatment to ongoing health management and well-being; supporting changes in the ecology of place and lifestyle behaviors [10]. This approach also considers the needs of physicians to engage them as champions who can help co-design collaboration and integration efforts, encourage agency in patients and their families, and support parents to advocate as role models and change agents. For more information regarding systems approach and analysis, also see CHAPTER 19: Life-Course Approach to Obesity Management: The Role of Family and Environment.

New models of care will require that physicians take a proactive approach to managing patients' health and wellness, collaboratively. Physicians are curators of their patients' data and will need to coordinate services and deliver care where they will have different roles, responsibilities and accountability; teams will not be organized vertically around the physician, but rather horizontally around the patient's needs [11], as illustrated in Fig. (**3**). Physician training will need to include new communication and leadership skills to better manage the whole patient, in some cases with multiple diseases. Care will need to be responsive and accessible to patient preferences, needs and values, so that they can actively participate in their treatment, decision-making and care [12].

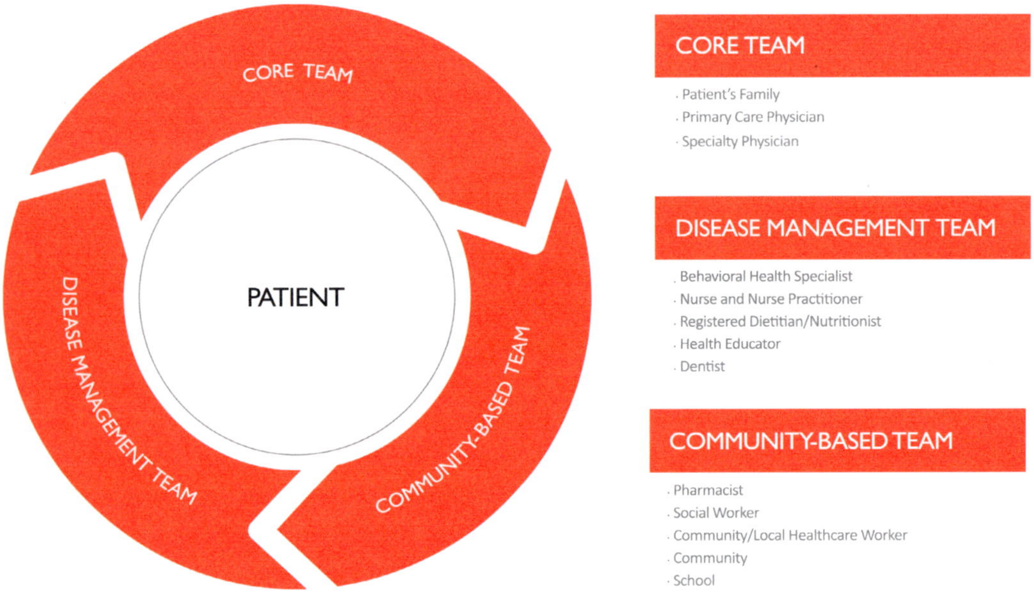

Fig. (3). Pediatric-centered framework of care.

Health Information Technology: Where Are We Now?

Although immunizations have proven to be one of the most effective healthcare innovations to prevent epidemics of infectious and preventable diseases, Mobile Health or mHealth is anticipated to be the next healthcare innovation to transform public healthcare worldwide. Maximizing medical technology capabilities has been an ongoing priority. "In 2005, a World Health Assembly resolution acknowledged e-health's potential for improving health systems and safety, quality and efficiency in health care" [13]. As more capabilities are developed, providers are embracing the technology and integrating it into their workflow, re-conceptualizing how and where they deliver quality healthcare.

In response to the anticipated healthcare workforce and physician shortage worldwide, eHealth and mHealth afford the opportunity to deliver real-time care to more patients, particularly those most at-risk, who live in remote and healthcare resource-poor communities. With an aging population living with chronic diseases, there is increased demand for health information including self-management and decision support tools to enable patients to age in place, without sacrificing quality of life and quality of care. The result should be more efficient and more cost-effective care.

The definition of health information technology (HIT) is rapidly changing as new capabilities are being introduced. These include institutional systems, systems that facilitate clinical practice, and systems that facilitate care at a distance [14]. Information technology has increased communication of educational and clinical information including diagnostic data among providers who are integrating the use of technology in the daily treatment and care of patients. This chapter focuses on communicating and providing care between practitioners and patients and discusses four domains: telemedicine, patient web portals, social media and mobile health [15].

Electronic Medical Records/Electronic Health Records

Electronic Medical Records/Electronic Health Records (EMRs and EHRs) are improving the quality and quantity of care provided by facilitating documentation and communication of patient information and diagnoses when patients present to their providers. Large information systems enable the entry and subsequent access of centralized patient data, including basic patient information, treatment records, diagnostic testing, and medication lists. Multiple access points connect providers and patients so care can be delivered in multiple settings including in the patient's community so that the patient no longer needs to travel to receive care. Point-of-care devices enable care coordination and delivery to patients particularly in remote and difficult to reach areas. Such access to patient data can also improve care across healthcare settings and patient hand-offs.

Telemedicine

Telemedicine is the use of communications technology to exchange information between providers (between provider sites) or between providers and patients who may not be within a geographic proximity, to improve patients' health status. The term refers to a variety of modalities including telephones, clinical call centers, two-way video, email, smart phones, videoconferencing, digital retinal cameras, secure messaging, wireless tools, store-and-forward imaging, streaming media, and remote monitoring [16-18]. Telemedicine and telehealth are sometimes used synonymously although telehealth does not always include clinical services. Regardless, information is communicated in real-time or stored-and-forwarded (such as use of Picture Archiving Communication System (PACS) for digital imagery). Patient education videos provide information regarding procedures, treatment protocols, and preadmission instructions; demonstrate healthy lifestyle behaviors and medication management. Data can be analyzed using decision support software or physician consultation, and a care plan is then developed and implemented. Telemedicine has been shown to improve access (especially to specialty providers), decrease costs (especially through chronic disease management), improve quality, and enable chronically ill and elder patients to live independently *versus* having to live in institutional settings.

Patient Web Portals

Patient web portals (PWPs) integrate EMRs. The web-based systems enable patients to communicate with their providers as well as provide access to educational materials to help them manage their disease, conditions, and wellness. Patients and providers have access to the patient's complete medical history *via* internet access. Patients can set up appointments, request refills for prescriptions, submit claims, make payments, receive reminders and alerts, and obtain specialist referrals. After users log in to a secure site, they navigate through their dashboard to access information on their health, disease, and healthcare services, to better manage their health and wellness.

Social Media

Social media refers to a wide range of online forums, blogs, collaborative websites (Wikis), social networking sites, video and photo sharing, chat rooms, and virtual communities where patients live through avatars. In addition to accessing information about their condition, patients connect with other patients and receive support through their communication.

Available resources include: Incorporating social networks: http://www.patients likeme.com/ and http://www.wellapps.com/patients-helping-patients-help-docto rs-help-patients

Mobile Health or mHealth

Mobile health or mHealth is the fastest growing and most significant of the health information technology innovations, particularly for chronic disease management and especially for socially disadvantaged populations [19]. mHealth involves using wireless technologies such as Bluetooth, GSM/GPRS/3G/4G, Wi-Fi, WiMax … to transmit and enable various eHealth data content and services. This enables chronic disease management and reporting of patient indicators such as vital signs, weight and behavioral health, and diagnostics remotely and in real-time. Usually these are accessed by the health worker through devices such as mobile phones, smart phones, PDAs, laptops and tablets [20].

According to a 2012 Pew Research Study on mobile health usage, 31% of cell phone owners and 52% of smart phone owners used phones to look up health or medical information. Further, young adults, Latinos, and African Americans lead the trend [21]. Emerging technologies such as smartphone applications (with email and text messaging (SMS) capabilities), two-way pagers and the internet have improved patient care and self-management of their conditions through monitoring and engagement in protocols that incentivize both the provider and the patient.

mHealth applications have been categorized into the following groups:

- Education and Awareness
- Remote Data Collection
- Remote Monitoring

- Communication and Training for Health Care Workers
- Disease & Epidemic Outbreak Tracking
- Diagnostic and Treatment Support [22]

Multiple studies worldwide indicate that SMS messages and other reminders have improved health behaviors and adherence to treatment guidelines resulting in improved physiological outcomes. mHealth applications have improved the efficiency and effectiveness of care delivery worldwide with corresponding reductions in infant mortality, and the spread of diseases. In rural areas, mobile health applications have effectively been used for surveillance and disease tracking and to improve population health through timelier public health information, increased access to healthcare and healthcare information, expanded access to medical education, and training for healthcare workers [23]. A large-scale and ongoing evaluation of the efficacy of these tools on behaviors and health outcomes is needed [24]. Interim outcome data should be evaluated and shared.

Available resources include:

Epocrates: http://www.epocrates.com/

PubMed Mobile: http://www.ncbi.nlm.nih.gov/m/pubmed/

AHRQ's Electronic Preventive Services Selector (ePSS): http://epss.ahrq.gov/PDA/index.jsp

Community Health Data Initiative: http://www.hhs.gov/open/plan/opengovernmentplan/initiatives/initiative.html

http://www.impakhealth.com/emmett-the-robot

http://www.imedicalapps.com/

Where it is Working

Successful uses of health information/communication technology in both the US and abroad integrate technology into the care delivery process *vs* as an add-on. They consider the cultural, human and environmental factors that will ensure utilization and improved health outcomes. These include culturally sensitive language, health literacy, user capability and comfort with the technology. The goal is to engage the patient and their family so they can manage their health and well-being.

Some examples of what is working include learning networks, virtual grand rounds [25], and chronic disease management tools that include interventions for self-management and decision support such as sites for smoking cessation, compliance alerts, and instant access to health information. This creates a system of healthcare without walls [26].

Text4baby/Text4kids

Building on the success of Text4baby, Bright Futures™ launched Text4kids, a mobile health messaging system to address children's changing health needs from birth to age 21. Personalized messages are sent to children and parents to remind them to set up and show up at scheduled appointments, comply with immunization guidelines, and provide information on various topics throughout the child's development. Personalized supportive messages are sent to the child to reinforce good choices and healthy decisions. It also provides links to helpful community resources. In 2012 a randomized control study [27] reported that vaccination rates doubled (from 18% to 36%) when parents received text reminders *versus* just paper reminders. More information can be found at: http://connect4health.net/text4kids.html or http://brightfutures.aap.org/.

Blood Glucose Monitoring Systems (BGMs)

Blood Glucose Monitoring Systems (BGMs) are wireless blood glucose meters capable of collecting HbAlC levels and sending the data to a server where they are forwarded to a cloud-based web application. The data can then be viewed by patients, families, and providers on their tablets, smartphones, or computers. BGMs have an alert when levels are too high or too low and recommend corrective action [28].

Care Coordination/Home Telehealth (CCHT)

The need to improve access by United States (US) veterans to the Veterans Health Administration (VHA) healthcare system, a focus on independent *versus* institutional living, and increasing demands of those with chronic disease, drove the conceptualization and development of the VHA investment in information and communication technologies. Care Coordination/Home Telehealth (CCHT) uses telehealth and decision-making points to care for its patients and support their independent living. The key to its success is the algorithm that the VHA developed to match their patients based on their ability to use technology, access, and care needs [29]. Active case management includes utilizing videophones, messaging devices, biometric devices, and digital cameras to monitor patient health data and update treatment protocols when needed. Case managers educate their patients on how to manage their health at home. Key components include a strong health information infrastructure, strong relationships with technology vendors, staff engagement, extensive training of care coordinators and integrating the technology into the ongoing care and management of the patients and their diseases [30]. More information can be found at: http://www.telehealth.va.gov/ ccht/.

Project ECHO (Extension for Community Healthcare Outcomes)

Project ECHO (Extension for Community Healthcare Outcomes) was started in 2004 through funding by the Agency for Healthcare Research & Quality. Since its initial year it has been funded through the state and also through the Robert Wood Johnson Foundation. It is based at the Health Science Center at the University of New Mexico School of Medicine and was created to extend/expand treatment for hepatitis C patients who live in rural and medically underserved areas. In New Mexico, access to care remains a huge challenge. Using teletechnology, Project ECHO trains primary care physicians, nurse practitioners, and community health workers in rural and underserved areas through virtual grand rounds and mentoring using a case-based approach. Through video conference clinics and additional training, patients have access to specialty care for their chronic and complex healthcare needs. The result is a virtual knowledge network with real-time transfer of knowledge and best practices and treatment for patients in rural and underserved communities. Project ECHO's disease management model has expanded to chronic diseases including 19 areas of specialty care. Recently they were funded by GE to integrate behavioral health services into primary care [31]. Click here for more information.

HealthLine Project

The HealthLine Project takes a different approach to communicating medical information. As models of care that include community health workers (CHW) expand in both developed and developing nations, there is concern regarding the availability and capability of available workers. In some countries the concern is with low and illiterate CHWs, who are willing to provide care in rural and underserved communities. Researchers at Carnegie Mellon University and Aga Khan University in Pakistan partnered to address the literacy issue with funding from Microsoft Research. They developed a speech-based telephone information system, HealthLine to provide medical information. The only technology that the CHW needs is access to a telephone (neither smart phones nor landlines are required, and in many cases they are unavailable). The worker calls a toll-free number and using verbal prompts, can access recorded information on a variety of health topics, in their native language. Still in its early stages, HealthLine continues to expand the topics covered from maternal and child health to sexually transmitted infections. More information can be found at: http://www.health line.com/.

Barriers to Widespread Use and Efficiencies

Implementation of EMRs, particularly in the United States has been slow. As of 2012, only 44% of hospitals had adopted EMRs and 29% participated in Health Information Organizations (HIO) [32]. Global healthcare systems are plagued by interoperability issues which prevent providers from accessing important patient information, especially regarding diagnostics, that results in duplication and overuse of services. Additionally, the majority of the mHealth apps are not connected to the existing EMR systems or internet-based systems and therefore the information remains siloed. Limited bandwidths constrain data transfer. An information technology infrastructure to connect these different communication systems must be developed to maximize the capability to provide real-time, cost-effective care. Further, information needs to be communicated over secure exchanges, and from multiple sources and systems. Globally accepted standards need to be adopted, using open architecture, standardized terminology, abbreviations, messaging, and vocabulary so that data can move effectively across systems and applications, transmitted securely to ensure patient privacy. Encryption and authentication protocols need to be employed worldwide.

Socio-economic barriers continue to isolate uninsured or underinsured groups despite healthcare reform efforts [33]. These barriers include infrastructure and transportation challenges, availability and accessibility of specialty providers, including long wait time for appointments, insufficient capacity and resources at community health centers which provide safety-net care, poor health literacy coupled with cultural barriers to access, use and follow-up care [34]. Although applications of mHealth technologies are beginning to address those barriers to health and well-being, inequalities in access and utilization of healthcare are reinforced by *the great digital divide*.

The biggest challenge facing providers who want to incorporate technology into their practice and care delivery is the *digital divide* where disparities in access to technology mirror healthcare disparities. Patients with lower socioeconomic status, minorities, the elderly, those who are disenfranchised, geographically isolated with poorer health and low health literacy, are less likely to have adequate access to eHealth technologies. In other words, there is a gap between people who have and those who do not have access to internet technology. The World Health Organization (WHO) defines health literacy as "the cognitive and social skills which determine the motivation and ability of individuals to gain access to, understand and use information in ways which promote and maintain good health"[35]. It is the ability to read healthcare materials such as prescription bottles, physician orders, discharge orders, care and treatment plans.

Healthy People 2020 refers to the capacity to interpret and understand basic health information and services, and the competence to use such information to make informed decisions about care [36]. Even those of lower socioeconomic status, who have access, may not be able to assess the accuracy or quality of the information or understand the information itself. Further, this demographic group obtains their information from passive sources such as television *versus* searching the internet. They do not ask the question, "Can I trust this source?" In a 2013 survey, only 35% of adults had gone online to determine a diagnosis for themselves or someone else, and only 54% of them followed up with a medical professional. Whites tend to search for health information online more than Blacks and Hispanics [37]. mHealth technology, using smartphones and mobile apps is reducing this divide and improving access to information and health care. However, the ability to assess and differentiate among accurate and trustworthy websites and mobile apps persists. Additionally, many patients indicate frustration with using the websites or apps including lack of user-friendly navigation, lack of confidence in the functionality, and confidentiality concerns which inhibits access and utilization.

Patients want to be more connected to teams of physicians who coordinate and collaborate their care. Physicians also like the flexibility of responding to patient needs *via* email, patient web portals, or mHealth. However, privacy, confidentiality, and cost are still a huge factor as reimbursement standards and methods for costing services provided have still to be created. Further, protocols need to be developed to ensure that documentation of the communication is included in the patient's medical record (either paper or electronic) so that patient data and treatment plans are up-to-date. Evaluation of systems developed including cost/benefit analysis and the impact of these innovations on population health is required so best practices can be adopted system-wide and costs can be reduced.

The Solution: From Intervention to Innovation

A 2009-2010 survey by NHANES (National Health and Nutrition Examination Survey) [38] reported prevalence for overweight and obesity was 26.7% for children ages two to five years and an alarming 32.6% for children ages six to eleven years. Racial disparities continue to exist as the rates of obesity for Hispanic children were significantly higher, 33.1% and 39.7% respectively. This further reinforces the urgency for action and to develop culturally-specific innovations-both content and delivery.

Taking a systems approach to improvement, the first step is to understand the existing delivery system by documenting the patient's experience; identifying barriers and obstacles to engaging them in their care and well-being. These barriers need to be addressed to improve access to providers, improve communication and collaboration among care teams, and improve adherence to recommended protocols and treatment plans in the community. As we consider new models of patient-centered care, we need to shift our approach from an encounter or episodic care to a life-course approach. The community in which the patient and the patient's family lives including environmental factors must be incorporated into care plans. Solutions include aligning the necessary systems (such as the technology, analytics, and infrastructure) to support healthy behaviors. Those who live in rural areas or medically underserved communities need to be connected to care.

As we move toward family-centered care, physicians will have new roles and leadership responsibilities. Environmental, social, and economic barriers must be addressed so that patients can take ownership of their health and well-being. Healthcare encounters should be leveraged as opportunities to educate and reinforce wellness and well-being and empower patients and their families. Patient data collection forms (questionnaires) should include questions about the patient's living and built environments such as: access to fresh air (do the windows open?), number of smokers in the home, screen time, after school care, typical breakfast, lunch, and dinner, access and use of playgrounds and what activities they participate in. This information can guide recommendations for management of chronic illnesses and wellness planning. For example, children who live in single-parent homes and those with two working parents generally eat more meals prepared outside the home, which impacts choices and what the child eats. They will trade off nutrition-rich foods for cost, taste, and convenience. Clever advertising influences snacks and meal choices. Further, this household environment also results in more screen time and sedentary lifestyle.

Communities must support improving health and well-being. Solutions require multi-sector collaboration (partnerships between private corporations and governments). Internationally this is being done through partnerships like the United Nations Foundation and the Vodaphone Foundation, where the carrier is providing network capabilities to programs in healthcare resource-poor and difficult to reach communities. Such partnerships need to be expanded in the U.S. Google Loon is an ambitious new project that aims to provide web access to rural and remote areas. This is being implemented by putting a network of solar air balloons into space to provide access to the internet. Click here to find out more information about Google Loon. In addition, Facebook partnered with Samsung, Ericsson, MediaTek, Nokia, Opera, and Qualcomm, to launch Internet.org. This project aims to provide affordable access to internet for two thirds of the world population who are not yet connected.

This project features three main goals:

- Making access affordable through cheaper smartphones;
- Using data more efficiently so people do not run up high costs; and
- Companies/partners working together to help mobile devices support more languages to demolish barriers to usage [39].

As Mark Zuckerberg states, "I believe connectivity is a human right, and that if we work together we can make it a reality" [40].

Health information technology is changing the way we deliver quality care, and improves our ability to access and treat patients, particularly those in remote or in health resource-poor communities and those most at-risk. The possibilities are endless. Physicians are utilizing tablets in surgery to guide them through procedures (click here to see the example), while other surgeons are using Google

Glass to stream the procedures to physicians and medical students in remote locations (more information can be obtained from: Google glass article on Mashable). As providers, we should embrace these tools and capitalize on our relationships with our patients building trust, so they will use the technology and actively engage in their own care. Privacy, confidentiality, security, and accessibility are key concerns. Prompts and training should facilitate good decisions, goal achievement and provide real-time feedback and support.

Tackling the epidemic of pediatric obesity requires a systems approach to the socioeconomic, psychosocial, behavioral and lifestyle factors that affect our patients' health and well-being. This includes addressing barriers in the living and built environments, and acccss to health information technology. Designing innovations and treatment plans, must move the patient from awareness to actualization of their care, facilitate success and engage them in their health and well-being. Designing the patient experience and leveraging the positive and prosocial effects of media [41] is key to compliance and participation.

"Design thinking is actually a systematic approach to problem solving" [42]. Design combines the "How", the "What" and the "Who". Poor design means that the patient will not utilize the technology, and will feel frustrated because he/she cannot get things to work. "Innovation is usually not about producing ideas nobody has ever thought of before; it's about creating better value for customers-and profit for ourselves-by combining elements into innovative business designs" [43]. Delivering patient-centered care in the digital age enables us to transform patient interactions, both virtual and face-to-face. All systems must be aligned to support improved outcomes. As healthcare providers we need to ensure the requisite support including infrastructure and analytics to encourage access, utilization, and decision-making.

CONCLUSION

The key to ongoing participation and engagement is developing healthcare innovations in a format in which the patient is familiar and comfortable. The design of these innovations should promote competence and confidence, and provide the requisite level of functionality required by the patient. Personalized interventions that incorporate elements of Gamification, Phygital™, and Social Engagement will be most effective in motivating behavior change and improved health and well-being. It must be fun! Healthcare providers must leverage their expertise with regard to content, and enlist designers to focus on creating messages that will improve health and well-being.

Additional Resources & Links:

American Academy of Pediatrics. Prevention and Treatment of Childhood Overweight and Obesity: About Childhood Obesity

http://www.aap.org/obesity/about.html

CDC eHealth Metrics Dashboard

http://www.cdc.gov/metrics/cdc-info/

CDC Foundation

http://www.cdcfoundation.org/blog-entry/tackling-obesity-one-school-time

CDC. Overweight and Obesity: Basics About Childhood Obesity

http://www.cdc.gov/obesity/childhood/basics.html

CDC, Overweight and Obesity: Causes and Consequences

http://www.cdc.gov/obesity/causes/index.html

National Child Care Information and Technical Assistance Center

http://www.icfi.com/insights/projects/families-and-communities/national-child-care-information-center

WHO eHealth Programmes

http://www.who.int/ehealth/programmes/en/index.html

EMR capabilities

http://www.healthit.gov

Health Information Technology

http://healthit.ahrq.gov/

Health Alliance-works with mHealth community

http://www.mhealthalliance.org/

Health Unbound- online knowledge resource center and interactive network for the mHealth community

http://www.hoohub.org/

eHealth Initiative

http://www.ehidc.org/

ACKNOWLEDGEMENTS

Declared none.

CONFLICT OF INTEREST

The authors confirm that this chapter contents have no conflict of interest.

REFERENCES

[1] American Academy of Pediatrics. Policy Statement: Children, Adolescents, and the Media 2013. [Cited 2013 Nov 3]. Available from: http://pediatrics.aappublications.org/content/132/5/958.full.pdf+html

[2] Madden M, Lenhart A, Duggan M, Cortesi S, Gasser U. Pew Internet & American Life Project: Teens and Technology 2013. [Cited 2013 Oct 30]. Available from: http://www.pewinternet.org/reports/2013/teens-and-tech.aspx

[3] Emarketer. Social Networking Reaches Nearly One in Four Around the World 2013. [Cited 2013 Nov 3]. Available from: http://www.emarketer.com/Article/Social-Networking-Reaches-Nearly-One-Four-Around-World/1009976#JYTF7B4xsgG1RJgV.99

[4] Voight J. Welcome to the New Face of Big Pharma. Advertising & Branding 2013. [Cited 2013 Nov 3]. Available from: http://www.adweek.com/topic/brandweek-report

[5] Nielsen NetView, Nielsen Smartphone Analytics 2012. [Cited 2013 Nov 3]. Available from: http://www.nielsen.com/us/en/reports/2012/state-of-the-media-the-social-media-report-2012.html

[6] Emarketer. Social Networking Reaches Nearly One in Four Around the World 2013. [Cited 2013 Nov 3]. Available from: http://www.emarketer.com/Article/Social-Networking-Reaches-Nearly-One-Four-Around-World/1009976#JYTF7B4xsgG1RJgV.99

[7] Fell J. Mark Zuckerberg on Facebook's Triumphs and Tribulations. Entrepreneur 2012. [Cited 2013 Nov 3]. Available from: http://www.entrepreneur.com/blog/224415#ixzz2f2PEaldo

[8] Laird S. Mobile Site or Mobile App: Which Should You Build First? 2012. [Cited 2013 Nov 3]. Available from: http://mashable.com/2012/06/06/mobile-site-mobile-app-infographic/

[9] Perna G. Patients Interested, But Not Accessing EHRs *via* Web. Healthcare Informatics 2013. [Cited 2013 Oct 15]. Available from: http://www.healthcare-informatics.com/news-item/study-patients-interested-not-accessing-ehrs-web

[10] Tahara D, McBride M. Chronic diseases and the strategic design of patient care (not published) 2013.

[11] Tahara D, Green R. Strategic re-Design of Team-based Patient-Focused Healthcare Services. Advances in Healthcare Management: Population Health Management in Health Care Organizations, 2014; 16: 3-22
[12] Ogden CL, Carroll MD, Kit BK, Flegal KM. Prevalence of obesity and trends in body mass index among US children and adolescents, 1999-2010. JAMA.2012; 307(5): 483-490.
[13] Van Gemert-Pijnen JEWC, Wynchank S, Covvey HD, Ossebaard HC. Improving the credibility of electronic health technologies. Bull World Health Organ 2012; 90:323-323A.
[14] Piette JD, Lun KC, Moura Jr LA, *et al*. Impacts of e-Health on the Outcomes of Care in Low- and Middle-Income Countries: Where do we go from Here? Bull World Health Organ 2012; 90:365-377.
[15] eHealth Initiative. An Issue Brief on eHealth Tools and Diabetes Care for Socially Disadvantaged Populations 2012. [Cited 2013 Oct 23]. Available from: http://www.ehidc.org/resource-center/publications/view_document/208-brief-an-issue-brief-on-ehealth-tools-and-diabetes-care-for-socially-disadvantaged-populations-chronic-disease
[16] Health Resources and Services Administration. Rural Health. n.d. [Cited 2013 Oct 23]. Available from: http://www.hrsa.gov/ruralhealth/about/telehealth/
[17] American Telemedicine Association. What is telemedicine? 2012. [Cited 2013 Oct 23]. Available from: http://www.americantelemed.org/learn/what-is-telemedicine
[18] eHealth Initiative. An Issue Brief on eHealth Tools and Diabetes Care for Socially Disadvantaged Populations 2012. [Cited 2013 Oct 23]. Available from: http://www.ehidc.org/resource-center/white-papers-and-briefs.html
[19] eHealth Initiative. An Issue Brief on eHealth Tools and Diabetes Care for Socially Disadvantaged Populations 2012. [Cited 2013 Oct 23]. Available from: http://www.ehidc.org/resource-center/publications/view_document/208-brief-an-issue-brief-on-ehealth-tools-and-diabetes-care-for-socially-disadvantaged-populations-chronic-disease
[20] Vita Wave Consulting. United Nations Foundation and the Vodafone Foundation Technology Partnership. mHealth for Development: The Opportunity of Mobile Technology for Healthcare in the Developing World 2009: 8.
[21] Fox S, Duggan M. Mobile Health 2012. Pew Internet and American Life Project 2012; 8.
[22] Vita Wave Consulting. United Nations Foundation and the Vodafone Foundation Technology Partnership. mHealth for Development: The Opportunity of Mobile Technology for Healthcare in the Developing World 2009.
[23] Vita Wave Consulting. United Nations Foundation and the Vodafone Foundation Technology Partnership. mHealth for Development: The Opportunity of Mobile Technology for Healthcare in the Developing World 2009.
[24] Piette JD, Lun KC, Moura Jr, LA, *et al*. Impacts of e-Health on the Outcomes of Care in Low- and Middle-Income Countries: Where do we go from Here? Bull World Health Organ 2012; 90:365-377.
[25] Arora S, Kalishman S, Dion D, *et al*. Partnering urban academic medical centers and rural primary care clinicians to provide complex chronic disease care. Health Aff 2011; 30(6): 1176-1184.
[26] Arora S, Kalishman S, Dion D, *et al*. Partnering urban academic medical centers and rural primary care clinicians to provide complex chronic disease care. Health Aff 2011; 30(6):1176-1184.
[27] Stockwell MS, Kharbanda EO, Martinez RA, *et al*. Txt4Health: impact of text message reminder-recalls for pediatric and adolescent immunizations. Am J Public Health 2012; 102(2): e-15-21.
[28] eHealth Initiative. An Issue Brief on eHealth Tools and Diabetes Care for Socially Disadvantaged Populations 2012. [Cited 2013 Oct 23]. Available from: http://www.ehidc.org/resource-center/publications/view_document/208-brief-an-issue-brief-on-ehealth-tools-and-diabetes-care-for-socially-disadvantaged-populations-chronic-disease
[29] Broderick A. The Veterans Health Administration: Taking Home Telehealth Services to Scale Nationally, The Commonwealth Fund Case Study Series 2013.
[30] Broderick A. The Veterans Health Administration: Taking Home Telehealth Services to Scale Nationally, The Commonwealth Fund Case Study Series 2013.
[31] Robert Wood Johnson Foundation (n.d.) Using ECHO (Extension for Community Healthcare Outcomes) to Train Primary Care Providers in Best Practices for Complex Health Conditions. [Cited 2013 Nov 18]. Available from: http://www.rwjf.org/en/grants/grant-records/2009/02/using-echo--extension-for-community-healthcare-outcomes--to-trai.html

[32] Furukawa MF, Patel V, Charles D, Swain M, Mostashari F. Hospital Electronic Health Information Exchange Grew Substantially In 2008-12. Health Aff 2013; 32(8): 1346-1354.

[33] Crilly JF, Keefe RH, Volpe F. Use of Electronic Technologies to Promote Community and Personal Health for Individuals Unconnected to Health Care Systems. Am J of Public Health 2011; 101:7: 1163-1167.

[34] eHealth Initiative. An Issue Brief on eHealth Tools and Diabetes Care for Socially Disadvantaged Populations 2012. [Cited 2013 Oct 23]. Available from: http://www.ehidc.org/resource-center/publications/view_document/208-brief-an-issue-brief-on-ehealth-tools-and-diabetes-care-for-socially-disadvantaged-populations-chronic-disease

[35] Nutbeam D. WHO Health promotion glossary. Health Promotion International 1998. [Cited 2013 Nov 18]. Available from: http://whqlibdoc.who.int/hq/1998/WHO_HPR_HEP_98.1.pdf

[36] Bodie GD, Dutta, MJ. Understanding Health Literacy for Strategic Health Marketing: eHealth Literacy, Health Disparities, and the Digital Divide. Health Mark Q 2008; 25(1/2):175-203.

[37] Fox S, Duggan M. Pew Internet & American Life Project: Health Online 2013. 2013. [Cited 2013 Nov 18]. Available from: http://pewinternet.org/reports/2013/health-online.aspx

[38] Zoorob R, Buchowski MS, Beech, BM, *et al.* Healthy Families Study: Design of Childhood Obesity Prevention Trial for Hispanic Families. Contemp Clin Trials 2013; (35): 108-121.

[39] Internet.org 2013. [Cited November18]. Available from: www.internet.org

[40] Interview with Mark Zuckerberg, CNN August 21, 2013. [Cited November18]. Available from: http://money.cnn.com/2013/08/20/technology/social/facebook-zuckerberg-5-billion/index.html

[41] American Academy of Pediatrics. Policy Statement: Children, Adolescents, and the Media 2013. [Cited 2013 Nov 3]. Available from: http://pediatrics.aappublications.org/content/132/5/958.full.pdf+html

[42] Liedtka J, Ogilvie T. Designing for Growth: A Design Thinking Toolkit for Managers. New York: Columbia Business School Publishing 2011; p. 14.

[43] Liedtka J, Ogilvie T. Designing for Growth: A Design Thinking Toolkit for Managers. New York: Columbia Business School Publishing 2011; p. 194.

Index

Judith Wylie-Rosett & Sunil S. Jhangiani (Eds)

D

E

F

S

T

U

V

W

Made in the USA
Las Vegas, NV
03 November 2026

57424409R00266